PLAY IN HEALTHCARE FOR ADULTS

PLAY. We all do it: wordplay, love play, role-play; we play cards, play sport, play the fool, and play around. And that's just the grown-ups! It features in every aspect of our lives, whether we call it by that or another name. We all do it, but why do we do it? What does it mean to play and what, if any, difference does it make to our lives? Most crucially, and central to the theme of this book, is the question, 'Does play have a positive impact on our health and wellbeing, and consequently a role in modern healthcare delivery?'

The contributors to this book provide a comprehensive overview of how play and play-based activities can be used throughout the adult lifespan to promote health and wellbeing within the context of healthcare service delivery for patients, their families and communities, and for the staff involved in their care. Responding to current global health concerns such as obesity, coronary heart disease, dementia and mental health, the book argues that play and playfulness offer a means of protection, promotion and recovery of positive health and wellbeing. The human tendency for play and playfulness as essential to personal growth and development lie at the heart of the discussion.

This book will be of interest to all those working in health or social care settings, including nursing, social work and allied health students and professionals, and to those working in the therapeutic disciplines of art therapy, music therapy and recreation alliances.

Alison Tonkin looks after the Higher Education provision at Stanmore College, which includes two foundation degrees and a BA (Hons) top up, all of which focus on children and young people. With a research background in health promotion for pre-school children, and having worked as both a diagnostic and therapeutic radiographer, the extension of play service provision to cover adult healthcare is a current area of interest, especially as the college offers the FdA in Healthcare Play Specialism.

Julia Whitaker has worked therapeutically with children and families in both public and private sectors for the past 30 years. Originally trained as a social worker and family therapist, Julia is also a registered Healthcare Play Specialist with wide-ranging clinical and teaching experience in the field. Julia is now interested in exploring ways in which the knowledge and skills associated with healthcare play might be used to benefit patients 'from the cradle to the grave'.

PLAY IN HEALTHCARE FOR ADULTS

Using play to promote health and wellbeing across the adult lifespan

Edited by Alison Tonkin and Julia Whitaker

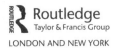

LONDON AND NEW YORK

First published 2016
by Routledge
2 Park Square, Milton Park, Abingdon, Oxon OX14 4RN

and by Routledge
711 Third Avenue, New York, NY 10017

Routledge is an imprint of the Taylor & Francis Group, an informa business

© 2016 A. Tonkin and J. Whitaker

The right of the editors to be identified as the author of the editorial material, and of the authors for their individual chapters, has been asserted in accordance with sections 77 and 78 of the Copyright, Designs and Patents Act 1988.

All rights reserved. No part of this book may be reprinted or reproduced or utilised in any form or by any electronic, mechanical, or other means, now known or hereafter invented, including photocopying and recording, or in any information storage or retrieval system, without permission in writing from the publishers.

Trademark notice: Product or corporate names may be trademarks or registered trademarks, and are used only for identification and explanation without intent to infringe.

British Library Cataloguing-in-Publication Data
A catalogue record for this book is available from the British Library

Library of Congress Cataloging in Publication Data
Names: Tonkin, Alison, 1962- , editor. | Whitaker, Julia, editor.
Title: Play in healthcare for adults : using play to promote health and wellbeing across the adult lifespan / edited by Alison Tonkin and Julia Whitaker.
Description: Abingdon, Oxon ; New York, NY : Routledge, 2016. | Includes bibliographical references and index.Identifiers: LCCN 2015050455|
ISBN 9781138931237 (hardback) | ISBN 9781138931244 (pbk.) |
ISBN 9781315679846 (ebook)Subjects: | MESH: Play Therapy |
AdultClassification: LCC RC489.P7 | NLM WM 450.5.P7 |
DDC 616.89/1653--dc23LC record available at
http://lccn.loc.gov/2015050455

ISBN: 978-1-138-93123-7 (hbk)
ISBN: 978-1-138-93124-4 (pbk)
ISBN: 978-1-315-67984-6 (ebk)

Typeset in Bembo
by Fish Books Ltd.
Printed in Great Britain by Ashford Colour Press Ltd

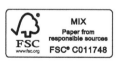

To the memory of Bob Wright (Bobbo)
Thank you for inspiring my love of the seashore
and research
A.T.

and

For Bernard Sands Martin,
my grandfather,
who showed me that you are never too old to play
J.W.

CONTENTS

List of illustrations	x
Foreword	xiii
Acknowledgements	xv
Contributors	xvii

	Introduction	1
1	Playing for health *Julia Whitaker and Alison Tonkin*	5
2	Conceptualizing play in healthcare provision *Alison Tonkin and Julia Whitaker*	18
3	Lifespan development *Julia Whitaker and Alison Tonkin*	32
4	Creating and growing a family *Julia Whitaker*	45
5	The concept of health and wellbeing across the lifespan *Rachel Bayliss and Jenni Etchells*	59
6	Using play as a means to widen access to health and wellbeing *Julia Whitaker and Claire Weldon*	70

viii Contents

7 Lifestyle trends and their impact on health 85
Claire Weldon, Denise Baylis and Alison Tonkin

8 Playing for mental wellness 99
Julia Whitaker and Alison Tonkin

9 Music as medicine 115
Rachel Bayliss

10 The game of chamber music in dementia music therapy 124
Emilie Capulet

11 Drama, dance and play: creative play as therapy 135
Leanne Grundy

12 Art for health 143
Julia Whitaker

13 Play and social therapy 152
Eric Fleming

14 Playing with words 160
Sandie Dinnen and Alison Tonkin

15 Playing with technology 173
Debbie Tonkin and Alison Tonkin

16 Aspire Leisure Centre: inspiration through integration 186
Claire Weldon

17 The facilitation of play and playfulness through
alternative healthcare provision 199
Julie Dakin and Alison Tonkin

18 Playful design 212
Alison Tonkin

19 Playing together: festivals and celebrations 226
Alison Tonkin and Shereen Jameel

20 Playing for spiritual health 238
Catherine Hubbuck

21	Using play for lifelong learning *Jeremy Weldon and Claire Weldon*	249
22	Playing politics *Carol Sullivan-Wallace and Alison Tonkin*	263
23	Playing for health, wealth and happiness *Julia Whitaker and Alison Tonkin*	277
	Index	287

ILLUSTRATIONS

Figures

1.1	An invitation to rail passengers passing through Brighton Station, summer 2014	13
2.1	The Health Model (Barton and Grant 2006 – reproduced by kind permission of Barton)	20
6.1	A feeling of joyfulness arises from the celebration of creative achievement	77
6.2	A respectful attitude for the natural world adds quality and meaning to everyday life	78
9.1	Apollo, God of literature, plays his harp; a town goes about its rituals (van der Straet 1594, produced courtesy of the Wellcome Library under Creative Commons Licence CC BY 4.0)	116
13.1	Serious play marks an attitude of experiment and invention	155
13.2	A sense of play re-emerges in the celebration of festivals	158
14.1	Integrated model of Health Literacy (Sorensen *et al.*, 2012, kindly reproduced under Creative Commons Attribution License)	162
14.2	Giant microbes provide a playful approach to sexual health	165
15.1	Weekly use of home internet connections to visit social networking sites (Ofcom 2013)	175
16.1	Joe setting out on a 'long push'	194
16.2	Joe carrying the Olympic torch during the Torch Relay prior to the London Olympics	195
16.3	Graham instructing a Spin class	197
18.1	Double Diamond Design Process (Better Services by Design 2015c, based on work by the UK Design Council)	216

18.2	Design for the dementia lounge – a quiet space for patients, family members and staff (Boex 2015a)	218
18.3	A sensory board featuring interactive panels which can be changed to reflect patients' individual life-stories (Boex 2015a)	220
18.4	The large kitchen table 'providing lots of space for collaboration, activities and playing games' (Boex 2015b)	221
18.5	Mapping the flow of patients and staff: a high-tech version of the knitting wool game (Boex n.d.)	222
21.1	Playing 'Whose shoes?'	259
22.1	Comparing behavior change funnels for tobacco quitting and eating five portions of fruit and vegetables a day (Department of Health 2009: 30)	272

Tables

1.1	Definitions of leisure, play and recreation (Hurd and Anderson 2011)	9
2.1	Linking the aspects of health to motivational theory (adapted from Barrett 2010)	22
3.1	An overview of periods of the lifespan (adapted from Singleman and Rider 2015)	33
3.2	Major perspectives on lifespan development (adapted from Feldman 2011)	35
5.1	Adapted from Bruce and Meggitt (2005)	60
8.1	Variation according to region (Office for National Statistics 2015)	100
8.2	Variation according to age (Office for National Statistics)	101
8.3	Variation according to gender (Office for National Statistics 2015)	101
8.4	Longitudinal incidence of feelings associated with anxiety and depression (Office for National Statistics 2015)	102
8.5	'Five ways to mental wellbeing' (quoted from Foresight Mental Capital and Wellbeing Project 2008b)	109
8.6	Ten practical ways to stay mentally well (adapted from the Mental Health Foundation n.d.)	110
17.1	Simplistic overview of differences between traditional medical and CAM approaches to treatment and the promotion of health and wellbeing	200
17.2	Main benefits to health and wellbeing of a selection of CAM techniques	205
17.3	The five phases (Liang 2004)	207
19.1	Components of the Indivisible Self Model (adapted from Myers and Sweeney 2008)	228
22.1	Key elements of Bandura's Social Learning Theory (Allen and Gordon 2011)	267
22.2	MINDSPACE elements (Dolan et al. 2010)	268

xii Illustrations

Boxes

4.1	Alice's story	49
4.2	Connor's story	50
4.3	Margaret's story	51
4.4	Emma's story	53
18.1	Summary of a conversation with Sam Boex exploring the design of two different wards for people with dementia	219
20.1	The use of Lego play to facilitate safe exploration of feelings that cannot be expressed	240

FOREWORD

This is a radical book. It argues that play is important for grown-ups.

There is something about such a claim that sits uncomfortably with the modern Western world. Play feels trivial, indulgent, silly, childish. To suggest that we should prioritise it within our professional systems – investing in it, writing it into policy, designing interventions around it – sounds somehow preposterous. Play certainly seems irrelevant to the goals of the system on which this book focuses: a progressive, effective, efficient healthcare system.

Yet, studies show that play is central to our biological makeup and our evolutionary history. It is crucial for all mammalian species, from dogs to elephants to dolphins. Some biologists have suggested that play is present even in the behavior of birds, reptiles and octopuses. When it comes to the human species, our hunter-gatherer ancestors may well have depended on play for their very existence. Peter Gray (2009: 479) has argued on the basis of anthropological evidence that 'play [was] used not to escape from, but to confront and cope with, the dangers and difficulties of a life that is not always easy'.

Intuitively, we recognize that play is important in adult lives. The most enjoyable moments in our relationships tend to be those in which we are laughing together. We seek out and pay large sums of money for entertainment. Holidays and down-time are an established element of employment law. Most people prefer to work in environments where colleagues laugh a lot together. When you have had an argument with a loved one, it is only when the two of you are once again spontaneously joking that you know the rift has truly been healed.

We know these truths instinctively. However, we relegate them to our private lives and personal relationships. Contemporary culture does not reserve an official role for play in our public, professional lives. Work is serious. Play is not.

That's why this book is radical. Its editors have been willing to shout loudly about the importance of play in professional contexts. They have been willing to

xiv Foreword

bring theory, empirical evidence, and practical examples to their claim. They have been brave enough to make the case that without enough play, our healthcare system will always be ineffective. Their publisher, Routledge, is courageous too, because they have taken the risk of publishing a volume the vision of which is so counter-cultural that sales could be at risk.

Yet the contents of this volume show the need to paint such a vision. Our sedentary lives are leading to chronic health conditions such as obesity, diabetes, and heart disease. Technological interventions strip the psychological-spiritual elements from our experience of our bodies. The normative treatment for mental health problems, loss, substance abuse and other emotional challenges has become pharmaceutical drugs, rather than human connection.

This is an academic volume that argues there is another route to health: dance, drama, ritual, relaxation, laughter, merriment. It provides the theoretical explanation and empirical evidence as to why these solutions should be effective. It illuminates the financial waste we create by failing to incorporate these solutions within our approach to health. It does all this whilst anticipating the doubt that many readers will experience when they encounter the argument that our healthcare system suffers because it doesn't include enough fun.

The editors of this volume have joined a growing band of academics who are trying to do something delightfully grandiose: bring our twenty-first-century society to its senses. It is both ironic and fitting that Julia Whitaker and Alison Tonkin should be attempting this through something as trivial and ordinary as play.

The core message of this book is that we grown-ups create positive social change every time we choose to play. That is a profound scientific-spiritual message.

Suzanne Zeedyk
Research Scientist and Honorary Fellow, University of Dundee
Founder of *connected baby*
Dundee, Scotland

Reference

Gray, P. (2009) Play as a foundation for hunter-gatherer social existence. *American Journal of Play*, Spring: 476–521.

ACKNOWLEDGEMENTS

We would like to thank:

All the contributors to this book, who have given their time so generously, in order to share their enthusiasm, knowledge and expertize; once again, we have written this together.

Suzanne Zeedyk for generously giving her time and energy to write the Foreword to this book and for her enthusiastic endorsement of playfulness as a means of making connections.

Grace McInnes, Commissioning Editor, Routledge, for giving us the opportunity to write this second exploration of play in healthcare.

Louisa Vahtrick, Senior Editorial Assistant, Health and Social Care, Routledge for guiding us through this process and trusting us to complete it.

Alison would like to thank:

The Senior Management Team at Stanmore College who enabled this project to be undertaken and completed under their care.

Julia – an inspirational choice of co-editor, who has so eloquently promoted the value of play and provided objectivity with such gentleness.

Claire Weldon for always listening and still saying 'yes'.

Kath Evans from NHS England for her infectious positivity and 'Can do' attitude.

Christina Freeman from the Society of Radiographers for allowing us to 'spread the word'.

My lovely family who have helped in so many ways to complete this book.

Julia would like to thank:

Healthcare Play Specialist colleagues working in the NHS and elsewhere who continue to promote the value of play during challenging and changing times.

xvi Acknowledgements

The National Association of Health Play Specialists who have worked tirelessly for over 40 years to put play on the health agenda and to keep it there.

Richard Klein, Eric Fleming and everyone at Orwell Arts for offering an insight into the Garvald community; with special thanks to the members of Garvald Edinburgh who appear in the photographs.

Meg Faragher and Helen Monaghan at the National Museum of Scotland; Natalie McFadyen White at Impact Arts; Janis Mackay at the Scottish Storytelling Centre and the Life Stories storytellers and contributors.

Frances Barbour for her friendship and invaluable support; Freya and Alex for their patience and love.

Alison, my intrepid co-editor, for engaging me in this wonderful project and for your cheerful optimism throughout.

Claire Weldon would like to thank:
The Aspire National Training Centre and in particular, Brian Carlin, Laura Haynes, Joe Gilbert, David Morphew and Graham Burns.

Photographs

Thank you to the photographers and the subjects
Alison Tonkin: Figures 1.1 and 14.2.
Douglas Bride: Figure 6.1 (Callum and Jane)
Douglas Bride: Figure 6.2 (Alison and Dominic)
Wellcome Library: Figure 9.1 (under Creative Commons Licence CC BY 4.0)
Eric Fleming: and 13.2 (Callum, Flora and Jenny)
Figure 13.1 (Alison and Joseph)
Figure16.1 (Joe Gilbert)
Figure16.2 (Joe Gilbert)
Figure16.3 (Graham Burns)
Sam and Will Boex: Figures 18.2, 18.3, 18.4 and 18.5
Gill Phillips: Figure 21.1

Figures

Thank you for permission to share the following Figures
Figure 2.1: Professor Hugh Barton, University of the West of England
Figure 14.1: Sorensen *et al.* 2012, kindly reproduced under Creative Commons Attribution License http://creativecommons.org/licenses/by/2.0
Figure 22.1: Department of Health – Open Government Licence 3.0 www.nationalarchives.gov.uk/doc/open-government-licence/version/3/

CONTRIBUTORS

Denise Baylis Information and Advice Officer, Age UK Norwich

Rachel Bayliss Core Medical Trainee, South London NHS Trust

Emilie Capulet Senior Lecturer and Head of Classical Performance Studies, London College of Music, University of West London

Julie Dakin Traditional Chinese Acupuncturist, Meon Valley, Hampshire

Sandie Dinnen Trustee, Healthcare Play Specialist Education Trust

Jenni Etchells Clinical Facilitator, Children's Community Nursing team, Hertfordshire Community NHS Trust

Eric Fleming Glass Studio Leader, Garvald Edinburgh

Leanne Grundy Drama and Applied Theatre Specialist, Assistant Principal, Stanmore College

Catherine Hubbuck Registered Health Play Specialist (Freelance)

Shereen Jameel Lecturer in Health and Social Care, Stanmore College

Carol Sullivan-Wallace Health Play Specialist, Queen Elizabeth Hospital, Woolwich

Alison Tonkin Head of Higher Education, Stanmore College

xviii Contributors

Debbie Tonkin PA and Project Administrator

Claire Weldon Mentor, Stanmore College

Jeremy Weldon Consultant Radiographer, London North West Healthcare and University of Hertfordshire

Julia Whitaker Health Play Specialist (Freelance), Registration Co-ordinator, Healthcare Play Specialist Education Trust

INTRODUCTION

The complexities and expectations of modern life leave us with little time, energy or inclination for rest and recreation – for PLAY. We are working longer hours, for more years, and are experiencing unprecedented levels of stress. Yet, play has been at the heart of human existence since the earliest times and was once considered too great a privilege for the young. There now exists a valuable body of knowledge, supported by research and clinical evidence, to suggest that play not only makes us feel better but holds benefits for our physical and mental health, with positive social repercussions for individuals, communities and society as a whole.

Furthermore, experts across a variety of disciplines are tapping-into this knowledge to apply what we know about play and its actual and potential benefits to help vulnerable groups in our society and those who are at risk of developing, or currently living with, serious or long-term health conditions. The global health challenges associated with the unprecedented rise in obesity and diabetes as a consequence of a sedentary lifestyle, factors associated with an aging population and the prevalence of diagnoses of age-related dementia, and a growing awareness of the personal and societal implications of unrecognized and untreated mental illness, mean that healthcare services are being obliged to explore creative options for tackling these 'hot potatoes'. Advancements in medical science, unimaginable even a few decades ago, have raised the demands and expectations of our health services at a time when global fiscal austerity means that these expectations cannot always or easily be met.

PLAY is an effective, low-cost, low-impact option for improving the health and wellbeing of the international community. This volume, a companion to the earlier *Play in Healthcare: Using Play to Promote Child Development and Wellbeing,* will present and explore the evidence for play in a healthcare context. With contributions from an eclectic range of specialists in their fields, it will prompt questions about how we value and promote positive health for all, regardless of their cultural identity, abilities or social circumstances.

2 Introduction

The aim of the book is to draw together various approaches to health and wellbeing from a play perspective. It is written as a contribution to the growing awareness of the value of play in all aspects of our lives. Whilst originally conceived for the healthcare professions, the book offers a much broader perspective which will appeal to a wide readership.

A socio-ecological perspective has been used to loosely structure the main content of the book, recognizing the contribution of play and playfulness for individuals, communities and for society as whole. The book is divided into three main sections.

Play for individual health and wellbeing

Chapter 1 explores the meaning of play in adult life and how this complements the developmental process throughout the lifespan.

Chapter 2 looks at the conceptualization of play in the context of healthcare provision.

Chapter 3 explores the concept of lifespan development. The book has purposefully avoided categorization according to age as the play concepts and strategies discussed are not themselves age-specific.

Chapter 4 looks at the adjustments involved when family units are formed and the role of play in forging and maintaining relationships. Play can be particularly effective at times of challenge, such as separation, loss and physical or mental illness, and lends itself as a tool to enhance engagement and communication during difficult times.

Chapter 5 looks at the conceptualization of health and wellbeing across the lifespan and at how play can make a significant contribution to health and wellbeing, according to individual needs and capabilities.

Chapter 6 then explores how play may be used when individual differences make access to services problematic. It discusses the use of play as a communication and therapeutic tool for adults who may have different needs, such as sensory impairment, learning difficulties and autism.

Chapter 7 examines current lifestyle concerns arising from the increasingly sedentary patterns of behavior which have led to chronic health conditions such as obesity, type 2 diabetes and coronary heart disease. Concerns relating to sexual health across the age range are explored along with substance abuse and the increasing problem of alcohol consumption. The emphasis is on the role of play and recreational activities for the promotion of positive lifestyle choices.

Chapter 8 discusses the contribution that play can make to the mental health and emotional wellness of individuals. Play as a route to resilience is exemplified with reference to contemporary projects designed to promote mental wellness.

The art of play for health

Chapter 9 explores how music offers enjoyment and pleasure, which contribute to positive health and emotional wellness throughout the lifespan, both at participatory and spectator levels.

Chapter 10 provides a detailed commentary on how a series of classical chamber music workshops were used with a small group of patients with early-onset dementia for facilitating creativity, spontaneity and playfulness in a shared 'space of play'.

Chapter 11 covers the use of dance and drama as tools for personal and group expression. These areas of the expressive arts are increasingly being used to explore personal relationships and social situations, enabling participants to enhance feelings of self-esteem and personal self-awareness. In the healthcare context, dance and drama are particularly effective within the mental health arena and for working with people with learning disabilities.

Chapter 12 examines the therapeutic use of art as an integral feature of the healthcare environment throughout history. Today, the notion of 'art for health' is firmly established and there is a strong evidence base for the use of art as a means of creating and supporting the healing environment.

Chapter 13 represents a social therapy perspective and the meaningful application of craft-based learning opportunities and festival celebrations. A case study approach is used to show how 'serious play' can lead to personal engagement and healthful development.

Playing together for a healthy society

Chapter 14 explores the significance of health literacy as a means of engagement for those working in healthcare services and as a route to empowerment for those who use these services. Exploring play-based examples of effective health literacy strategies, the role of humor and storytelling are advocated as effective means of tailoring health-related information to optimize the messages being conveyed.

Chapter 15 demonstrates how technological advances have changed the face of healthcare provision. The utilization of play-based technology has enabled the development of games for health education and rehabilitation, and of facilities for tracking health and fitness. The use of social media is also explored as a means of social interaction and peer support.

Chapter 16 investigates the potential for integrated recreational facilities for disabled and non-disabled people with reference to how these facilities make adult play-based activities accessible to all.

Chapter 17 looks at the role of alternative and complementary medicines and their contribution to a holistic approach to health and wellbeing. The chapter focuses on Traditional Chinese Medicine and how the pursuit of playfulness and joy is promoted for optimal wellbeing.

Chapter 18 discusses the use of play and playfulness within the design process, from the initial concept and planning phase, through to the completed project, and how this approach benefits many aspects of healthcare provision, at both individual and community levels.

Chapter 19 reflects on the contribution made by celebrations and seasonal festivities to the health of the community. Play is a significant feature of many

4 Introduction

festivals and embracing the playful nature of celebration as part of healthcare provision is shown to be particularly effective for strengthening emotional wellbeing and a sense of community.

Chapter 20 explores how spirituality is being promoted within healthcare provision as an integral part of a caring, people-focused service. It is argued that play and sprituality share a common purpose in helping people to explore their own paths to wellness.

Chapter 21 discusses how the use of play and playfulness is equally important for health-givers as for those who receive their care. This chapter focuses on enabling health-givers to acknowledge their own need to play and to find ways of incorporating play into their Continuing Professional Development. Play is discussed as a means of reducing stress and work-related burn-out.

Chapter 22 investigates how policy can be used to promote play-based strategies within healthcare provision. It reviews the role of policy for developing innovative practice and how, in times of global fiscal restraint, play-based techniques have been used as a positive means of engaging people at local, national and international levels as part of the current health agenda.

Chapter 23 concludes the book by drawing together the major themes that have emerged from the preceding chapters. The scope of play and how it has been applied across a range of healthcare contexts is discussed, before glimpsing into a future in which play is seen as essential to the provision of healthcare and to the attainment of personal and societal wellness.

Much has been written on the subject of play and we hope that this book represents a novel contribution to the debate. The body of evidence for the value of play in healthcare, as reflected in the content of this book, is now such that play's value cannot be denied. We hope the book will be both an inspiration and a challenge to all those with a vested interest in health and wellbeing, whether service users or providers.

1

PLAYING FOR HEALTH

Julia Whitaker and Alison Tonkin

Play, we all do it: wordplay, love play, role-play; we play cards, play sport, play the fool, and play around. And that's just the grown-ups! Play features in every aspect of our lives, whether we call it by that or another name. We all do it, but why do we do it? What does it mean to play and what, if any, difference does it make to our lives? Most crucially, and central to the theme of this book, is the question, 'Does play have a positive impact on our health and wellbeing, and consequently a role in modern healthcare delivery?'

Exploring play in an adult world

There have been many and various attempts to define the meaning of play – mostly in the context of childhood development and learning. Definitions include: play as an innate characteristic necessary for the survival of the species (Groos 1901); play as an outlet for surplus energy (Schiller 1795 [2012]); play as a means of achieving mastery or power (Freud 1920); and play as a key stage of social and cognitive learning (Piaget 1962; Erikson 1965). The definitions of play are as diverse as the variety of play phenomena that fall under that heading – from daydreaming (playing with thoughts and ideas), military re-enactment (playing at soldiers), stand-up comedy (playing with convention), to skate-boarding (playing at youthfulness).

> Almost anything can allow play to occur within its boundaries.
>
> *(Sutton-Smith 1980)*

What all theorists seem to agree upon is that play is a crucial feature of both animal and human existence, endowing life with an essential element of self-determined pleasure, creativity and generalized enhancement (St Clair 2005). Brown and Vaughan (2009) re-state for the twenty-first century the notion that play is as important to the human condition as breathing, an energizing life-force that maintains its importance throughout the lifespan.

> I sometimes compare play to oxygen – it's all around us, yet goes mostly unnoticed or unappreciated until it is missing.
>
> *(Brown and Vaughan 2009: 6)*

Kets de Vries (2012) proposes that play has been essential to the survival and evolution of man from his earliest emergence in prehistoric times, as depicted in the cave drawings found in France and Spain. Noting the care and attention to detail within these drawings, Kets de Vries (2012: 3) explores the motivation behind them, asking 'were these ancient scrapings and paintings the sophisticated creations of serious artists or merely the playful graffiti of Palaeolithic teenagers?'

Play theorists of the modern age, since the time of the European Enlightenment and the Romantic period, have tended to emphasize play as a means to personal growth and development at the *start* of life. Rousseau (1712–78), Pestalozzi (1747–1827) and Froebel (1782–1852) have all contributed to an understanding of play as a learning tool belonging to the early years, yet play 'inhabits all spheres of human activity' (Huizinga 1949). Play and playfulness are evident in our cultural legacy from the most primitive times and the earliest portrayals were certainly not childish matters. The play depicted in word (e.g. Shakespearean comedies), art (e.g. the Kama Sutra) and architecture (e.g. the grotesque gargoyles of medieval church architecture) are distinctly adult representations of play.

If we accept the popular premise that play is about growth and adaptation to one's social and emotional environment, we might also question why adults continue to play once fully grown and adapted. This might be explained by Erikson's (1965) playful suggestion that, whilst children move forwards in their play, adults move sideways. Sutton-Smith (1997) offers a complementary construction of play: as a waiting game, a pastime and as a means of generating positive feelings at times of hardship and adversity.

Play is also a means by which the individual seeks personal actualization or the attainment of existential completeness. In the fifteenth letter of 'On the Aesthetic Education of Man', written in 1795, Friedrich Schiller (1795 [2012]: 80) writes of play,

> man only plays when in the full meaning of the word he is a man, and he is only completely a man when he plays.

Schiller proposes that play represents the supreme expression of the human spirit, reconciling the artificial divisions for which civilization is responsible. Schiller (1797 [2012]) divides the creative impulse into three sense drives: the desire for sense, the desire for form and the desire for play. He calls play (*Spieltrieb*) the 'salvation' of the other two in that it integrates reason and sensation and synthesizes from their union the true essence of humanity.

We play because we want to and because we can, not because we have to. What seems to make an action or activity playful is the absence of functional necessity and a creative disregard of the established order. Consider the commonality of theme and style in the rough-and-tumble play of young mammals and the hilarious clowning of the great comics of the silent screen.

In *The Ambiguity of Play*, Sutton-Smith (1997) offers one of the most comprehensive reviews of the literature on play in the form of *Seven Rhetorics* of play which serve to organize and extort the meaning of play in all its various forms. This attempt to create some coherence in the field of play theory, by clarifying the cultural rhetorics, or ideological narratives, that underlie the various popular play theories is a concept which lends itself to the consideration of play as concomitant to health and wellbeing.

1 *Play as progress* generally applies to the play of children and is seen primarily in terms of imitative development rather than pure pleasure. This includes theories of play as adaptation, training for life and socialization.

2 *Play as fate or destiny* contrasts with the popular notion that play incorporates an element of free choice. This, the oldest rhetoric in historical terms, is reliant on a belief that both human life and play are in the hands of the gods or of Fate – except through the use of magic or prayer to achieve mastery over life's circumstances. The current popularity of games of chance (office sweepstakes, lotteries and online gambling) would fall in this category and implies that play can be passively voluntary even when it involves risk-taking.

3 *Play as power*, as a route to glory, status and belonging (Huizinga 1949). This is play as usually applied to sports, athletics and interpersonal competition and relies on the notion of conflict as a route to hero-status. This bracket might also include Freudian intrapersonal explanations for play as mastery over both emotions and the other.

4 *Play as identity* as it applies to traditional community and seasonal festivals and celebrations, confirming and promoting membership or 'belonging' within a community.

5 *Play as a representation of the imaginary* embraces playful improvization in literature and the arts, as well as play as a route to creativity and imagination. Sutton-Smith includes in this rhetoric the fantasy play of childhood, highlighting the inversion and irrationality that is typical of play's flexibility. This is enacted in the clowning and nonsensical performance evident in contemporary comedic displays.

6 *Play as self-satisfaction*, as a form of fun, relaxation and escapism: hobbies and high-risk sports fall into this category.

7 *Play as frivolous*, as a deviation from the 'work ethic' view of play as significant and purposeful. Historically tricksters and fools, 'the frivolous', were protagonists who enacted playful protest against the status quo; the court jester, the heckler, the class clown.

8 Julia Whitaker and Alison Tonkin

Play and the playful

A distinction is often made between *play* (which is well organized, eagerly pursued and valued) and *playfulness* (which refers more to a mood of light-heartedness, recklessness and humor). Play may incorporate the playful but playfulness is not necessarily fundamental to a definition of play. Whitehead (cited in Moyles 1994), writing in the context of childhood education, outlines the dichotomy between play and fun and questions whether or not all play needs to include an element of the latter. This view contrasts with a growing recognition of the need to incorporate fun into the delivery of healthcare for children (Carter *et al.* 2011) and the emergence of clown doctors within both pediatric and elderly care over the last five years (Ford *et al.* 2014). There is a growing evidence base of efficacy which suggests that fun is a necessity rather than an optional extra (Tonkin 2014a). The idea of play as fun suggests an element of light-heartedness and superficiality, which is now being utilized to boost productivity and innovation in the workplace, enabling workers to take more creative risks (Robinson *et al.* 2014).

However, the evidence also exists to suggest that much play can be quite the opposite of fun (Henricks 2008). Consider the intensity of a chess game or the risk inherent in certain adult role-play scenarios. This so-called 'deep play' (Geertz 1976) which subverts authority and often makes a play for power, as exhibited in many forms of creative activity as well as in games of chance and the high-risk play of gamblers and sky-divers, might not be included in the lexicon of 'fun' activities yet this pushing of acceptable boundaries may be critical to what it is that makes life meaningful and worthwhile. Deep play distances the individual from the practical demands and constraints of their particular circumstances, creating a separate and personal space – what Winnicott (1971) calls a 'third area' where one can truly be oneself.

What becomes evident is that definitions of play may lie in the experience of the player or within the characteristics of the play itself (Smith and Vollstedt 1985). Children – the experts in this field – tell us that play is about pleasure, voluntariness, friends, and the outdoors – and not about work (Nicholson *et al.* 2014).

Defining play

Despite the rich history and the celebrated diversity of adult play (Henricks 2008), its value and associated benefits are often 'vastly underrated' (St Clair 2005). For many commentators, the difficulty lies in the use of the term 'play' and how the definition of play links to the associated activities. For example, Kuschner (2010) questions Brown and Vaughan's (2009) conceptualization of play noting that 'the activity of climbing cliffs or baking bread may be satisfying, rewarding, enjoyable [and] intrinsically motivated … all qualities that can be associated with play – but are they necessarily examples of play' (Kuschner 2010: 375). This shows how trying to provide a single working definition of play can lead to an overextension of play as a concept which ultimately minimizes its clarity and usage. Climbing and baking

Playing for health **9**

bread have much to offer in terms of the enjoyment and therapeutic value they provide for the individuals concerned and supply a rationale for the integration of leisure and recreational activities when considering what may contribute to the health and wellbeing of adults.

Broadening the scope of activities beyond play still results in difficulties when it comes to providing standard definitions. Hurd and Anderson (2011) suggest that the benefits of defining the concepts of leisure, recreation and play lie in the provision of firm foundations on which services, facilities and programs can be built. Hurd and Anderson provide a useful overview of the differing concepts, which also necessitates the breaking down of leisure into three primary areas, as defined in Table 1.1.

Although the clear differentiation of what constitutes play, leisure and recreation has been made, it is still difficult to compartmentalize the differing concepts. This may also detract from the content that is being explored and in many ways is unnecessary for a book of this nature. Therefore, whilst acknowledging there is conceptual variation, the word *play* is predominantly used herein as a generic term, unless the terms *leisure* and/or *recreation* are specifically used for contextual purposes.

The benefits of play for health throughout the adult lifespan

Play is considered to be 'fundamental to the health and wellbeing of individuals and communities' (Playwork Principles Scrutiny Group 2005). This 'principle' relates to children and young people but there is an emerging body of evidence that demonstrates the efficacy and necessity of play for adults.

TABLE 1.1 Definitions of leisure, play and recreation (Hurd and Anderson 2011)

Concept	Definition
Leisure as time	Leisure is a time free from obligation, work (paid and unpaid), and tasks required for existing (sleeping, eating).
Leisure as activity	Leisure is a set of activities that people engage in during their free time – activities that are not work-orientated or that do not involve life maintenance tasks such as housecleaning or sleeping.
Leisure as state of mind	Leisure depends on a participant's perception. Perceived freedom, intrinsic motivation, perceived competence, and positive affect are critical to the determination of an experience as leisure or not leisure.
Play	Play is imaginative, intrinsically motivated, non-serious, freely chosen, and actively engaging. Play is typified by spontaneity, joyfulness, and inhibition and is done not as a means to an end but for its inherent pleasure.
Recreation	Recreation is an activity that people engage in during their free time, that people enjoy, and that people recognize as having socially redeeming values. The activity performed is less important than the reason for performing the activity, which is the outcome.

10 Julia Whitaker and Alison Tonkin

Physical play for health

Play is probably most noticeably associated with physical health and there is global recognition of the need to promote physical activity across the age range (World Health Organization 2014), with a proportionate variation in intensity matching the age of the participant (Cox 2012). The World Health Organization (2014) has produced a set of physical activity fact sheets, dividing the adult population into those aged 18 to 64 years of age and those aged 65 years and upwards. These provide global recommendations that apply to everyone 'irrespective of gender, race, ethnicity or income level' and the benefits include lower levels of the so-called modern mortality conditions such as 'coronary heart disease, high blood pressure, stroke, type 2 diabetes, metabolic syndrome, colon and breast cancer and depression' (World Health Organization 2011). Activity can include playing sport and, although this is associated with adults under 40 years of age, there have been recent adaptations to encourage participation across a much broader age range with the introduction of new versions of popular sports such as walking football (The FA (Football Association) 2014), walking basketball (Basketball England 2013), walking netball or walking rounders (Green 2014). However, this goes beyond purely the physical, as the benefits of exercise are known to be enhanced when it can involve other people as well (Cox 2012). Socialization after the event is also an important aspect and the *FA Mars Just Play* sessions, which include walking football are:

> Recreational, light-hearted and most importantly – fun! The cup of tea after the game and the post-match banter is another enjoyable part of the sessions – adding a social element to a thoroughly enjoyable experience.
>
> *(The FA 2014)*

There are particular benefits of physical activity for older adults, aged 65 and over, and these include improvement in 'cardiorespiratory and muscular fitness, bone and functional health... [and a reduction] in the risk of non-communicable diseases, depression and cognitive decline' (World Health Organization 2014). Play is specifically mentioned as one of the activities that contributes to physical activity, but this is not elaborated upon. Other activities include walking, dancing, gardening, hiking, cycling, swimming, household chores, games or planned sports 'in the context of daily, family and community activities' (World Health Organization 2014). For 'community dwelling older adults', preventing falls is particularly important in order to minimize the occurrence of fractures. Low-intensity physical activity that strengthens muscles and/or enhances balance, through activities such as Tai Chi, has been shown to be effective in reducing falls (Cox 2012).

Adults enjoy opportunities to play on structured play apparatus such as playground equipment, but this can be problematic when they use equipment that is designed for children. For example, firefighters from Somerset and Devon were called out 13 times over a five-year period to assist adults stuck in children's play equipment (*The Western Morning News* 2014). As part of a TED conversation, Morris (2012) asks,

'Why aren't there playgrounds for adults?' stating that 'Adults will readily play when given the permission and opportunity. I think adult playgrounds could be one step towards making society more approving of play.' There are examples of play provision for adults, such as PlayZone (2014) in Portsmouth, UK, with 'adult only' nights twice a week, enabling access to 'huge slides, rope walk ways, fireman's poles, web climber, tumble towers, up and overs pads [and] bish bash bags, etc.' Other examples include 'tone zones' or 'outdoor gyms' which, although suitable for all ages, provide equipment that is 'particularly usable by the more mature members of society' (Kilkenny People 2012).

Steen (2012) in response to Morris (2012) suggests, 'In my perception, we have playgrounds all around us … rivers, lakes, mountains, bike paths, gardens, etc. My toys are a kayak, bicycle, skis, garden tools, etc.' The influence of the natural environment has attracted wide-ranging research across the continents. Specific benefits are attributable to 'green exercise' whereby activities are conducted in the presence of nature, combining the benefits of both physical activity and enhanced mental health (Cox 2102). This effect is heightened near natural water environments, known as 'blue space' and research is currently being undertaken by the European Centre for Environment and Human Health (2014) looking at the efficacy of the 'Blue Gym'. This will be discussed in more detail in Chapter 4.

Play and mental wellness

Additional benefits arise when play is 'felt to be exciting or fun' (Henricks 2008: 162) and the links between play, emotional wellbeing and mental health are attracting considerable interest. The so-called 'dot.com' companies recognize the link between a fun working environment and productivity and many now provide opportunities for 'employees to play and let off steam' (Robinson *et al.* 2014). Play is known to engage the creative side of the brain and according to Kets de Vries (2012), learning and creativity will not happen without the input of play.

However, Kets de Vries (2012) also suggests that societal changes throughout the last four centuries, brought about first by farming, then industrialization and now the digitization of modern life may have caused a 'misfit between our modern life and our evolutionary make up [and asks] are the present day diseases of civilization (obesity, cardiovascular disorders, metabolic disturbances, allergies, depression, chronic stress) due to a hitch in our evolutionary progression over time?' (Kets de Vries 2012: 5). On a global level, Basu (2012) comments on the 'dot.com' boom from a different perspective and explores the drive for the manufacture of electronic components in countries such as China and Mexico. With most of the components made by hand by migrant workers, one of the major health impacts has been the increase in mental health problems due to the repetitive nature of the work and long hours. Contrasting this with the dot.com companies where play is encouraged, one might reasonably ask whether the promotion of play could contribute to the reversal of these global issues. As demonstrated in childhood, it is sometimes the deficit of play opportunities that provides the most visible testimony to the benefits that play provides (Care Quality Commission 2014).

The previous coalition government in the UK has recognized the significant effect of the economic recession on the wellbeing of the population and clearly stated that 'we need to heal emotional wounds, which means that we are looking for a psychological recovery alongside our economic recovery' (Department of Health 2011: 2). The role of play and recreational activity is noted as a contributor for maintaining good mental health but also as a treatment for people with mild depression. 'Exercise on prescription' is now offered alongside traditional treatments such as talking therapies and medication (NHS Choices 2014a). This is discussed more fully in Chapter 8.

Perhaps play's greatest contribution to positive health is through developing and maintaining positive mental wellbeing, which enables us to feel good about ourselves and to engage with the opportunities life has to offer (NHS Choices 2014b). There is an obvious link to socialization and to how people interact with those around them; the role of play, and of the light-hearted approach to life that is often associated with playful people, can be particularly effective in achieving and maintaining positive health (Robinson *et al.* 2014).

NHS Choices (2014b) suggest there are five steps to mental wellbeing. All can be promoted through play-based activities.

Connectedness – play provides opportunities to connect and develop relationships that can promote and protect individuals and whole communities. This is exemplified through the development of play-orientated programs by library services in America, which have managed to engage the hard to reach 19–50 year age range, turning them into avid library users in the process (Barbakoff 2014).

Being active – not just physical activity, but participation in activities that are enjoyed by the individual themselves, such as singing and the expressive arts. For example, Figure 1.1 is of a piano for the public to play on the concourse at Brighton Railway Station.

Learning – the acquisition of new tasks is easier when an element of play is involved, particularly in social situations where ideas can be shared and explored together. Barbakoff (2014) suggests:

> Experiential, playful learning should not end with childhood. If you want your adult patrons to learn, create a space for fun. Give them an environment to dream, grow, invent, jump, and try. Let them play with your existing services and materials in a new way by providing them in unexpected places.

Giving to others – time is a precious commodity but finding the time to play with other people not only helps the recipients but also boosts the self-esteem and sense of wellbeing in the person who volunteers. This was demonstrated by the 'Games Makers' at the London Olympics in 2012.

Playing for health 13

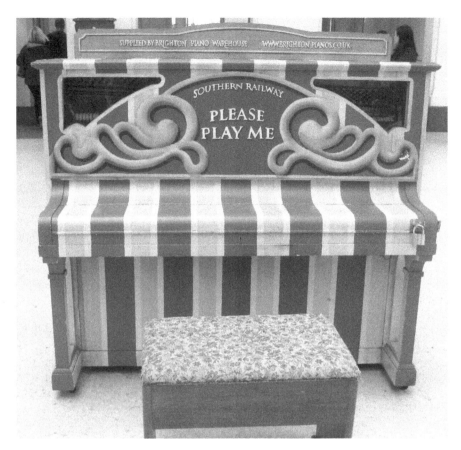

FIGURE 1.1 An invitation to rail passengers passing through Brighton Station, summer 2014

Taking notice – particularly of the environments that surround us. Humans have a natural affinity with nature (Lester and Maudsley 2007) and playscapes that incorporate natural features are known to promote 'a sense of self and wellbeing' (Goldstein 2012).

Play within healthcare

Accepting Sutton-Smith's (1980) assertion that play is key to 'the potentiation of adaptive variability', suggests a premise for the role of play in healing and rehabilitation and in the promotion and evolution of the concept of positive health. There is an important distinction to be made here between play and the more solution-focused occupational and recreational therapies, although these may ultimately metamorphose into behavior that can be re-categorized as play. For example, art therapy as a route to creative self-expression pursued for its own sake; or physical

14 Julia Whitaker and Alison Tonkin

rehabilitation after serious injury resulting in a new-found passion for an olympic sport. The Invictus Games (2014) are a prime example of how rehabilitative therapies can transmute into self-motivated and self-affirming recreational pursuits which are undertaken for reasons of personal pleasure and pride, whilst at the same time giving injured servicemen and servicewomen a new-found route to self-fulfilment.

The individual who is born with, or who encounters, a challenge to their physical, mental or social health will be required to adapt to the situation and set of personal circumstances in which they find themselves. Ideally this is a reciprocal endeavour in which society and its members are also required to find adaptive means of living with difference (Universities of Hull, Staffordshire and Aberdeen 2010). The form this adaptation takes will vary with the individual and the nature of the context. Play is both of its time and of its culture. An individual's survival or recovery demands that they identify ways of living and being which maintain their status and function within the group, whilst preserving their own sense of personal identity and integrity. Play serves to deliver status (Asher and Coie 1990) and belonging (Corsaro 1995) as well as to establish a sense of self-worth and identity (Taylor 1989), independent of the individual's capacity for work and full social integration. For example, the Universities of Hull, Staffordshire and Aberdeen (2010) provide the case-study of an individual with dementia for whom a holistic 'biographical approach' to care-planning provided a vehicle for communication which focused on the subject as a valued individual rather than solely a service user.

Playing to learn and learning through play

Moyles (2010) offers a tripartite pedagogy of play which addresses three main concepts inherent in play and playfulness. This 'playful pedagogy' offers a fruitful framework within which to consider the role of play in health-giving and is outlined here as it relates to the adult service user in the healthcare context.

Pure play – this is play which is under the control of the individual. It is self-initiated, sustained and developed for the purposes of the self – defined or otherwise. It refers to an act of will, to activities selected by the individual and engaged with according to their own discretion. Pure play is generally intuitive, creative and unrestrictive.

Chapter 10 explores engagement in the expressive arts which can be understood as a creative form of pure play, undertaken for its own sake whilst also serving the secondary function of evoking a sense of wellbeing and positivity. The role of the health-giver in pure play is one of enabler, to make resources available, to show interest and to engage, only if invited to do so – without interrupting the private play agenda of the main player. This demands open-ended planning and a willingness to accept a transfer of power and control to the service user.

Playful learning – This can be interpreted in the adult healthcare context as referring to learning experiences that are initiated or inspired by the health-giver, which engage the individual in playful activity and which endeavour to reflect the instinctive nature of play. Children often learn from one another in this way and it is a model evident in the use of play with adults with health needs. The caregiver's role is to be sensitive to the individual's playful learning modes and to make planned provision to address these, to actively interact, participate and model the activity within the frame of a set of clear learning objectives.

In Chapter 4, a case study is used to illustrate how the health play specialist uses playful learning in the context of a parenting assessment of a young couple with learning difficulties. By first observing their instinctive play-style and then using this information to create playful scenarios in which their problem-solving and decision-making skills might become evident, the play specialist is able to assess the couple's learning needs and to link this to planning.

Playful teaching – teaching that draws on the light-heartedness of play and a sense of fun can be labelled 'playful teaching'. Learning new tasks in a relaxed manner is known to be a more effective method of teaching (Robinson *et al.* 2014) and educators have long realized that a study-day or workshop that incorporates an element of fun can have more impact than a purely instructive model (Tonkin 2014b).

In playful teaching, learning objectives are presented in active and imaginative formats and allow for some unpredictability in terms of outcome, but the intention is determined by what the player/service user needs to do or learn. Whilst such teaching will utilize resources perceived as 'playful', participants will be aware that this is not pure play and recognize the difference between the two. The role of the health-giver in this context is to ensure that tasks are planned and presented in an enjoyable but meaningful way and to engage the service user in a reflective evaluation of learning outcomes. A playful approach to teaching and learning is discussed in more detail in Chapter 21.

Health interventions in all their forms, ranging from medical and nursing care, psychological, social and spiritual support and guidance, education and rehabili-tative training – even when expertly delivered and co-ordinated – may leave the individual (whether health-giver or recipient) with little time, means, or inclination for the 'pursuit of pure pleasure' for its own sake, be it in the form of playful fun or risky 'deep play'. A holistic approach to health and wellbeing must surely acknowledge and incorporate the human instinct for play in its various guises and recognize its role in the discovery or recovery of the true self.

References

Asher, S.R. and Coie, J.D. (1990) *Peer Rejection in Childhood*, New York: Cambridge University Press.

Barbakoff, A. (2014) *Learning Through Play in Adult Programs,* Online. Available at www.ebsco host.com/novelist/novelist-special/learning-through-play-in-adult-programs (accessed 22 February 2016).

Basketball England (2013) *Ball Again Walking Basketball Session in Surrey,* Online. Available at www.basketballengland.co.uk/news/default.aspx?newsid=5049 (accessed 4 December 2015).

Basu, S. (2012) Occupational health in the electronic age: disease in the new sweatshop, *EpiAnalysis Blog.* 23 January 2012. Online. Available at http://epianalysis.wordpress.com/2012/01/23/esweat/ (accessed 4 December 2015).

Brown, S. and Vaughan, C. (2009) *Play, How it Shapes the Brain, Opens the Imagination and Invigorates the Soul,* London: Penguin.

Care Quality Commission (2014) *Alder Hey Children's Hospital Quality Report,* Care Quality Commission.

Corsaro, W.A. (1995) *Friendship and Peer culture in the Early Years,* New York: Ablex.

Cox, S. (2012) *Game of Life: How Sport and Recreation Can Make Us Healthier, Happier and Richer,* Sport and Recreation Alliance. Online. Available: This Is not stated on the pdf 0 but can be accessed through the following link… www.sportandrecreation.org.uk/sites/sportandrecreation.org.uk/files/web/Game_of_Life/3310_SRA_literary%20review_v9%20WITH%20HYPERLINK.pdf

Department of Health (2011) *Talking Therapies: A Four-year Plan of Action. A Supporting Document to No Health without Mental Health: A Cross-government Mental Health Outcomes Strategy for People of all Ages,* London: Department of Health.

Erikson, E. (1965) *Childhood and Society,* Harmondsworth: Penguin.

European Centre for Environment and Human Health (2014) *Interdisciplinary Research: Blue Gym.* Online. Available at www.ecehh.org/research/#!blue-gym (accessed 4 December 2015).

Ford, K., Tesch, L. and Carter, B. (2011) FUNdamentally important: humour and fun as caring and practice, *Journal of Child Health Care* 15 (4): 247–249.

Ford, K., Courtney-Pratt, H., Tesch, L. and Johnson, C. (2014) More than just clowns – Clown Doctor rounds and their impact for children, families and staff, *Journal of Child Health Care* 18 (3): 286–296.

Freud, S. (1920) *Beyond the Pleasure Principle,* New York: Norton.

Geertz, C. (1976) Deep play: a description of the Balinese cockfight. In Bruner, J.S., Jolly, A. and Sylva, K. (eds) Play: It's Role in Development and Evolution. New York: Viking Penguin: 656–676.

Goldstein, J. (2012) *Play in Children's Development, Health and Wellbeing,* Brussels: Toy Industries of Europe.

Green, S. (2014) *Walking Sports: All You Need to Know,* Online. Available at www.saga.co.uk/health/fitness/walking-sports.aspx (accessed 4 December 2015).

Groos, K. (1901) *The Play of Man.* New York: Appleton.

Henricks, T. (2008) The nature of play: an overview, *The American Journal of Play,* 1 (2): 157–180.

Huizinga, J. (1949) *Homo Ludens: A Study of the Play Element in Culture,* London: Routledge and Kegan Paul.

Hurd, A. and Anderson, D. (2011) *The Park and Recreation Professional's Handbook,* Champaign, IL: Human Kinetics.

Invictus Games (2014*) Invictus Games 2014,* Online. Available at http://invictusgames.org/ (accessed 4 December 2015).

Kets de Vries, M.F.R. (2012) *Going Back to the Sandbox: Teaching CEOs How to Play,* INSEAD.

Kilkenny People (2012) Adults at play in Kilkenny's linear walk. *Kilkenny People,* 30 March 2012, Online. Available at www.kilkennypeople (accessed 4 December 2015).

Kuschner, D. (2010) Book review for *Play:* how it shapes the brain, opens the imagination, and invigorates the soul, *The American Journal of Play,* 2 (3): 374–376.

Lester, S. and Maudsley, M. (2007) *Play, Naturally: A Review of Children's Natural Play,* London: Play England.

Morris, C. (2012) *TED: Why Aren't there Playgrounds for Adults?* Online. Available at www.ted.com/conversations/11969/why_aren_t_there_playgrounds_f.html (accessed 4 December 2015).

Moyles, J. (1994) *The Excellence of Play*, Maidenhead: Open University Press.

Moyles, J. (2010) *Thinking about Play: Developing a Reflective Approach*. Maidenhead: Open University Press.

NHS Choices (2014a) *Exercise for Depression*, Online. Available at www.nhs.uk/conditions/stress-anxiety-depression/pages/exercise-for-depression.aspx (accessed 4 December 2015).

NHS Choices (2014b) *Five Steps to Mental Wellbeing – Stress, Anxiety and Depression*, Online. Available at www.nhs.uk/conditions/stress-anxiety-depression/pages/improve-mental-wellbeing.aspx (accessed 4 December 2015).

Piaget, J. (1962) *Play, Dreams and Imagination in Childhood*, New York: Norton.

Playwork Principles Scrutiny Group (2005) *Playwork Principles,* Playwork Principles Scrutiny Group, Cardiff 2005.

PlayZone (2014) *PlayZone: Fizzical Fun for Everyone!* Online. Available at www.theplayzone.co.uk/ (accessed 4 December 2015).

Robinson, L., Smith, M. and Segal, J. (2014) *Why Play Matters for Adults,* Online. Available at www.helpguide.org/life/creative_play_fun_games.htm. (accessed 4 December 2015).

St Clair, M. (2005) *The Top Ten Benefits of Play,* Online. Available at www.creativity-portal.com/bc/other/play.html (accessed 4 December 2015).

Schiller, F. (1795 [2012]) *On the Aesthetic Education of Man*, New York: Dover Publications.

Smith, P. K. and Vollstedt R. (1985) On Defining Play: An Empirical Study of the Relationship between Play and Various Play Criteria, *Child Development*, 56 (4): 1042–1050.

Sutton-Smith, B. (1980) *Play and Learning*, Hoboken, NJ: John Wiley & Sons, Inc.

Sutton-Smith, B. (1997) *The Ambiguity of Play*, Cambridge, MA: Harvard University Press.

Taylor, C. (1989) *Sources of the Self: The Making of Modern Identity*. Cambridge, MA: Harvard University Press.

The FA (2014) *Mars Just Play Walking Football Sessions Prove to be a Hit,* Online. Available at www.thefa.com/news/my-football/players/2014/jun/walking-football-fa-mars-just-play#XLDR48Cf2VLbgbWk.99 (accessed 2 November 2014).

The Western Morning News (2014) Adults stuck in play equipment, *The Western Morning News,* 1 July 2014: 21.

Tonkin, A. (2014a) *The Provision of Play in Health Service Delivery*, The National Association of Health Play Specialists.

Tonkin, A. (2014b) Promoting the Use of Evidence through a Teddy Murder Mystery, *Working Together: Building Respectful and Responsive Relationships. Proceedings of the 2014 7th Biennial International Conference held in Auckland*. Hospital Play Specialists Association of Aotearoa/New Zealand.

Universities of Hull, Staffordshire and Aberdeen (2010) *Spiritual Care at the End of Life. A Systematic Review of the Literature,* London: Department of Health.

Winnicott, D.W. (1971) *Playing and Reality*, Harmondsworth: Penguin.

World Health Organization (2011) *Global Recommendations on Physical Activity for Health: 18–64 Years Old,* Online. Available at www.who.int/dietphysicalactivity/physical-activity-recommendations-18-64years.pdf?ua=1 (accessed 2 November 2014).

World Health Organization (2014) *Physical Activity and Older Adults*, Online. Available at www.who.int/dietphysicalactivity/factsheet_olderadults/en/ (accessed 2 November 2014).

2

CONCEPTUALIZING PLAY IN HEALTHCARE PROVISION

Alison Tonkin and Julia Whitaker

Conceptualization refers to the formation of ideas or concepts (Oxford Dictionaries 2015a) which, for the purpose of this chapter, will incorporate theoretical perspectives to demonstrate why play for adults may be utilized within healthcare provision.

Introduction

When exploring the subject of adults and play, the use of theoretical frameworks that lend themselves to adaptation helps to focus attention on the key elements under consideration. Trudge *et al.* (2009: 198) suggest that 'the meaning of theory in any scientific field is to provide a framework within which to explain connections among the phenomena under study and to provide insights leading to the discovery of new connections'. These connections can be visualized through the use of modelling to represent a system or process (Oxford Dictionaries 2015b). Play is considered by many psychologists to be a process, particularly in relation to the emotional and mental processes involved when play occurs (Henricks 2008). Therefore, play can be *represented* within other complex systems, such as health, which also incorporates concepts from differing theoretical perspectives (Grzywacz and Fuqua 2000).

The social ecology of health

Kurt Lewin (1939), considered by many to be the 'father of modern social psychology', advocated the use of scientific concepts from divergent fields for solving problems, providing they could be applied in practical ways. Lewin (1939) utilized the concepts and laws of physics to develop the *field-theoretical approach* as a practical research tool to explore the interdependence of physiological, psychological and sociological factors on human development. This work is considered to be the forerunner to Bronfenbrenner's *Bioecological Theory of Human Development* (Härkönen 2007).

Bronfenbrenner (1994: 37) stated that 'ecological models encompass an evolving body of theory and research concerned with the processes and conditions that govern the lifelong course of human development in the actual environments in which human beings live'. Bronfenbrenner mapped a wide range of human developmental influences as a series of concentric circles, showing the interconnectedness between environmental settings that can directly and indirectly contribute to the development of the individual (O'Donoghue and Maidment 2005). Since then, Bronfenbrenner's original bioecological theory has been applied as the theoretical foundation for research across a wide range of disciplines. Health, as a multidisciplinary construct that applies across many differing levels through the lifespan, has adapted ecological theory to identify its influential dispositions, resources and characteristics (Grzwaka and Fuqua 2005). The most enduring and effective example of this is the representation by Dahlgren and Whitehead (NHS Education for Scotland n.d.). This model from 1991, 'shows how individual determinants including a person's age, sex and hereditary factors are nested within the wider determinants of health which include lifestyle factors, social and community influences, living and working conditions and general socio-economic cultural and environmental conditions' (Local Government Association 2010).

Barton and Grant (2006: 1) suggest that over the past century, 'we have been literally building unhealthy conditions into our local human habitat and this has contributed to the current problems linked to obesity, asthma and reduced levels of physical activity'. They have consequently adapted Dahlgren and Whitehead's model, keeping all the original elements but spreading them out and linking in the global ecosystem, as shown in Figure 2.1. For the first time, play is explicitly mentioned within a health specific ecological model, as an activity that determines health and wellbeing. This suggests that play and health share characteristics that can be explored at both an individual and community level, and both can be represented through a biopsychosocial approach that integrates key features together as opposed to separating them out into different disciplines.

Grywacz and Fuqua (2000) view heath as a 'developmental phenomenon' and suggest that an ecological theory of human development should be used to provide an 'overarching framework', enabling equal focus to be placed on the environment and the person. This suggests that the developing person is an active player who can change and restructure the environment to accommodate their role within it (O'Donoghue and Maidment 2005). Piaget (1962, cited Henricks 2008: 161) noted the role of assimilation and accommodation when describing play, whereby people need to impose their own 'personal ideas and behavioral strategies on the world', which in turn utilize play to gain an element of control and self-direction. Piaget identified this as an opportunity to build skills and to practise them, for future use within a wider context (Henricks 2008).

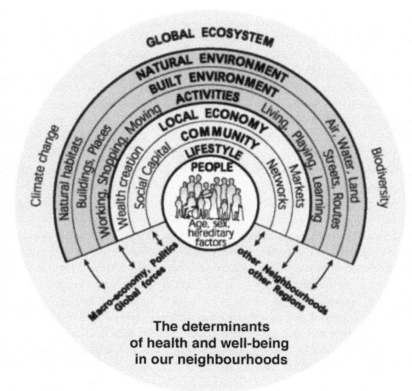

FIGURE 2.1 The Health Model (Barton and Grant 2006 – reproduced by kind permission of Barton)

Using play as a motivational tool to address individual needs

Lewin (1939) developed the formula B = f(PE) where behavior (B) is the result (f) of the interaction between the person (P) and the environment (E) (Härkönen 2007). Saarinen *et al.* (1994, cited Härkönen 2007) later noted that this influence occurs in both directions: the person influences the environment and the environment influences the person. Bandura's (1986) work demonstrates this through the concept of *reciprocal determinism* whereby interactions between our thoughts, the environment and our behavior constantly change the way we think and feel (Allen and Gordon 2011). Boyd and Bee (2012) extend this by suggesting three components – the external environment, individual behaviors and cognitive/personal factors – influence, and are influenced by each other on a reciprocal basis (Boyd and Bee 2012).

Abraham Maslow (1943: 371) acknowledged the situation or field in which organisms react, noting that 'while behavior is almost always motivated, it is also

Conceptualizing play in healthcare provision **21**

almost always biologically, culturally and situationally determined as well'. However, Maslow noted that field theory could 'rarely serve as an exclusive explanation for behavior' and proposed *A Theory of Human Motivation*, which he described at the time as a 'fusion or synthesis' of a number of pre-existing theoretical perspectives.

Maslow (1943: 370) described human motivation as 'a channel through which many basic needs may be simultaneously expressed or satisfied'. These needs are arranged in hierarchies of 'pre-potency' whereby 'the appearance of one need usually rests on the prior satisfaction of another, more pre-potent need' (Maslow 1943: 370). These needs, in order of pre-potency, are physiological needs, safety needs, love needs, esteem needs and the need for self-actualization (Table 2.1). This means that if all needs are unsatisfied, physiological needs dominate until they are satisfied and all other pursuits that do not contribute to meeting these needs lie dormant and become of secondary importance. However, once physiological needs have been satisfied, more social needs emerge, particularly the need for love, affection and belonging. Maslow (1943) suggests that social needs are treated with ambivalence in society due to a lack of awareness, noting that restrictions and inhibitors that prevent love needs being met can be detrimental to the health of the individual. Within the realms of public health, Freeman (2012) recognizes the significance of family and friends within a complex web of factors that contribute to 'being healthy, but notes this is not something that can be "offered on the NHS"'. However, Relate (2015) identify this lack of recognition of the significance of relationships as a serious issue, stating that 'our relationships are often ignored in the NHS [and] this needs to change ... by putting '"relationships at the heart of the NHS"'. This is one area where play can definitively be effective.

Play can be used as a 'powerful catalyst for positive socialisation [fostering] a sense of belonging and connection to other people' (St Clair 2005). Playfulness in the form of banter between colleagues and between staff and patients is seen as a cultural necessity within the context of healthcare provision in the NHS (Payne 2002). This is exemplified by an innovative scheme run by the Oxford University Hospitals NHS Trust whereby new nurses from overseas were offered 'courses in colloquial English and lessons in what makes Britons laugh' as part of their induction program because many nurses failed to understand their patients' 'quaint and curious colloquialisms' and did not understand their humor (Payne 2002). The Elderflowers program in Scotland (Hearts and Minds 2015) also uses humor to promote participation in the performing arts for people with dementia who are in full-time hospital care. The program utilizes the patient's own humor and personality to engage in 'playful banter' which encourages interaction and laughter whilst stimulating creativity and mental capacity.

Maslow (1943) originally proposed his theory as a framework for future work and Barrett (2013) has subsequently adapted Maslow's hierarchy into the *Seven Levels of Consciousness Model*. This can also be linked to the six aspects of health as defined by Ewles and Simnett (2003).

Barrett (2010) replaced Maslow's concept of pre-potency needs with a focus on underlying anxieties and subconscious fears as the determinants of the level of

22 Alison Tonkin and Julia Whitaker

TABLE 2.1 Linking the aspects of health to motivational theory (adapted from Barrett 2010)

Maslow (1943) hierarchy of needs	Barrett (1997) seven levels of consciousness	Ewles and Simnett (2003) six aspects of health
Need for self-actualization	Service	Spiritual
	Making a difference	Societal
	Internal cohesion	
	Transformation	Mental
Esteem needs	Self-esteem	Emotional
Love needs	Relationship	Social
Safety needs	Survival	Physical
Physiological needs		

consciousness currently being experienced. Barrett (2013) identified humor and fun as part of the 'internal cohesion' level for personal consciousness, suggesting that these are necessary for finding meaning in existence and a sense of purpose in life. This endorses the view that 'It is play that is the universal … and that belongs to health' (Winnicott 1971: 41).

Play deprivation

The significance of play and of its contribution to human development and self-actualization have been exposed and explored within these opening chapters. There inevitably follows the question of what happens when play is absent or deficient and what the consequences of this might be for the health of the individual and for the wellbeing of society as a whole.

Recent statistics suggest the following:

- In a Workplace Quality of Life Index (WQLI) survey of employee wellbeing, the UK achieved a low ranking in a comparison of 27 countries (Newcombe 2013).
- Reported stress levels have increased by 18 per cent (women) and 25 per cent (men) in US employees over the past 25 years (Cohen and Janicki-Deverts 2012).
- Forty-eight per cent of UK employees reported being more stressed than 12 months previously (YouGov 2012).
- One in four adults (Mind 2013) and one in ten children and young people, have been diagnosed with a mental illness in the past year. More than half of the adults with a diagnosed mental illness were diagnosed in childhood (YoungMinds 2015).

At the same time, additional research indicates that:

- Over the past decade, employees in the UK are working longer hours (Institute for Employment Studies 2015).

Conceptualizing play in healthcare provision **23**

- Families in the UK spend an average of just 49 minutes a day together (BBC News 2010).
- The average UK adult spends more time using digital communications technology (8 hours 41 minutes) than they do sleeping (8 hours 21 minutes) (Ofcom 2014).

It is not unreasonable to examine whether play – or the lack of it – might be a variable in the relationship between these research findings. Could it be that twenty-first-century adults are paying the price for longer working hours and the increased use of digital media with a resultant reduction in the time and motivation available for the pursuit of playfulness?

Bergen and Pronin Fromberg (2006) postulate that technological advances and an increase in leisure time might raise the status of play such that it is re-positioned in the adult domain. They suggest that,

> play will become so valued by adults, who will have the leisure, health and technological resources to engage in more play themselves, that the value of play for children will be more widely recognised ... Play will be taken over by adults [who] will require children to earn the right to play, after they have mastered some authoritatively determined body of knowledge.
>
> *(Bergen and Pronin Fromberg 2006: 418)*

The link between play and technology is discussed in Chapter 15.

It is perhaps more conceivable that our wealth-driven, achievement-driven, civilization denies a space to activities that lack the seriousness of clearly recognizable outcomes – with discernible consequences for the health of both individuals and of society in general. As the twenty-first century unfurls, our school children are more intensively tested that at any earlier time in history, resulting in a 200 per cent increase in children suffering exam stress (TES 2015) and 'playtime' or recess being reduced in many schools (Children's Play Information Service 2010). The widespread performance management of adult workers is matched by increased sickness absence (Taylor 2012) and record levels of the prescription of anti-depressive/anti-anxiety medication (Spence *et al.* 2014). Retirement is an ever more distant milestone for many as pension entitlements are pushed further and further into the future.

As the space for play and playfulness is squeezed-out of our children's lives, we are minded to re-visit the evidence for the lifelong consequences of a play-deprived start in life. Hughes (2003: 67) speculates, 'is it possible that because some children are deprived of play generally, or of specific types in particular, they are harmed in some way…?'

Hughes (2000) differentiates between *play deprivation* which is defined in terms of a lack of sensory interaction with the world or sensory deprivation, and *play bias* which is characterized by a loading of a certain type of sensory or playful

24 Alison Tonkin and Julia Whitaker

experience over another. The underlying assertion is that individuals need to experience play which includes a range of stimuli, both positive and negative, if it is to fulfil its adaptive and enriching potential. 'Growing up' tends to be associated with the leaving-behind of purely pleasure-driven recreation in favour of that which serves a discernible purpose (fitness, skill acquisition, social enhancement). The perceived risks of a playful pursuit of pleasure for its own sake are challenging to our concept of ourselves as responsible, superior beings capable of self-regulation and restraint.

Our increasingly risk-averse society (Gill 2007) means that many young adults of today have grown-up as the subjects of parental and societal fear and paranoia and have therefore never learnt to take risks, to experiment, to make mistakes, or to choose to deviate from expected and accepted behaviors. They have not known what it is to immerse themselves in 'deep play' (Geertz 1976) and thus lack the confidence to 'lose themselves' in playful pursuit.

Healthcare professionals who may themselves have been subject to a cautious approach to play are less likely to appreciate that play, including playful approaches to healing and rehabilitation (Ward-Wimmer 2003), need to include the full spectrum of sensory stimulation in order for the player to experience the freedom of unpredictable outcomes and the creative potential for change.

The *stimulation theory* of play evolved from Suomi and Harlow's (1976) now ethically questionable work with rhesus monkeys, which explored the effects of sensory, social and spatial deprivation on the animals' behavior. The results of their work, entitled *Monkeys without Play*, demonstrated that the absence of play is associated with social disturbance, social incompetence in adulthood, aggressively antisocial and self-harming behavior. This research, and parallel findings by Jane Goodall (1990) and others, imply a causal relationship between deprivation of what in humans might be defined as 'play' and the subsequent disintegration of the physical and psychological processes essential for meaningful survival.

Just as the importance and value of play has long been recognized for children, the deprivation of play experiences in childhood has long been identified as a predictive precursor to asocial and antisocial behavior in those affected by it (Frost and Jacobs 1995). Psychological profiles of some of the most notorious recent cases of violent aberration have highlighted the extreme lack and/or distortion of play experiences in the lives of those responsible (Jennings 1995; Josephs 1993).

Brown and Lomax (1969) examined the causal link between play and the psychological states of young murderers, leading Brown (2009: 26) to conclude that 'the absence of play in their childhood was as important as any other factor in predicting their crimes'.

Whilst it cannot be construed that those deprived of meaningful play in childhood will emerge as disturbed adults, research into the damaging effects of play deprivation invites reflection on the potential implications of a lack of play for both individuals and for the wider society. Statistics for the occurrence of mental ill-health, including suicide rates, may be used to emphasize this point. It is notable that in countries such as Japan, with a strong work ethic and where young people

Conceptualizing play in healthcare provision **25**

and adults experience a significant imbalance between the hours devoted to work and to leisure, suicides rates are among the highest in the world (Milosevic 2011).

Early work on brain development and the environment in the 1960s and 1970s offered an explanation for the observed impact of play deprivation and play bias. Studies by Bennett *et al.* (1964) and Rosenzweig (1971) demonstrated the impact of the sensory environment upon both the levels and distribution of neuro-chemicals in the brain and upon the brain's anatomical structure. Rosenzweig *et al.* (1972) proposed the concept of neural 'plasticity', that the size and activity of the brain and its neural pathways expand and contract dependent on its use. The implications for play theory are that individuals who are deprived of play, or whose experience of play is limited in its focus, may experience negative plasticity whereby their brain size is contracted and neurochemical activity is reduced. The current work of Zeedyk (2014) and colleagues at Dundee University has reinforced these early findings that the way in which our brains develop is inextricably linked to our lifelong connections with each other and with the social world.

Hughes (2003) cautions against any assumption that play deprivation is exclusively associated with social or economic deprivation; it is the stressful or limited nature of the opportunities for play that have more of an impact than any material factors. It may be that social or emotional isolation or deviation (including physical or emotional neglect, abuse or disability, or any form of severe trauma) may have a greater link to play deprivation or bias than material poverty or economic disadvantage (McEwen 1999).

In a comprehensive study of the play of Roma children, Brown (2012) demonstrated that even those growing-up in extreme material poverty could benefit from a rich and diverse play experience. The freedom of the Roma to explore and experiment, together with the extreme physical nature of their play, was evidenced in highly developed motor skills and strikingly creative imaginative skills. Studies such as these suggest that, whilst play reflects its host culture, it is not necessarily defined by its limitations. As Green (2005: 11) suggests:

> 'there is no culture without play: there are no periods in history from which play has been absent … this universal activity belongs to an innate attribute of the mind that takes different shapes, not only in various groups, but also for different individuals'.

Research on the benefits of play, taken together with evidence of the impact of play-deprived early years, make a strong and powerful case for play as essential not only to individual development but to the evolution of the species (Kets de Vries 2012).

Nevertheless, despite strong evidence for the effects of play deprivation and play bias, evidence also exists for the curative effect of play on those adversely affected by its lack. Harlow and Suomi (1971) found that the negative effects of sensory deprivation could be rapidly overcome by the re-introduction of normal play

26 Alison Tonkin and Julia Whitaker

opportunities. This early research has been reinforced time and again by examples of the effects of therapeutic play work with stimulus deprived groups (Perry and Szalavitz 2006; Webb and Brown 2003).

It is this remedial or therapeutic potential of play that has resulted in the emergence and growth of the play professions.

Playing for health and wellbeing

The notion that there is a job to be done in supporting, enabling and guiding children's play is manifest in the concept of *Playwork* (Skills Active 2013).

The idea that there is a role for adults in this respect pre-dates most of the research described above. Originally arising in the context of church-based voluntary work in the late Victorian period, early play provision served both to draw children and families towards the church and to model desirable domestic and leisure pursuits. In the late 1860s, the social housing reformer Octavia Hill showed what might be achieved through play by including a children's playground in a housing scheme for the first time and later by employing a supervisor to oversee children's play (Darley 1990). In 1898, Mary Ward precipitated the establishment of the Evening Play Centre Committee (EPC), the forerunner of contemporary playwork provision, with the opening of a centre for children in London's inner-city which made provision for play six days a week and during school holidays (Trevelyan 1920).

The influence of early play theory and evidence from the EPC, coupled with the impact of war on the need for formally supervised play and recreation, resulted in the responsibility for play provision being assumed by local authorities in the early part of the twentieth century. Adventure playgrounds where 'children's freedom to come and go as they please was seen as important' and where they were 'free to explore their capacity for doing things themselves' (Chilton 2003: 116) were the focus of playwork until the mid-1980s. The introduction of After-School Clubs, for political and economic purposes, changed the focus from freely chosen, intrinsically-motivated and personally-directed play towards closely-supervised and regulated play provision for the most part. Some might say that playwork has returned to its historical origins, with children's leisure being organized and delivered by well-meaning adults for their own purposes.

Whilst playwork was originally seen as a preventive and proactive measure designed to steer children away from deviant leisure-time pursuits and the dangers of the streets, there developed in parallel the idea that play could also be used therapeutically, as a 'cure' for those having experienced emotionally damaging relationships and experiences.

Play therapy

Play therapy derives from the creation of an intense relationship between therapist and client in which play – as opposed to talking – is used as the primary means of

Conceptualizing play in healthcare provision **27**

communication and problem resolution. The aim of play therapy is to bring-about the recovery of an appropriate level of social and emotional functioning in order that normal developmental progress may be resumed (O'Connor and Schaefer 1994). The role of the therapist in play therapy is to accept, understand and interpret the symbolic content of the child's play, free from the censorship of reality, acknowledging Freud's assertion that 'the opposite of play is not what is serious but what is real' (Freud 1908: 132).

Anna Freud (1946) developed her father's concept of play as an instrument of catharsis, whereby the negative feelings and behaviors associated with traumatic events (internal or external) could be 'played-out', using a variety of play media (sand, water, art, symbolic figures). The contributions of Freud, and later Melanie Klein (1963), reverberate in the work of those subsequently working with society's most damaged children including Virginia Axline (1976) whose widely-read case study, *'Dibs. In Search of Self'*, brought play therapy to the attention of the wider public. Axline described play as a naturalistic expressive form:

> play therapy is based on the fact that play is the child's natural medium of self-expression. It is an opportunity which is given to the child to 'play out' his feelings and problems just as, in certain types of adult therapy, an individual 'talks out' his difficulties.
>
> *(Axline 1987: 9)*

Although play therapy has long been recognized as an effective approach with children, there is a growing body of evidence that adults can also benefit from a play therapy approach. Research has demonstrated that play therapy techniques can be usefully incorporated into therapy for adult service-users including those with developmental disabilities, mental health disorders, and those who have experienced early emotional trauma (Schaefer 2003). These are user groups who might find it more difficult to access traditional *talking therapies* (Donaldson 1993) and therefore 'play continues as an important vehicle because it fosters numerous adaptive behaviors, including creativity, role reversal and mind/body integration' (Ward-Wimmer 2003).

Inner-child work is a contemporary branch of popular psychological therapy and often incorporates creative aspects including drama, art and play elements. It holds that psychological symptoms in adulthood can be addressed with reference to the experiences, and learnt behaviors of childhood (Schaefer 2003).

A feature of most (although not all) play therapy is that it is non-directive and that, like pure play, its focus is determined by the healthcare-user rather than the health-giver — albeit within carefully defined boundaries.

'Play is a process that enables change' (Rennie 2003: 31) but change is rarely straightforward; it may have unexpected and far-reaching consequences that do not necessarily sit comfortably with all those within the sphere of its influence.

Conclusion

Linking the provision of play in adult healthcare into varying theoretical frameworks, enables the modelling of integrated systems that demonstrate how play can contribute to the healing process, as well as being a means of prevention and protection from the stresses and strains associated with modern life. However, Ward-Wimmer (2003: 10) reminds us, through the adaptation of a quote from Jung to:

> Learn your theories as best you can, but lay them aside when you touch the miracle of the human soul. Lay them aside and play!

References

Allen, S. and Gordon, P. (2011) *How Children Learn 4: Thinking on Special Educational Needs and Inclusion,* Bournemouth: Practical Pre-School Books.

Axline, V. (1976) *Dibs. In Search of Self,* Harmondsworth: Penguin.

Axline, V. (1987) *Play Therapy,* New York: Ballantine.

Bandura, A. (1986) *Social Foundations of Thought and Action: A Social Cognitive Theory,* Upper Saddle River, NJ: Prentice-Hall.

Barrett, R. (2010) *From Maslow to Barrett,* Online. Available at www.valuescentre.com/uploads/2010-07-06/From%20Maslow%20to%20Barrett.pdf (accessed 25 May 2015).

Barrett, R. (2013) *Seven Levels of Consciousness: Personal, Organisational, Community/society,* Online. Available at www.valuescentre.com/uploads/2013-03-19/Barrett 7 Levels of Consciousness – personal organisation society 2013 v3.pdf (accessed 25 May 2015).

Barton, H. and Grant, M. (2006) A health map for the local human habitat, *The Journal of the Royal Society for the Promotion of Health,* 126 (6): 252–253.

BBC News (2010) *Parents Spend '49 Minutes' a Day with Their Children,* Online. Available at http://news.bbc.co.uk/1/hi/education/8703010.stm (accessed 26 May 2105).

Bennett, E.L, Diamond, M.C., Krech, D. and Rosenzweig, M.R. (1964) Chemical and anatomical plasticity of brain, *Science,* 146 (3644): 610–619.

Bergen, D. and Pronin Fromberg, D. (2006) Epilogue: emerging and future contexts, perspectives and meanings for play, in Pronin Fromberg, D. and Bergen, D (eds), *Play from Birth to Twelve: Contexts, Perspectives and Meanings,* 2nd ed., New York: Routledge.

Boyd, D. and Bee, H. (2012) *The Developing Child,* 13th ed., Harlow: Pearson.

Bronfenbrenner, U. (1994) Ecological models of human development, in Gauvain, M. and Cole, M. (eds) *Readings on the Development of Children,* 2nd ed., New York: Freeman: 37–43.

Brown, F. (2012) The play behaviours of Roma children in Transylvania, *International Journal of Play,* 1 (1): 64–74. 1..

Brown, S. (2009) *Play, How it Shapes the Brain, Opens The Imagination and Invigorates the Soul,* London: Penguin.

Brown, S. and Lomax, J. (1969) *A Pilot Study of Young Murderers,* Hogg Foundation Annual Report: Austin, Texas.

Children's Play Information Service (2010) *Factsheet No.15: The Benefits of School Play time,* London: NCB.

Chilton, T. (2003) Adventure playgrounds in the 21st century, in Brown, F. (ed.) *Playwork – Theory and Practice,* Buckingham: Open University Press: 114–127.

Cohen, S. and Janicki-Deverts, D. (2012) Who's stressed? Distribution of psychological stress in the United States in probability samples from 1983, 2006, 2009, *Journal of Applied Social Psychology*, 42 (6): 1320–1334.

Darley, G. (1990) *Octavia Hill*, London: Constable.

Donaldson, F. (1993). *Playing by Heart,* Florida: Health Communications.

Ewles, L. and Simnett, I. (2003) *Promoting Health: A Practical Guide*, 5th ed. The Netherlands: Baillière Tindall.

Freeman, C. (2012) Public health: Who cares? *Synergy News*, December 2012.

Freud, A. (1946) *The Psychoanalytical Treatment of Children*, London: Imago.

Freud, S. (1908) *Creative Writers and Day-Dreaming. The Standard Edition of the Complete Psychological Works of Sigmund Freud,* vol. IX (1906–1908): Jensen's 'Gradiva' and Other Works. London: Hogarth Press141–154.

Frost, J.L. and Jacobs, J. (1995) Play deprivation: a factor in juvenile violence, *Dimensions*, 3 (3): 6–9.

Geertz, C. (1972) *Deep Play: Notes on the Balinese Cockfight*. Louisville, KY: Contre Coup Press.

Geertz, C. (1976) Deep play: a description of the Balinese cockfight. In Bruner, J.S., Jolly, A. and Sylva, K. (eds) *Play: It's Role in Development and Evolution*. New York: Viking Penguin: 656–676.

Gill, T. (2007) *No Fear: Growing Up in a Risk Averse Society,* London: Gulbenkian Foundation.

Goodall, J. (1990) *Through a Window: 30 Years Observing the Gombe Chimpanzees,* London: Weidenfield and Nicolson.

Green, A. (2005) *Play and Reflection in Donald Winnicott's Writings*, London: Karnac.

Gryzwacz, J. and Fuqua, J. (2000) The social ecology of health: leverage points and linkages, *Behavioural Medicine,* 26 (3): 101–116.

Härkönen, U. (2007) The Bronfenbrenner ecological systems theory of human development, Scientific Articles of V International Conference: Person, Colour, Nature, Music. October 17–21, 2007. Saule: Daugavpils University.

Harlow, H.F. and Suomi, S.J. (1971). Social recovery by isolation-reared monkeys, *Proceedings of the National Academy of Science of the United States of America,* 68 (7): 1534–1538.

Hearts and Minds (2015) *The Elderflowers Programme*, Online. Available at www.heartsminds. org.uk/the-elderflowers/ (accessed 27 May 2015).

Henricks, T. (2008) The Nature of Play: An overview, *The American Journal of Play*, 1 (2): 157–180.

Hughes, B (2000) A dark and evil cul-de-sac: has children's play in Belfast been adulterated by the troubles? Unpublished MA dissertation, Anglia Polytechnic University.

Hughes, B. (2003) *Play Deprivation: Play Bias and Playwork Practice*, in F. Brown (ed.) *Playwork – Theory and Practice*, Open University Press: Buckingham.

Institute for Employment Studies (2015) *Report summary: Working Long Hours: a Review of the Evidence, Volume 1 – Main Report,* Online. Available at www.employment-studies.co.uk/report-summary-working-long-hours-review-evidence-volume-1-%E2%80%93-main-report (accessed 26 May 2015).

Jennings, S. (1995) Playing for real, *International Play Journal*, 3 (2): 132–141.

Josephs, J. (1993) *Hungerford: One Man's Massacre*, London: Smyth Gryphon Publishers.

Kets de Vries, M. (2012) *Going Back to the Sandbox: Teaching CEOs How to Play*, Fontainebleau: INSEAD.

Klein, M. (1963) *The Psychoanalysis of Children*, Hogarth: London.

Lewin, K. (1939) Field theory and experiment in social psychology: concepts and methods, *American Journal of Sociology*, 44 (6): 868–896.

30 Alison Tonkin and Julia Whitaker

Local Government Association (2010) *Understanding and Tackling the Wider Social Determinants of Health,* Online. Available at www.local.gov.uk/health/-/journal_content/56/10180/3511260/ARTICLE (accessed 15 May 2015).

McEwen, B.S. (1999) Stress and hippocampal plasticity. *Annual Review of the Neurosciences*, 22: 105–122.

Maslow, A. (1943) A theory of human motivation, *Psychological Review,* 50 (4): 370–396.

Milosevic, T. (2011) *Japan: The Psychology Behind Dignity*, Online. Available at www.huffingtonpost.com/tijana-milosevic/japan-psychology-behind-dignity_b_840901.html (accessed 30 May 2015).

Mind (2013) *Mental Health Facts and Statistics,* Online. Available at www.mind.org.uk/information-support/types-of-mental-health-problems/statistics-and-facts-about-mental-health/how-common-are-mental-health-problems/ (accessed 26 May 2015).

Newcombe, T. (2013) Exclusive: UK Has Some of the Worst Employee Wellbeing Scores in the World, *HR Magazine*, 12 February 2013. Online. Available at www.hrmagazine.co.uk (accessed 26 May 2015).

NHS Education for Scotland (n.d.) *Introducing the Wider Determinants of Health.* Online. Available at www.bridgingthega:scot.nhs.uk/understanding-health-inequalities/introducing-the-wider-determinants-of-health.aspx (accessed 17 May 2015).

O'Connor, C. and Schaefer, C. (1994) *Handbook of Play Therapyvol. 2: Advances and Innovations,* New York: John Wiley & Sons, Inc.

O'Donoghue, K. and Maidment, J. (2005) The ecological system metaphor in Australasia, in Nash, M., Munford, R. and O'Donoghue, K. (eds), *Social Work Theories in Action.* London: Jessica Kingsley Publishers: 32–49.

Ofcom (2014) *The Communications Market Report: United Kingdom*, Online. Available at http://stakeholders.ofcom.org.uk/market-data-research/market-data/communications-market-reports/cmr14/uk/ (accessed 26 May 2015).

Oxford Dictionaries (2015a) *Conceptualization,* Online. Available at www.oxforddictionaries.com/definition/english/conceptualization?q=conceptualisation (accessed 27 May 2015).

Oxford Dictionaries (2015b) *Model,* Online. Available at www.oxforddictionaries.com/definition/english/model (accessed 27 May 2015).

Payne, S. (2002) Foreign nurses learn to banter with the English, *Daily Telegraph*, 14 January 2002. Online. Available at www.telegraph.co.uk/news/uknews/1381399/Foreign-nurses-learn-to-banter-with-the-English.html (accessed 24 May 2015).

Perry, B.D. and Szalavitz, M. (2006) *The Boy Who Was Raised as a Dog,* New York; Basic Books.

Relate (2105) *The Best Medicine,* Online. Available at www.relate.org.uk/policy-campaigns/our-campaigns/best-medicine (accessed 24 May 2015).

Rennie, S. (2003) Making play work: the fundamental role of play in the development of social relationship skills, in Brown, F. (ed.) *Playwork – Theory and Practice*, Buckingham: Open University Press: 18–31.

Rosenzweig, M.R. (1971) Effects of environment on development of brain and behaviour, in Tobach, E. (ed.) *Biopsychology of Development*, New York: Academic: 303–342.

Rosenzweig, M.R., Bennet, E.L. and Diamond, M.C. (1972) Brain changes in response to experience, *Scientific American*, 226 (2): 22–29.

Schaefer, C. (2003) *Play Therapy with Adults,* New York: John Wiley & Sons, Inc.

Spence, R., Roberts, A., Ariti, C. and Bardsley, M. (2014) *Focus On: Antidepressant Prescribing Trends in the Prescribing of Antidepressants in Primary Care*, London: Nuffield Trust and Health Foundation.

St Clair, M. (2005) *The Top Ten Benefits of Play,* Online. Available at www.creativity-portal.com/bc/other/play.html (accessed 29 September 2014).

Skills Active (2013) *The Pocket Guide to Playwork*, Online. Available at www.outdoorplayan-dlearning.org.uk/uploads/2/8/9/1/2891140/pocket_guide_to_play_work.pdf (accessed 29 May 2015).

Suomi, S.J. and Harlow, H.F. (1976) Monkeys without play, in Bruner, J.S., Jolly, A. and Sylva, K. (eds) *Play: Its Role in Development and Evolution*, New York: Basic Books.

Taylor, P. (2012) *Performance Management and the New Workplace Tyranny. Report for the Scottish Trades Union Congress*, Online. Available at www.stuc.org.uk/files/Document%20 download/Workplace%20tyranny/STUC%20Performance%20Management%20Final% 20Edit.pdf (accessed 27 May 2015).

TES (2015) 200 per cent increase in children suffering exam stress, *TES magazine*, 14 May 2015. Online. Available at www.tes.co.uk/ (accessed 26 May 2015).

Trevelyan, J.P. (1920) *Evening Play Centres for Children: The Story of their Origin and Growth*, London: Methuen.

Trudge, J., Mokrova, I., Hatfield, B. and Karnk, R. (2009) Uses and misuses of Bronfen-brenner's Bioecological Theory of Human Development, *Journal of Family Theory and Review*, 1: 198–210.

Ward-Wimmer, D. (2003). Introduction: the healing potential of adults play, in Schaefer, C.E. (ed.) *Play Therapy with Adults*. Hoboken, NJ: John Wiley & Sons, Inc.: 1–13.

Webb, S. and Brown, F. (2003) Playwork in adversity: working with abandoned children. in, Brown, F. (ed.) (2003) *Playwork: Theory and Practice*, Buckingham: Open University Press: 157–175.

Winnicott, D. (1971) *Playing and Reality*, London: Tavistock.

YouGov (2012) *Workers 'More Stressed' Now*, Online. Available at www.yougov.co.uk/news/ 2012/02/16/workers-more-stressed-now/ (accessed 26 May 2015).

YoungMinds (2015) *Mental Health Statistics*, Online. Available at www.youngminds.org.uk/ training_services/policy/mental_health_statistics (accessed 26 May 2015).

Zeedyk, S. (2014) *The Science of Human Connection*, Online. Available at www.suzanne zeedyk.com (accessed 1 November 2015).

3

LIFESPAN DEVELOPMENT

Julia Whitaker and Alison Tonkin

The development of play during the course of the lifespan changes over time and in relation to cultural and societal trends. Contemporary thinking is influenced by historical, generational and international perspectives and these will be explored in relation to the potential contribution of play as a feature of healthcare provision. As Moya (2014) suggests:

> 'The desire for playful activities is universal, and in the human species it transcends age'.

Introduction

Lifespan development theory centers on human development, exploring the patterns of growth and change that occur as people mature over the course of their lives (Feldman 2011). The concept of lifespan development is not a new one, with roots firmly established in the eighteenth and nineteenth centuries (Hoyer 2002). This short introduction to lifespan development theory presents a selective overview of some of the key themes linking play and lifespan development. For a more robust and detailed coverage of this topic, there are a number of excellent resources which cover the subject in greater detail, such as the ten volumes of research edited by Baltes covering 'lifespan development and behaviour' (Stassen Berger 2011).

Nowadays, lifespan development is considered to be a 'meta theory' due to the number of differing themes and approaches that contribute to the study of development (Hoyer 2002) with fields such as anthropology, sociology, genetics, neuroscience and psychology all contributing to our biological understanding of human life (Stassen Berger 2011). The developmental pathway generally follows a

Lifespan development **33**

predictable pattern for all members of the human species, despite life-altering experiences and events that can affect the health and wellbeing of people as they grow older (Feldman 2011). These experiences may include opposing influences, such as relative wealth or deprivation; experiences of harmonious living or war; and societal issues that impact on the family unit and their associated communities. However, all development is inextricably linked to the process of aging (Hoyer 2002) and the way lifespan development and aging are portrayed will be dependent on who is defining it and the purpose behind the definition (Heckhausen and Wrosch 2010).

Categorising lifespan development

All developmentalists identify development as a continuing process that occurs over the entire course of the lifespan (Feldman 2011). However, there are fundamental differences in the way lifespan development is explored and defined.

Age as a categorising framework

Chronological age is almost universally used as a defining characteristic that 'anchors accounts of change over the lifespan' (Sugarman 2001: 7). There are significant differences between individuals in terms of the timings associated with these events (Feldman 2011) and presenting development within distinct age ranges is considered to be conceptually more useful as an 'indicator of developmental status' (Singleman and Rider 2015: 5).

Emerging adulthood is a new developmental stage, reflecting the fact that, increasingly, adolescents have been taking longer to become adults (Singelman and Rider 2015). Indicative of this is the extension of support offered to young people who have a Special Educational Need or Disability (SEND) who can now continue to access help and support through integrated health and care packages

TABLE 3.1 An overview of periods of the lifespan (adapted from Singleman and Rider 2015)

Period of life	Age range
Pre-natal	Conception to birth
Infancy	First two years of life
Pre-school period	Two to five (or six) years of age
Middle childhood	Six to about ten years (or the onset of puberty)
Adolescence	Approximately ten to 18 years (puberty to relative independence)
Emerging adulthood	18 to 25 years or even later (transitional period)
Early adulthood	25 to 40 years (adult roles are established)
Middle adulthood	40 to 65 years
Late adulthood	65 years and older

up to the age of 25 years. This follows legislative changes through the Children and Families Act 2014 in England (Department for Education and the Department of Health 2015). The introduction of an integrated approach extending beyond the traditional age of transition at 18 years demonstrates the relative contribution of different disciplines which dictates the necessity for 'framing' the changes that occur as we grow and mature, enabling the application of what is discovered.

Classically, the development of children is categorized in terms of their physical, cognitive, linguistic, emotional and social development (Boyd and Bee 2012). However, it is noted that development is a holistic process, and change in one area will usually impact on the process of development in other areas (Singleman and Rider 2015). In the study of adulthood, emphasis is also placed on the role of *personality*, which is linked to social development (Feldman 2011). The study of personality development explores the enduring characteristics that make us unique as individuals and provides a useful example of one of the most contentious issues when discussing development across the lifespan – the relative importance of innate characteristics (nature) that people are born with, compared to the influence of an individual's interaction with the environment (nurture).

The nature/nurture debate

Laberge (2006) states that our personality derives from ongoing interactions between temperament, the environment and character. Temperament is determined by a set of genetically determined traits, which appear to be particularly important for self-control, social skills, the ability to learn and an individual's sense of purpose (Collins 2012). This is suggestive of the significance of *nature* as a defining feature of personality. However, interaction with the environment also influences how we think and what we feel, which affects our behavior through the process of reciprocal determinism (Bandura 1986). This leads to adaptive patterns of development (Laberge 2006). As people grow and mature, environmental factors change as the individual's circumstances and responsibilities change. Adaptation allows us to retain the enduring characteristics that define us as individuals, providing compelling evidence that *nurture* is a significant factor in personal development. Character evolves throughout life and relies on innate traits as well as early experiences (Laberge 2006). This suggests that both nature *and* nurture have significant contributions to make (Singleman and Rider 2015), through a synergistic effect which optimizes the developmental process (Hoyer 2002). This is demonstrated by research into epigenetics, which focuses on mechanisms that act as switches for genetic regulation, many of which originate within the environment and are known to contribute to differentiation in the aging process (Kanherkar *et al.* 2014).

What is known is that stability of temperament, character and the environment throughout life, as change occurs, is a key issue for the developmental process (Feldman 2011). Sugarman (2001: 2) notes that 'the life course is characterized by continuity' with behaviors and temperaments from the past being useful predictors for the future. For example, a playful disposition as a child is likely to be carried through and utilized as an adult, provided that the satisfaction of pre-potency needs allows this disposition to be expressed (Maslow 1943). This suggests that the regulation of motivation is a key determinant of adaptation through the lifespan, in response to opportunities that present themselves, demonstrating humans to be active agents of change (Heckhausen and Wrosch 2010).

Theoretical considerations linked to lifespan development

Comparative theories enable us to look at things from differing perspectives and, in the case of developmental theories, these can provide statements outlining general principles (Boyd and Bee 2011) which can be applied across the lifespan. Feldman (2011) offers six major theoretical perspectives that are applicable to the study of lifespan development and these are summarized in Table 3.2.

TABLE 3.2 Major perspectives on lifespan development (adapted from Feldman 2011)

Perspective	Description and associated theorists
Psychodynamic	*Freud* (1856–1939) focused on the individual, suggesting inner forces motivate many aspects of behavior. These include memories and conflicts, which the person may not be aware of or able to control. These *unconscious* aspects of personality continue to influence behavior throughout the lifespan. In contrast, *Erikson* (1902–1994) emphasized the role of social interaction with other people, noting that humans are shaped by the challenges they face from both culture and society. Erikson proposed that development occurs throughout the lifespan, through a psychosocial eight-stage framework.
Behavioral	Rejecting the notion of a staged theory of development, behaviorism holds that observable behavior is linked to external stimuli in the environment. According to behaviorists, if you know the stimuli, you can predict the behavior. *Watson* (1878–1958) believed that virtually any behavior could be produced if you were able to control the person's environment, suggesting that the concept of classical conditioning can be used to explain how we learn emotional responses. *Skinner* (1904–1990) advocated the concept of operant conditioning as responsible for modifying behavior. Voluntary responses, when associated with positive or negative consequences, can strengthen or weaken the tendency to repeat behavior through a process of reinforcement or punishment. *Bandura's* (1925–) social-cognitive learning theory stated that behavior is learned through observation and modelling. In order to repeat behavior that is modelled, the observed must be motivated to learn and imitate that behavior. This requires mental activity whereas classical and operant conditioning rely solely on responses to external stimuli.

36 Julia Whitaker and Alison Tonkin

Table 3.2 Continued.

Perspective	Description and associated theorists
Cognitive	*Piaget* (1896–1980) proposed a four stage developmental, discontinuous model of development whereby each stage was self-contained and a person could not move onto the next stage without completing the previous one. However, recent research suggests that development is a continuous process and the age at which differing cognitive skills occur varies across differing cultures. Throughout the lifespan, schema formation through the process of assimilation and accommodation enables 'representational change over time' enabling understanding of new experiences and changes in thinking.
Humanistic	Humanists believe that decisions are made as a result of free will, and that humans have a natural capacity for decision making. As people mature, they are motivated to behave in a way that enables them to reach their full potential. *Maslow* (1908–1970) proposed that behavior is motivated by the fulfilment of pre-potent needs which rely on the satisfaction of basic needs, before the individual can reach the primary goal in life – self–actualization. *Rogers* (1902–1987) believed humans have a need for 'positive regard', which can be achieved by being loved and respected by other people.
Contextual	People's development cannot be seen in isolation from the social and cultural context within which they operate. *Bronfenbrenner* (1917–2005) identified the interconnectedness of development and introduced a bioecological approach to our understanding of development. Five levels of environmental factors operate simultaneously to influence development of the individual. As individuals mature, the significance of the differing levels alter – a notion that allows for the flexibility to map this model to lifespan development. *Vygotsky* (1896–1934) also advocated the influence of society and culture as key determinants of development, noting that individuals do not develop within a cultural vacuum. However, critics suggest that biological makeup and the role of the individual in decision-making cannot be ignored.
Evolutionary	Genetic inheritance influences behavior, through the expression of traits, which include personality and social behavior. *Darwin* (1809–1882) suggested that individuals adapt to their environment through the creation of traits that contribute to the process of natural selection, resulting in an increase in survival rates. *Lorenz* (1903–1989) was a proponent of ethology whereby behavior is understood to be influenced by our biological makeup. Recently, this has resulted in the field of behavioral genetics.

If nothing else, Table 3:2 demonstrates the very broad and contentious nature of lifespan development theory. Developmental theorists note that there are no right or wrong theories when comparing and contrasting perspectives relating to human development, the usefulness of any particular approach being dependent on the context under examination (Boyd and Bee 2011).

Play as culture

All human development unfolds within a given cultural context, which both affects and is affected by that development, in a constant state of evolutionary flux. A culture-inclusive view of lifespan development is now recognized as essential to an understanding of the processes that shape both individual and group identities, including our attitudes, values and behavior as they relate to health and wellbeing.

The perception and practice of play throughout the lifespan both reflect and are reflected in its cultural context. It may be said that play is culture for it is the window to the biological, historical and social evolution of the group. According to Huizinga (1949: 1), 'play is older than culture, and all culture is a form of play'.

The developmental process of play

Early anthropological studies, such as those of Margaret Mead (1928) and Ruth Benedict (1934), shared the assumption that the relationship between cultural context and developmental outcome is one-directional: that culture influences behavior. Less attention was given to how individual differences, in the form of the varying needs, abilities, and interests of individuals (including health differentials) affect the way in which they might engage with, or respond to, cultural mores and values.

Our understanding of how attitudes to play and play practices are related to other aspects of development across the lifespan are more helpfully informed by the concept of the 'developmental niche' (Super and Harkness 1997) which recognizes development as comprising three integrated elements: physical and social environment; customs and child-rearing practices; and caretaker psychology (parental belief systems).

Cross-generational change and the perception of play

This three-dimensional model of the evolution of play perceptions is evidenced in Holmes' (2011) study of adult attitudes towards play on the Hawaiian island of Lana'I, in which Holmes considers the impact of a changing economic environment on lifestyle practices and beliefs and how changes in lifestyle have altered play behavior across the generations. When the island economy was based on long hours of physical labour on fruit plantations, play was seen as the antithesis of work, reserved for occupying children in the company of their peers whilst the adults were at work or resting. Parents' playful interactions with their children were limited to the weekends and tended to comprise the sharing of skills such as fishing or sports. In contrast, contemporary parents, mostly employed in service industries related to the tourist trade, rate play with their children highly, as beneficial to both development and health (Holmes 2011). Over the course of a generation, play has become a highly valued, shared experience, which reflects other aspects of cultural change

38 Julia Whitaker and Alison Tonkin

Another example of how perceptions of play metamorphose through time and place, in symbiosis with socio-cultural change, concerns the shifting status of the Brazilian 'game' of *capoeira* – an acrobatic form of martial art, which incorporates elements of both competition and musical composition (Lewis 1992). A seminal study by Lewis (1992) describes capoeira as both a dramatic representation of combat, in the style of Geertz (1973) 'deep play', and a liberating framework for managing social encounters. Originally identified with the lowest economic strata of Afro-Brazilian society, the practice of capoeira was outlawed at the end of the nineteenth century but subsequently found legitimacy in its increasing appeal to the urban middle and upper classes, becoming recognized as a national sport in 1972. Today, capoeira is practiced around the globe, with people of all ages, backgrounds and cultures attracted by its unique blend of the social, the artistic and the physical (Prytherch and Kraft 2015).

Many people are also attracted by capoeira's philosophical origins and communal spirit; unlike other martial arts, capoeira has no winners or losers. The 'playing' of capoeira is not about beating or getting beaten but about expressing playfulness and collaboration, endowing it with the quality of health-giving play for all generations (Prytherch and Kraft 2015).

Projects such as Bidna Capoeira (2011) in the Middle East, and Capoeira for Peace in the Congo (Mosikikongo 2015), are applying the communal benefits of this play-form to re-build communities decimated by conflict and displacement. In an inversion of the common assumption that play is a practice belonging primarily to childhood, capoeira has been transplanted from its adult origins in the Brazilian ghettos to become a seedbed of physical and emotional re-growth for young people whose lives have been affected by the trauma of war.

There is some irony that in Europe and the US, capoeira has become a popular health pursuit among a wholly different cohort of young people, as part of the collective drive to increase activity levels and reduce obesity among the young (de Novães 2006).

The play-element or disposition

Huizinga (1949) makes the significant distinction between the 'play-element' or a disposition for play, and 'play' as a separate activity or set of activities. It is this disposition for play as integral to health and wellbeing, which is evidenced in both the examples above. The play-element is characterized by the improvisation and innovation that derives from an open outcome; play is undertaken freely and in the absence of a pre-determined goal, in contrast to the functional drive of parallel experiences such as work, education or ritual.

Gadamer's (1975) discourse represents an analogous exploration of 'play as object', existing in space and time and belonging primarily to childhood, and 'play as subject', a dynamic movement back-and-forth, an experiment with randomness. Gadamer (1975: 93) speaks of play as a 'to-and-fro movement which is not tied to any goal which would bring it to an end'.

When play is regarded as disposition or 'subject', rather than as a specific form or type of activity or 'object', it can be embraced as a unifying medium for the development of wellbeing, regardless of cultural difference. To be open to the possibility of growth and change, without directly seeking it, empowers the player as an agent of that change, regardless of intent.

The role of play throughout the lifespan might best be understood in the acceptance of the philosophical notion that it is not so much the nature of the activity itself, but the playful quality of the concept, that takes play from childhood into the adult world.

> The contention here is that playing may be seen as such a movement away from order, stability and predictability. It is the process of being a child, becoming different and open to what it not yet is.
>
> *(Ryall* et al. *2013: 136)*

Three lifespan approaches

There follows an exposition of three contrasting cultural approaches to lifespan development which are reflected in the way that play is seen as integral to the health of the individual and of the community.

Rudolf Steiner's anthroposophical theory of human growth is one of many that describes development in terms of seven-year cycles of interrelated biological, psychological and spiritual features (Armstrong 2008; Lievegoed 1979). For Steiner, there is no externally defined state of optimum wellbeing but a recognition and respect for the uniqueness of the individual within his or her own developmental context.

> We should not ask 'What does a person need to be able to do in order to fit into the existing social order today?' Instead we should ask 'what lives in each human being and what can be developed in him or her?'
>
> *(Steiner, cited Alsop and Skonieczny 2001)*

Anthroposophy (literally, 'human wisdom') is an educational, therapeutic and creative system of thought which seeks to optimize physical and psychological health and wellbeing (Lievegoed 1979). Play, in all its various forms, is valued as inherent in the natural human disposition for self-discovery and personal fulfilment. This approach holds that each stage of childhood development has its parallel in adulthood, and that an interruption to the natural course of development will have consequences both for the individual and for society (Harwood 1958). For example, the fantasy world of the young child is thought to lay the foundations for creativity in the social and working life of the adult years. The child who is denied the freedom to immerse him- or herself in the world of the imagination (through poverty of opportunity, early intellectualization or exposure to worldly concerns, for example) will lack spontaneity and versatility in later life. The adult who has not known in childhood the personal release and pleasure which can be derived from play, may be helped to assimilate early disequilibrium through social and artistic therapies (Harwood 1958). In anthroposophy, the play-element is manifest in an appreciation of the aesthetic – through art, architectural design, music and the movement form eurhythmy. Eurhythmy, sometimes known as 'visible music' or 'visible speech', is a form of artistic expression which unites sound and movement with the associated feeling experiences and is purported to have a positive effect on health-related life functions. It is through the extension (or re-visiting) of the imaginative, creative, spirited play of early childhood that the individual can achieve the realization of the self in adulthood (Harwood 1958).

> More than anything else, art heals our senses and keeps them healthy.
>
> *(Salter 2015)*

The 'Art of Health' program at Taruna College, a Steiner-based adult education centre in New Zealand, explores the use of imaginative and creative processes in the understanding and treatment of illness and health. Exploring the meaning of color through the use of various artistic media, students experience an alternative holistic perspective to the traditional physiological construct of what constitutes 'positive health'.

A parallel construct which emphasizes the inter-relationship between individual characteristics, life-stage and routes to wellbeing, belongs to the Ayurvedic tradition. Ayurveda is a holistic philosophy conceived to maintain a state of positive health whilst realizing the full human potential and proffers guidelines on optimal daily and seasonal routines, nutrition, behavior and the precise use of the senses – acknowledging that health comprises the balanced and dynamic integration of environment, body, mind, and spirit (Aarogya 2015). Ayurveda recognizes that the playful disposition is present throughout the lifespan, although its expression will be influenced by individual and developmental factors.

The practice of yoga, espoused by the Ayurvedic tradition as a health-enriching pursuit, is not traditionally outcome-driven and incorporates many playful elements. Proponents of yoga traditionally see the practice as being intrinsically beneficial, leading to improved physical health, emotional wellbeing and joy in living. Yoga's organic and inverted poses and breathing exercises are reminiscent of the symbolic play of childhood whilst encompassing the energetic release of the playground with its accompanying feelings of freedom and exhilaration. The practice of yoga invites an openness to liberation from worldly concerns as well as a sense of physical release and, as in the case of capoeira referred to earlier, is a system which has evolved from its historical origins to become a custom widely practiced by old and young alike, with varying motivations (Aarogya 2015).

The play-element is an explicit feature of the curriculum of the International University of Laughter Yoga in Bangalore (Laughter Yoga n.d.). The core philosophy of laughter yoga is to cultivate joyfulness. The concept of 'joyfulness' is juxtaposed with 'happiness' which is described as a concept of the mind dependent on external variables, rather than internally driven. Advocates of laughter yoga propose that joyfulness can be triggered by simple physical activities like singing, dancing, laughing and playing, resulting in a release of mood-changing neuro-chemicals. By circumventing the intellectual processes that typically inhibit natural expressions of emotion in adulthood, laughter yoga generates feelings of 'childlike playfulness' which encourage the imaginative and creative response. Various academic studies have demonstrated the health benefits of laughter, including benefits to cardiovascular health (Dolgoff-Kaspar *et al.* 2012) and mood (Shahidi *et al.* 2011). Michael Miller, director of the Center for Preventive Cardiology at the University of Maryland Medical Center says:

> We know that exercising, not smoking and eating foods low in saturated fat will reduce the risk of heart disease. Perhaps regular, hearty laughter should be added to the list.
>
> *(Miller cited in Murray 2009)*

It is the characteristics of childhood play (imagination, creativity, energetic release, joyfulness) that re-emerge in these playful approaches to positive adult health and wellbeing – albeit enrobed in the conceptual frameworks of maturity.

Some of the earliest descriptions of the phases of human development may be found in the proverbs of ancient China and, for the Chinese, play has always featured unapologetically in day-to-day life.

> It is better to play than do nothing.
>
> *(Confucius, 551BC–479BC)*

In modern China, the playful disposition is evident throughout the lifespan with different generations sharing various playful pursuits, many of which are firmly rooted in the country's cultural history of productive activity. The inhabitants of the grasslands of Mongolia and Tibet, and of the Kazak region, enjoy pastimes that utilize their traditional skills in horsemanship, whilst those from communities which rely on agriculture and hunting for their existence, enjoy activities that involve hunting, wrestling and climbing. Singing, dancing and musical performance are popular features of the many traditional festivals, such as the intricate Bamboo Pole Dance of the Li people. Chapter 19 examines the playful features of festivals and celebrations. Skipping rope games are widely practised by both children and adults as a playful way of keeping fit and maintaining intergenerational harmony. Stilt-walking (gaoqiao) in the Hunan province, which derives from earlier times when people had to find a way of keeping their feet dry during the rainy season, is now a commonly practiced sport celebrating speed and balance (Travel China Guide 2015).

In contrast, the entrepreneurial ethic of members of the business community is echoed in the playing of the game *mahjong* among Chinese elders, affording opportunities for them to utilize' the skills acquired during a lifetime of market trading whilst re-experiencing the exhilarating, strategic play involved with gambling on uncertainties (Oxfeld 1993; Festa 2006).

Once again, play in China embodies both its origins in the culture of people and place as well as its power to reflect wider societal change. Play can be a way to connect with past generations and past versions of the self as well as being a path to present and future fulfilment. As Bergson (1911: 7) suggests, 'To exist is to change, to change is to mature, to mature is to go-on creating oneself endlessly'

Conclusion

In the cross-cultural context, a lifespan approach offers a framework within which to explore culture-specific approaches to play as it relates to concepts of positive health and wellbeing. Play may serve various functions at personal, social and historical levels but it is its voluntary nature, and the fact that it represents an acceptance of the randomness of future outcomes, that unites cultures and generations in the pursuit of meaning and fulfilment.

References

Aarogya (2015) *Ayurveda*, Online. Available at www.aarogya.com/complementary-medicine/ayurveda.html (accessed 6 December 2015).

Alsop, M. and Skonieczny, K. (eds) (2001) *Learning to Learn: Waldorf Alumni Reflections.* Fair Oaks, CA: AWSNA Pubs.

Armstrong, T. (2008) *The Human Odyssey: Navigating the Twelve Stages of Life,* New York: Sterling Publishing.

Benedict, R. (1934) *Patterns of Culture,* New York: Houghton Mifflin.

Bergson, H. (1911) *Creative Evolution,* New York: Henry Holt and Co.

Bandura, A. (1986) *Social Foundations of Thought and Action: A Social Cognitive Theory,* Upper Saddle River, NJ: Prentice-Hall.

Bidna Capoeira (2011) *Bidna Capoeira,* Online. Available at http://assets.sportanddev.org/downloads/bidna_capoeira_overview.pdf (accessed 1 November 2015).

Boyd, D. and Bee, H. (2011) *Lifespan Development,* 6th ed., Harlow: Pearson.

Boyd, D. and Bee, H. (2012) *The Developing Child,* 13th ed., Harlow: Pearson.

Collins, N. (2012) It's nature, not nurture: personality lies in genes, twins study shows, *Daily Telegraph,* 16 May 2012.

de Novães, J.J. (2006) Social support as mental health and obesity prevention: interventions through school settings play activities, *Arqivos Neuro-Psiquiatria,* 64 (2b).

Department for Education and Department of Health (2015) *Special Educational Needs and Disability Code of Practice: 0 to 25 Years,* London: Department for Education.

Dolgoff-Kaspar, R., Baldwin, A., Johnson, M.S., Edling, N. and Sethi, G.K. (2012) Effect of laughter yoga on mood and heart rate variability in patients awaiting organ transplantation: a pilot study, *Alternative Therapies in Health and Medicine,* 18 (5): 61–66.

Feldman, R.S. (2011) *Development Across the Lifespan,* 6th ed., Harlow: Pearson.

Festa, P.E. (2006) Mahjong politics in contemporary China: civility, Chineseness, and mass Culture, *Positions: East asia Cultures Critique,* 14 (1): 7–35.

Foresight Mental Capital and Wellbeing Project (2008) *Systems Maps*, London: The Government Office for Science.

Gadamer, H.G. (1975) *Truth and Method*, New York: Seabury Press.

Geertz, C. (1973) *Deep Play: Notes on the Balinese Cockfight*, in *The Interpretaion of Cultures: Selected Essays*. New York: Basic Books.

Harwood, A.C. (1958) *The Recovery of Man in Childhood*, New York: Myrin.

Heckhausen, J. and Wrosch, C. (2010) A motivational theory of life-span development. *Psychological Review*, 117 (1): 32–60.

Holmes, R.M. (2011) Adult attitudes and beliefs regarding play on Lana'I, *American Journal of Play*, Winter 2011: 356–384.

Hoyer, W. (2002) *Life Span Development: Encyclopaedia of Aging*, Online. Available at www.encyclopedia.com (accessed 9 June 2015).

Huizinga, J. (1949) *Homo Ludens*. Abingdon: Taylor and Francis.

Kanherkar, R.R., Bhatia-Dey, N. and Csoka, A. B. (2014). Epigenetics across the human lifespan, *Frontiers in Cell and Developmental Biology*, 2 (49): 1–19.

Laberge, M. (2006) *Personality Development*, Online. Available at www.encyclopedia.com/topic/Personality_development.aspx (accessed 12 June 2015).

Laughter Yoga (n.d) *The Front Page*, Online. Available at http://laughteryoga.org.nz/ (accessed 6 December 2015).

Lewis (1992) *Ring of Liberation: A Deceptive Discourse in Brazilian Capoeira*, London: University of Chicago Press.

Lievegoed (1979) *Phases. Crisis and Development in the Individual*, London: Rudolf Steiner Press.

Maslow, A. (1943) A theory of human motivation, *Psychological Review*, 50 (4): 370–396.

Mead, M. (1928) *Coming of Age in Samoa*, New York: William Morrow Paperbacks.

Mosikikongo, D. (2015) *Capoeira Is a Tool for Peace in the DRC*, Online. Available at https://blogs.unicef.org/blog/capoeira-is-a-tool-for-peace-in-the-drc/ (accessed 1 November 2015).

Moya, M.C. (2014) *Playful Thinking for Adults: Engaging the Brain without Gadgets*, [Kindle version]. Available at www.amazon.co.uk (accessed 9 June 2015).

Murray, M. (2009) *Laughter is the Best Medicine for Your Heart*, Online. Available at http://umm.edu/news-and-events/news-releases/2009/laughter-is-the-best-medicine-for-your-heart (accessed 3 November 2015).

Oxfeld, E. (1993) *Blood, Sweat and Mahjong: Family and Enterprise in an Overseas Chinese Community (Anthropology of Contemporary Issues)*, Ithaca, NY: Cornell University Press.

Prytherch, H. and Kraft, K. (2015) *The Psychosocial Impact of Capoeira for Refugee Children and Young People*, London: Capoeira4Refugees.

Ryall, E., Russell, W. and MacLean, M. (2013) *The Philosophy of Play*. London: Routledge.

Salter, J. (2015) *Certificate in Art of Health, Taruna*, Online. Available at www.taruna.ac.nz/programmes/certificate-in-art-of-health/ (accessed 4 November 2015).

Shahidi, M., Mojtahed, A., Modabbernia, A., Mojtahed, M., Shafiabady, A., Delavar, A. and Honari, H. (2011) Laughter yoga versus group exercise program in elderly depressed women: a randomized controlled trial, *International Journal of Geriatric Psychiatry*, 26(3): 322–327.

Singelman, C. and Rider, E. (2015) *Life-Span: Human Development*, 8th ed., Stamford, CT: Cengage Learning.

Stassen Berger, K. (2011) *Life-span Development*. Online. Available at www.oxfordbibliographies.com/view/document/obo-9780199828340/obo-9780199828340-0079.xml (accessed 9 June 2015).

Sugarman, L. (2001) *Life-Span Development: Frameworks, Accounts and Strategies,* 2nd ed., Abingdon: Routledge.

Super, C.M. and Harkness, S. (1997) The cultural structuring of child development, in Berry, J.W., Dasen, P. and Saraswathi, T.S. (eds), *Handbook of Cross Cultural Psychology, vol. 2: Basic Processes and Human Development,* Boston: Allyn & Bacon: 1–39.

Travel China Guide (2015) *Traditional Sports and Activities.* Online. Available at www.travelchinaguide.com/intro/focus/sport.htm (accessed 6 December 2015).

4
CREATING AND GROWING A FAMILY

Julia Whitaker

The determinants of health and wellbeing depend greatly upon what happens to us in our lives – even before those lives have been incarnated – and on how we integrate our life experiences into the self-concept, such that we can become the person that we choose to be. Huxley expressed this idea in his widely-quoted declaration that:

> Experience is not what happens to a man; it is what a man does with what happens to him.
>
> *(Aldous Huxley 1932)*

It is 'the family' that forms the scaffold for both the construction and the dismantling of lived experience and it is the interpretations of experience embodied in 'family life' that influence how we go forward on our personal journeys towards wholeness (White and Epston 1990).

Family has always meant different things to different people and never more so than in the possibility-rich twenty-first century. Derived from the Latin *familia,* meaning household, it suggests domestic *familiarity* with associated implications of closeness and connection. Yet there are clearly a multitude of ways in which people choose to live together (or not) and to arrange their lives in relation to others. In some cultures, the concept of 'family' might include deceased relatives as well as those yet to be born (Shorter 1998). According to the Japanese cultural tradition, successive generations are linked together by the idea of *keizu*, a bond of relationship which exists for the maintenance and continuance of the family as a valued social institution (Ariga 1954).

Recent scientific study (Cozolino 2006) has revealed new insights into our understanding of the growth and function of the human brain and underlines the importance of *relationships* for our health, happiness and wellbeing. Perhaps the

46 Julia Whitaker

single universal truth of family life is that it is about relationships – about how they are created and maintained throughout the lifespan. Family life – whatever shape it takes – also inevitably involves processes of adjustment and change. Research evidence shows that personal experiences of connection and belonging have an enduring impact on how people manage these regulatory processes with repercussions for their physical and mental health, self-esteem, and feelings of wellbeing or satisfaction with life (Handley *et al.* 2015).

The concept of the 'family life-cycle' was proposed by family systems theorists in the 1970s and 1980s as a way of representing the ever-changing nature of family life (Duval 1977; Carter and McGoldrick 1980). Common points of transition such as marriage, the birth of a child, leaving home, retirement, and bereavement are identified as trigger-points for renewed challenge and demands for adjustment. Family systems theory holds that the choices families make at these critical junctures (what family therapists call their *attempted solutions*) are influenced by the beliefs they hold about themselves as individuals, as a family, and as members of the wider community (White and Epston 1990). It is these beliefs which underpin the narratives that families create about themselves and their lives – stories which find their origins in the earliest experiences of infancy. Professor Colwyn Trevarthen (2009 and Trevarthen *et al.* 2014) has described the emotional dynamic of early interaction as a process of intersubjective 'story-telling' and has shown how this narrative form is a blueprint for all future communication, with an enduring influence on how we make connections with different parts of ourselves, with others, and with the natural world.

Family systems theory and research from the field of neuroscience come together in their recognition that the connections or relationships between people can be understood and influenced by the patterns of communication that are developed and maintained in a type of 'feedback loop' (Bateson 1958). Brain studies reveal that, rather than an event or action having a linear cause and effect, it is the feedback received in response to an occurrence or interaction that determines what follows, through a circular process of continual change (Siegel 1999). The story-telling model is useful here in understanding that, unlike words in a book, aspects of a family's narrative or 'story-making' are subject to constant review and revision. The ability to be playful in the sharing of our personal and family stories, to 'play around' with beliefs and attempted solutions, opens-up the possibility of new plot-lines and alternative endings.

Family life can be a source of great joy and satisfaction but it can also generate overwhelming stress, and strain personal resources to their limits. For most of us, it is something of a mixture of both. The everyday tasks and challenges involved in being part of a family will test a family's resourcefulness and resilience over the natural course of things. When the family story includes elements of trauma, or seemingly insurmountable problems, there are real implications for the health and wellbeing of individual family members and for the family group as a whole (Thoits 2011).

For the past thirty years, I have had the privilege of becoming part of the story-making of many families struggling to survive the gamut of life's stresses, including the universal challenges of developmental change; family disruption or re-configuration; mental and physical ill health, bereavement and displacement. Whilst originally trained in the appropriately-named 'talking therapies', it became apparent to me early-on in my career that more could often be achieved by actually talking less: by listening, by observing, by feeling and by sharing what remains unspoken. When words are hard to find, or inadequate to their intended purpose, a playful interaction or play intervention can open-up a different way of connecting and reveal hitherto hidden resourcefulness. Nachmanovitch (1990: 43) writes:

> This is the evolutionary value of play – play makes us flexible. By reinterpreting reality and begetting novelty, we keep from becoming rigid. Play enables us to rearrange our capacities and our very identities so that they can be used in unforeseen ways.

The anonymized case examples included in this chapter are taken from my own practice as social worker, family therapist and health play specialist and are offered in gratitude to all those who have found a way to play when they are feeling the least playful. Pseudonyms are used throughout.

Sowing the seed

In the preface to family life, before the seed of 'family' is even sown, there is a place for play and playfulness – and that place is the bedroom. However, in stark contrast to the ever-increasing accessibility of virtual sex, survey data suggests that, in real-life, sexual play has dropped-down the list of personal priorities in the context of the increasing demands and stresses of modern life (Mercer *et al.* 2013).

Desensitization to pornography and widespread virtual exposure to extreme sexual behaviors have had an irreversible impact on how individuals perceive their own sexuality and their intimate relationships. A 2015 survey by Relate in the UK shows that less than half of all adults are presently satisfied with their sex lives (Relate 2015).

In parallel to this, statistics suggest that as many as one in six, or 12–18 per cent, of couples are having difficulty starting a family (Thoma *et al.* 2013) with a steady increase in the number of people seeking treatment for infertility (HFEA 2012). Whilst there are various hypotheses for this increase in infertility rates, it is widely recognized that for many couples the pressures of austerity, uncertainty in the jobs market, and the struggle to secure a first home, mean that the sexual aspect can become routine or even absent from a relationship.

Life stress may interfere with pregnancy directly through its hormonal effects or indirectly by interfering with a couple's engagement with meaningful sexual relations. The logistical requirements for conception can take the fun out of what is supposed to be a pleasurable activity and the emotional impact of trying for a baby, or of infertility treatment, is recognized as a major factor in determining outcomes. Ellis (1922, cited in Ellens 2009) famously claimed that playfulness between romantic partners crafts a relationship in a manner akin to creating a work-of-art and that sexual playfulness is crucial to personal and relational healing.

Repeated unsuccessful attempts at conception can have a significant negative effect on a woman's health (Barnes 2014). Experiences of disappointment and discouragement create physical and psychological stress, including sleep disturbance, anxiety, and depression, which in turn affect fertility outcomes (Cousineau and Domar 2007). One study has shown that infertile women have global symptom scores equivalent to those of cancer patients (Domar *et al.* 1993).

A successful pregnancy is accompanied by its own set of health challenges and is 'a critical period for central nervous system development in mothers' (Glynn and Sandman 2011). Physical and psychological problems before and after childbirth are not uncommon and may have a significant negative and long-term impact on women's wellbeing and day-to-day functioning (National Perinatal Epidemiology Unit 2015). There is strong research evidence to show that the continuation of physical activity and social participation during pregnancy can have physical and psychological benefits (Gross 2007). The evidence suggests that a woman's experience of pregnancy is strongly affected by her expectations – by what her family story tells her about what it means to have a baby. Taylor (1989) and Taylor and Brown (1988) have shown that positive and negative beliefs are reflected, not just in how people feel but in what they do and how they behave in times of challenge.

And then there were three ...

Even after a successful pregnancy and the arrival of a new baby, the start of family life rarely matches the images portrayed in the media and reflected in our hopeful imaginings. Lack of sleep, inexperience, and a neglect of the couple relationship underlie the reality of the transition to parenthood and characterize the opening chapter of the family story. Personal integration or rejection of the family narrative will have a lasting influence on the subsequent life choices of the individual:

> You want to know someone? Heart, mind and soul? Ask him to tell you about when he was born. What you get won't be the truth: it will be a story. And nothing is more telling than a story,
>
> *(Setterfield 2007: 32)*

Differences in parental and familial attitudes to child-rearing can be the source of tensions in relationships, and the impact of a parent's own early childhood experiences will strongly influence their adaptation to the parenting role. A study by Hoffenaar *et al.* (2010), which explored the impact of starting a family on women's wellbeing, found no difference in reported wellbeing before and after the birth of a child, in contrast to the advertising industry's portrayal of maternal bliss. Likewise, there appeared to be no significant changes in reported mood, anxiety or depression – although there was a slight increase in the pleasure derived from participation in active leisure and being in the company of others.

In contrast, a German study by Margolis and Myrskyla (2015) found that, whilst 30 per cent of new parents report stable or increased feelings of wellbeing after the birth of a baby, the majority said that their levels of happiness reduced in the first two years after birth, placing parenthood higher up the stress scale than unemployment, divorce or the death of a partner (Cha 2015).

Yet it is the connections that are created and developed during these first weeks and months of family life that will determine how the family story unfolds (Crittenden 2015). Attention has long been paid to the importance of early interactional experience and the process of mother-infant attachment to the subsequent development of the child. The early studies by Bowlby and Ainsworth (Ainsworth and Bowlby 1991) have found resonance in contemporary developmental and neurobiological research, which is now positioned to explain how early experiences of emotional interaction impact on the maturation of brain structure and the systems involved in emotional regulation (Schore and Schore 2008). There is a growing realization that the impact of early attachment patterns and experiences of emotional connection endure long into adulthood, affecting an individual's ability to form relationships, to communicate effectively, and to manage life's inevitable challenges, with significant consequences for their health and wellbeing (Mikulincer and Shaver 2007).

The following case examples illustrate how differences in early play experiences have an impact on parental ability to be playful in the process of attachment and to play to create connections between the generations. Play and the playful exchange of 'stories' have been shown to represent the first line of communication between infant and parent-figure (Trevarthen 1999) and the adult's capacity for playful interaction can be seen to reverberate throughout all aspects of their own and their child's lives as a means of forging connections between them and with their social world.

BOX 4.1 ALICE'S STORY

When Alice discovered that she was pregnant, she was trapped in a pattern of heavy drinking calculated to numb the physical and emotional pain of an abusive relationship. Confinement in a neonatal unit after the premature birth of her son offered respite from both a stressful domestic set-up and Alice's self-destructive response to it and proved to be a seedbed of renewed hopefulness. Healthcare play specialists (HPS) have been working with the families of sick and hospitalized children in the UK since the post-war years (National Association of Health Play Specialists 2012) and they are now deploying their knowledge and skills in promoting resilience at times of stress across a range of health and educational contexts. A key element of baby Ben's treatment plan was a daily play session with an HPS, with the primary aim of providing opportunities for playful interaction whilst assessing and facilitating attachment between Ben and his mother. Regular play-times offered a valuable counterpoint to the artificiality of the clinical environment and provided a more naturalistic context within which Alice could adopt the role of 'mother' as opposed to that of 'patient'. Modelling by the HPS of appropriate and desirable interactive behaviors prompted Alice's own spontaneous interactions with her child and revealed a capacity for playful parenting which belied her antenatal history. The play sessions also became the setting for a renewal of the relationship between Alice and her own mother, representing an opportunity to reminisce about Alice's own infancy in the context of three-generational playful exchange. By the time Alice and her baby were transferred from the neonatal unit to the children's ward in preparation for discharge, Alice was sharing her recovered playfulness with other parents on the ward and planning to set-up a telephone support network for graduates from neonatal care.

This example in Box 4.1 shows how the introduction of a therapeutic play intervention can be as helpful to a parent as to the child itself. At a time when both Alice and the professional team working with the family questioned her suitability for the parental role, play opened-up a space within which she could reveal aspects of her true self which might otherwise have remained undiscovered. In a similar fashion, a specialized play program described in Box 4.2 proved key to the assessment of baby Connor and his parents – albeit with a very different outcome.

BOX 4.2 CONNOR'S STORY

Baby Connor's parents both have moderate learning difficulties and had formed a close relationship at the day centre they attended. After Connor's unexpected home-birth, mother and baby were admitted to a children's ward for observation and assessment, whilst the baby's father was encouraged to attend regularly. The healthcare play specialist visited the family daily to play with Connor and to offer support to this new triad. From the outset, both of Connor's parents displayed candid excitement at the arrival of the play specialist with her basket of playthings which they proceeded to explore with uninhibited enthusiasm. Following the play specialist's lead, they would use the play-props to interact with Connor but their interactions were of short duration and they swiftly moved-on from playing with Connor to playing with each other with the baby's toys. They would mimic the play specialist's utterances with the child but added no spontaneous vocalisations or gestures of their own, and seemed to indulge in the interactive play for the personal satisfaction they derived from it. It swiftly became evident that both of Connor's parents had unsatisfied play needs of their own. Each had been raised in residential care, with minimal contact with their own families, and their purposeful early care and education had allowed little space for the type of spontaneous playfulness which they were now exploring in the parental context.

The unprecedented rise in so-called 'parent education' and the superfluity of parenting manuals and other resources can give new parents the impression that the arrival of a third (or fourth or fifth) person in the family demands the acquisition of a whole new set of skills and behaviors. Whilst it may be true that nappy-changing and wriggly-baby-bathing take some practice and experience, the truly important components of child-raising – the giving and receiving of love and respect – are an intrinsic part of being human. For generations, and in most societies, families have survived on their own resourcefulness (Liedloff 1975). It would be disingenuous however to imply that this suggests that raising a family is a straightforward process; whilst our capacity for social connectedness may be present at birth, it is the unfolding of lived experience which determines what use we make of it.

Playful parenting

The earlier case studies have illustrated how differences in a parent's own early experience of play affect their play interactions with their own children and there are many other reasons why parents may need professional help to discover, or to re-discover, their natural aptitudes for making playful connections.

Furedi (2008) insists that parenting is not a complex science and decries the trend for so-called 'expert' intrusion in the process of raising children. He nevertheless endorses the view that the process of learning *how* to manage the parent–child relationship lies at the crux of effective parenting. Furedi's premise that parents know intrinsically what is best for their children does not concede to the fact that *knowing* and *feeling* are two very different concepts (Reddy 2010). A parent may *know* that playful interaction is important for a child's development but if they do not *feel* that playfulness, the knowledge is of little value.

BOX 4.3 MARGARET'S STORY

Margaret, a school-teacher in her thirties, knew just how important it was to the development of her young sons that she should engage in warm, playful interactions with them. However, following the death of her husband in military action, she also felt the enormous weight of grief that prevented her from doing so. Two years after their father's death, the boys seemed to be thriving: they were physically healthy, showed no problems at

> school and were well behaved. However, Margaret missed the closeness they had once shared and worried about the potential long-term effects of her prolonged grief and emotional unavailability. During the early stages of family therapy, the team explored what the loss of a husband and father meant to this family, how life was different without him. Both Margaret and the boys returned repeatedly to the matter of how they missed his stories – his letters from the front and the bedtime tales he would read when he was home on leave. The therapy team chose to develop this story-telling theme, working with the family to co-create the tale of a beautiful but sad princess trapped in a high tower beyond everyone's reach, and of the two young princes who came each day with a new idea to try to make her smile. The boys played the parts of the princes with knowing vigour, whilst Princess Margaret's tears continued to fall. At each of their meetings, the therapy team and family, working together, would add or re-write parts of the story until it reached the point at which the princess in the tower had cried for so long that she had run-out of tears. It was only when she could cry no more that she found the secret staircase leading to a beautiful garden which had grown-up around her during her long years of weeping.

This example of how storytelling can be incorporated into therapeutic work with families illustrates how the use of metaphor can contribute to the making or re-making of a family's own story. Crawford *et al.* (2004) write, 'Stories can powerfully communicate what it is like to be in the world and can provide opportunities to change our view of reality.' This is a playful concept that can be engaged with at both conscious and unconscious levels by all generations. The power of play as a medium for making and sharing stories derives from the fact that it does not need the accompaniment of verbal explanation or interpretation in order to have an impact on what happens in the real world of family life (Ariel 1992). Play and stories are each processed at an emotional – as well as a cognitive – level and, as such, make it possible to work with tricky content that resists being brought into full consciousness. Play and storytelling have long been used as a way of facilitating communication around emotionally challenging or problematic aspects of family life. From talk about the 'Birds and the Bees', the baby 'found under the gooseberry bush' through the 'in-jokes' that couples and families share, we all possess sophisticated mechanisms for playing around with ideas and emotions: mechanisms that are inherent from birth (Reddy 2001).

Story-making offers a safe arena within which to experiment with different perspectives on a situation whilst demonstrating the possibility of change. By externalising a problem in story form, its potency is reduced and it can be examined from different viewpoints (White and Epston 2009). The ability to view family life from different perspectives – to play with experiential perceptions – is essential for the family's successful adaptation to transitional demands and the

Creating and growing a family **53**

search for solutions to problems. Again, research from the field of neuroscience informs our understanding of how this capacity for tuning-into other people's point-of-view is inherent in the new-born and underlies the development of relational communication throughout the lifespan (Reddy 2010). In the extraordinary film *The Connected Baby* (2011) Zeedyk and Robertson reveal how babies come into the world ready-wired for empathic interaction. Contrary to received scientific wisdom that infantile behavior comprises a series of random reflex responses, up-to-date research evidence demonstrates how the ability to modify our behavior in relation to others and to what is going on around us, is a natural part of the human condition and a necessary requirement for healthy adaptation to life's ups-and-downs (Gerhardt 2005).

Adolescence: staying connected at a time of disconnection

The onset of adolescence poses interesting and often surprising challenges for many, if not most, families. Petersen (1988) describes adolescence as a phase of life beginning in biology and ending in society. Lerner (1999) offers reassurance that most adolescents possess the necessary biological, psychological and social resources to manage the transition from childhood to adulthood unaided. Yet where connections between family members are fragile or under stress, adolescence can be the time when a family's resilience is most tested and disconnection becomes a problematic issue.

BOX 4.4 EMMA'S STORY

Emma and her family were referred for therapy when she had just turned 14 years of age. Her parents had separated two years previously and her mother's new partner had recently joined the household. The adjustment demands of a change in domestic arrangement, coinciding with the biological and psychological demands of the onset of adolescence, had proved overwhelming for Emma who had reacted by withdrawing from family life, either by isolating herself in her bedroom or by staying away from home altogether. Communication between Emma, her mother and new partner consisted of tearful and angry exchanges with negative implications for the new couple relationship and for the family's ability to meet the needs of Emma's siblings. At the first family therapy session, it became clear that talking would get nowhere; the therapy team could barely make themselves heard above the raised voices, angry accusations and loud crying. So, instead of talking … they started to sing! The team had learned that Emma was a fan of Hip-Hop music and one team member (whose own child shared a similar musical inclination) started to 'rap', with the rest of the team providing amusingly ill-informed vocal and gestural accompaniment. The effect was immediate. The family were so taken-aback by this

> unexpected turn of events that they stopped shouting at one another and, after a moment of stunned silence, began to laugh. Within minutes, everyone was laughing helplessly at the ridiculousness of the situation and the mood shifted. The family were still laughing after a short session break, advocating the continuation of the playful mood. An agreement was made to postpone any discussion of the serious breakdown in family communication until the following week and in the interim the family were set a therapeutic task. They were asked to turn their home into 'a house of song' by substituting singing for every angry verbal exchange. When the adults wanted to ask something of Emma, they were to 'rap' their request or, failing that, to attempt to reproduce a few lines of the Hip-Hop music they had so often objected to. When Emma wanted to protest or complain about a perceived injustice in the demands made of her, she was to sing a refrain from one of the Rock 'n Roll numbers favoured by the adults. If either party still felt like questioning, nagging, complaining or protesting after they had sung their piece, that was fine – but they had to sing first! The family therapy team had identified this family's potential for playfulness and exploited it as a first step at connecting with them as well as suggesting a way in which they might re-connect with each other.

Play can often be used in this way to interrupt an unhelpful pattern of interaction. Parents commonly use playful interjections during a child's early upbringing – to encourage, to distract and to help the general flow of daily-life. When play and humor can be carried from the first phases of the family life-cycle to adolescence and beyond, healthful connections can be continuously maintained and re-made. Killick (2015: 15) speaks of playfulness as the 'unfettering of mind and body'. It applies equally to the young adult's drive for novelty and creative exploration (Siegel 2014), to the inventiveness and creativity that accompany the life-experience of maturity, and to the irreverent humor and emotional disinhibition of the older adult with dementia.

In the burgeoning field of positive psychology (Csíkszentmihalyi 1997), the concept of 'flow' is used to describe the state of intense involvement and enjoyment experienced when an individual is fully engaged and absorbed in a meaningful interactive exchange, such as play or storytelling. Flow may be used to describe the feeling of spontaneous joy or 'rapture' that accompanies complete immersion in play or a playful interaction (Goleman 1996) and resonates with Maslow's concept of self-actualization as the ultimate state of positive wellbeing.

Csíkszentmihalyi (1997) states that happiness is derived from this process of personal development and growth and that flow situations permit the experience of personal development. When a family finds itself with a cohesive and coherent family story, each member is separately and collectively open to the attainment of a state of 'flow' and the growth or 'flowering' of their potential. The concept of flow finds parallels in the therapeutic attainment of *insight* or *resolution* as a desired outcome of the therapeutic relationship.

Family life under stress

Our innate ability to make the relational connections necessary for healthy growth requires a fertile soil in which it can develop. Families can and do thrive in the most disadvantageous conditions – but they swim against the tide. When overwhelmed by adverse social or economic circumstances, the drive for physical, social and psychological survival supersedes emotional or playful motivations as the family story becomes one of survival rather than connection and flow. It seems only right, therefore, to conclude this chapter with respectful acknowledgement of the established benefits of so-called 'parenting education' programs which work with vulnerable families with the aim of anticipating and alleviating the potentially harmful effects of stress on family functioning (Child Welfare Information Gateway 2013).

Margaret Mead (1901–1978), a pioneering influence on our understanding of familial relationships, wrote: 'Nobody has ever before asked the nuclear family to live all by itself in a box the way we do. With no relatives, no support, we've put it in an impossible situation' (cited Auerbach 1979:18). There can be no denying that contemporary stresses on parents are numerous – whether living with the demands of a western, consumer-driven society or displaced by conflict and economic necessity. It is perhaps unsurprising that the evidence confirms that the greater the number and duration of stress factors present, the less able parents are to engage in the positive parenting of their children (Deater-Deckard 2005). Positive parenting is here defined as: 'parental behavior based on the best interests of the child that is nurturing, empowering, non-violent and provides recognition and guidance which involves setting of boundaries to enable the full development of the child' (Council of Europe 2006).

Socioeconomic status has been identified as a key variable in the capacity for positive parenting and the literature suggests that reduced socioeconomic circumstances are linked to inhibited child development (Bradley and Corwyn 2002), and that this association begins at the start of life. The combination of stresses resulting from socioeconomic disadvantage and the consequent increase in the likelihood of children experiencing poor parenting,

> have a detrimental effect on children's progression and wellbeing, which can impact right through into their adulthood, in turn affecting the subsequent generation. The way that disadvantage perpetuates is shaped by the experiences, attainment and outcomes of children growing up in socioeconomic disadvantage and by the way that negative parental activities experienced through childhood may repeat in adulthood.
>
> *(Department of Work and Pensions and Department for Education 2011: 15)*

It is this research, taken in conjunction with what we know about the development of neural pathways, that has driven widespread investment in parenting education. All parents, and particularly those living in actual or potentially stressful circumstances, can benefit from guidance and support in the parenting relationship (Department for Children, Schools and Families 2010). This is most importantly in the interests of the next generation, but with no less significant implications for personal development and wellbeing throughout the lifespan and for the health of society as a whole.

A healthy society is one in which all of its members have equal access to the personal knowledge and skills necessary for the attainment of a positive state of health and wellbeing. This refers not just to public information about ways of keeping physically and mentally 'fit', but to a public debate about the impact of family and other relationships on people's developmental potential and about the place of play in this developmental process.

References

Ainsworth, M.D.S. and Bowlby, J. (1991) An ethological approach to personality development, *American Psychologist,* 46: 331–341.

Ariel, S. (1992) *Strategic Family Play Therapy,* Chichester: John Wiley & Sons, Ltd.

Ariga, K. (1954) The family in Japan, *Marriage and Family Living,* 16 (4): 362–368.

Auerbach, S. (1979) *Confronting the Child Care Crisis,* Boston: Beacon Press.

Barnes, D. (2014) *Women's Reproductive Mental Health across the Lifespan.* New York: Springer.

Bateson, G. (1958) *Naven,* Stanford, CA: Stanford University Press.

Bradley, R.H. and Corwyn, R.F. (2002) Socioeconomic status and child development, *Annual Review of Psychology,* 53 (1): 371–399.

Carter, E. and McGoldrick, M. (1980) *The Family Life Cycle: A Framework for Family Therapy,* New York: Gardner Press.

Cha, A.E. (2015) *It Turns out Parenthood is Worse than Divorce, Unemployment – Even the Death of a Partner,* Online. Available at www.washingtonpost.com/news/to-your-health/wp/2015/08/11/the-most-depressing-statistic-imaginable-about-being-a-new-parent/ (accessed 7 October 2015).

Child Welfare Information Gateway (2013) *Parent Education to Strengthen Families and Reduce the Risk of Maltreatment,* Washington DC: U.S. Department of and Human Services, Children's Bureau.

Council of Europe (2006) *Recommendation Rec (2006) 19 of the Committee of Ministers to Member States on Policy to Support Positive Parenting,* Online. Available at https://wcd.coe.int/ViewDoc.jsp?id=1073507 (accessed 8 December 2015).

Cousineau, T.M. and Domar, A.D (2007) Psychological Impact of Infertility. Best Practice and Research, *Clinical Obstetrics and Gynaecology,* 21: 293–308.

Cozolino, L. (2006) *The Neuroscience of Human Relationships: Attachment and the Developing Social brain,* London: W.W. Norton.

Crawford, R., Brown, B. and Crawford, P. (2004) *Storytelling in Therapy,* Cheltenham: Nelson Thornes.

Crittenden, P.M. (2015) *Raising Parents: Attachment, Representation, and Treatment,* 2nd ed., London: Routledge.

Csíkszentmihalyi, M. (1997) *Finding flow. The Psychology of Engagement with Everyday Life,* New York: Basic Books.

Department for Children, Schools and Families (2010) *Parenting and Family Support: Guidance for Local Authorities in England,* Nottingham: DCSF Publications.

Department of Work and Pensions and Department for Education (2011) *A New Approach to Child Poverty: Tackling the Causes of Disadvantage and Transforming Families' Lives,* London: HM Government.

Deater-Deckard, K. (2005) Parenting stress and children's development: introduction to the special issue, *Infant and Child Development,* 14: 111–115.

Domar, A., Zuttermeister, P. and Friedman, R. (1993) The psychological impact of infertility: a comparison to patients with other medical conditions, *Journal of Psychosomatic Obstetrics and Gynecology,* 14: 45 –52.

Duval, E. (1977) *Marriage and Family Development,* Philadelphia, PA: Lippincott.

Ellens, H. (2009) *The Spirituality of Sex,* Santa Barbara, CA: Greenwood.

Furedi, F. (2008) *Paranoid Parenting,* London: Continuum.

Gerhardt, S. (2005) *Why Love Matters: How Affection Shapes a Baby's Brain.* London: Routledge.

Glynn, L.M. and Sandman, C.A. (2011) Prenatal origins of neurological development: A Critical period for fetus and mother. *Current Directions in Psychological Science,* 20 (6): 384.

Goleman, D. (1996) *Emotional Intelligence: Why It Can Matter More Than IQ,* London: Bloomsbury.

Gross, H. (2007) *Sanctioning Pregnancy: A Psychological Perspective on the Paradoxes and Culture of Research,* London: Routledge.

Handley, S., Joy, I., Hestbaek, C. and Marjoribanks, D. (2015) *The Best Medicine? The Importance of Relationships for Health and Wellbeing,* Doncaster: Relate.

Hoffenaar, P. J., van Balen, F. and Hermanns, J. (2010) The impact of having a baby on the level and content of women's well-being, *Social Indicators Research,* 97 (2): 279–295.

Human Fertilisation and Embryology Authority (2012) *Fertility Treatment in 2012. Trends and Figures,* London: HFEA.

Huxley, A. (1932) *Texts and Pretexts,* New York: Harper and Bros.

Killick, J. (2015) *Playfulness and Dementia.* London: Jessica Kingsley.

Lerner, R. (1999) *Social Interactions in Adolescence and Promoting Positive Social Contributions of Youth,* Abingdon: Taylor and Francis.

Liedloff, J. (1975) *The Continuum Concept,* London: Penguin.

Margolis R. and Myrskyla, M. (2015) Parental well-being surrounding first birth as a determinant of further parity progression, *Demography,* 52: 1147–1166.

Mercer, C.H., Tanton, C., Prah, P., Erens, B., Sonnenberg, P., Clifton, S., Macdowall, W., Lewis, R., Field, N., Datta, J., Copas, A. J., Phelps, A., Kaye Wellings, K. and Johnson, A. M. (2013) Changes in sexual attitudes and lifestyles in Britain through the life course and over time: findings from the National Surveys of Sexual Attitudes and Lifestyles (Natsal), *The Lancet,* 382 (9907): 1781–1794.

Mikulincer, M. and Shaver, P.R. (2007) *Attachment in Adulthood: Structure, Dynamics and Change,* New York: Guilford Press.

Nachmanovitch, S. (1990) *Free Play: Improvisation in Life and Art,* New York: Tarcher.

National Association of Health Play Specialists (2012) *National Association of Hospital Play Staff Milestones.* Online. Available at http://nahps.org.uk/index.php?page=history (accessed 8 December 2015).

National Perinatal Epidemiology Unit (2015) *Maternal Health and Wellbeing in the Perinatal Period,* Online. Available at www.npeu.ox.ac.uk/research/maternal-health-and-wellbeing-in-the-perinatal-period-212 (accessed October 2015).

Petersen, A.C. (1988) Adolescent development, *Annual Review of Psychology*, 39: 583–607.

Reddy, V. (2001) Infants clowns: the interpersonal creation of humour in infancy, *Enfance*, 53: 247–256.

Reddy, V. (2010) *How Infants Know Minds*, Cambridge, MA: Harvard University Press.

Relate (2015) *The Way We Are Now: The State of the UKs Relationships 2015*. Doncaster: Relate.

Schore, J.R. and Schore, A.N. (2008) Modern attachment theory: the central role of affect regulation in development and treatment, *Clinical Social Work Journal*, 36 (1): 9–20.

Setterfield, D. (2007) *The Thirteenth Tale*, New York: Simon and Schuster.

Shorter, A. (1998) *African Culture. An Overview*, Nairobi: East African Educational Publishing.

Siegel, D. (1999) *The Developing Mind*. New York: Guilford Press.

Siegel, D. (2014) *Brainstorm: The Power and the Purpose of the Teenage Brain*, New York: Tarcher.

Taylor, S.E. (1989) *Positive Illusions; Creative Self-deception and the Healthy Mind*, New York: Basic Books.

Taylor, S.E. and Brown, J.D. (1988) Illusion and well-being: a social psychological perspective on mental health. *Psychological Bulletin*, 103 (2): 193–210.

Thoits, P.A. (2011) Stress and health: major findings and policy implications, *Journal of Health and Social Behaviour*, 51: S41–S53.

Thoma, M.E., McLain, A., Louis, J.F., King, R., Trumble, A., Sundaram, R. and Buck Lewis, G. (2013) Prevalence of infertility in the United States as estimated by the current duration approach and a traditional constructed approach, *Fertility and Sterility*, 99 (5): 1324–1331.

Trevarthen, C. (1999) Musicality and the intrinsic motive pulse: evidence from human psychobiology and infant communication, in *Rhythms, Musical Narrative, and the Origins of Human Communication, Musicae Scientiae Special Issue*, 1999–2000: 157–213.

Trevarthen, C. (2009) The functions of emotion in infancy, in Fosha, D. (ed.), *The Healing Power of Emotion: Affective Neuroscience, Development and Clinical Practice*. London: W.W. Norton.

Trevarthen, C., Gratier, M. and Osborne, N. (2014) The human nature of culture and education, *Wiley Interdisciplinary Reviews: Cognitive Science*, 5, March/April: 173–192.

White, M. and Epston, D. (1990) *Narrative Means to Therapeutic Ends*, New York: W.W. Norton.

The Connected Baby (2011) Produced by Suzanne Zeedyk and James Robertson (DVD).

5

THE CONCEPT OF HEALTH AND WELLBEING ACROSS THE LIFESPAN

Rachel Bayliss and Jenni Etchells

Play has a significant – and not yet fully realized – contribution to make to the holistic health and wellbeing of individuals at each stage of their lifespan. This chapter will focus on the six aspects of health and how play can impact positively, respecting individual needs and capabilities. It will also signpost content, introduced within this chapter, for deeper exploration elsewhere in the book.

Introduction

The human need to achieve health and wellbeing is not exclusive to one period of life and it is increasingly recognized that the health and wellbeing of individuals impacts upon all other aspects of their lives. There is progressive emphasis put upon 'community-centred' approaches which increase people's control over their health and wellbeing (NHS England 2015) and consideration is being given to how this health autonomy can be achieved across the lifespan. Although the notion of play may 'sit' more comfortably within the early periods of life, it has a role throughout the whole of the lifespan. The National Institute for Play (2015) cites play 'as basic and as pervasive a natural phenomenon as sleep'. However, the notion of play does not conform to a 'one size fits all' model and it is therefore important to understand how play can have a positive health impact which is responsive to, and supportive of, individual needs and capabilities.

Background context

Positive health is an evolving and fluctuating concept that incorporates a variety of important strands. A holistic view recognizes that the idea of health and wellbeing changes throughout the lifespan and that people at different stages of life have different notions of what constitutes good health and the factors that may affect it.

60 Rachel Bayliss and Jenni Etchells

There are various ways to represent the breakdown components of health and wellbeing; the one used to scaffold this chapter is the six aspects of health as identified by Bruce and Meggitt (2005) and outlined in Table 5.1.

TABLE 5.1 Adapted from Bruce and Meggitt (2005)

Aspect	Description
Physical	How the body functions
Emotional	The expression of emotions and being able to deal with thoughts and feelings e.g. fear, frustration, happiness
Social	Interacting and relating with other people; forming and maintaining friendships and relationships
Spiritual	Associated with a quest for 'inner peace' and personal principles and conduct
Mental	The organization of thoughts and being able to think clearly
Environmental	Factors linked to the environment which influence the health of individuals e.g. pollution or social housing concerns

Within these six core aspects, play has a pivotal role in positively contributing to the means of achieving and facilitating each aspect. The spontaneity, creativity and flexibility of play allows it to percolate through the layers of health, enabling adaptation to meet individual needs and capabilities.

The six aspects of health

Physical health

Physical health is perhaps the most readily identifiable aspect of overall health and wellbeing. The importance of maintaining and conditioning the body and its functions throughout the lifespan is at the epicentre of health and medical care. It is globally recognized that regular physical activity reduces morbidity and mortality and, in the UK alone, it has been quoted that 'physical inactivity costs the NHS an estimated £0.9 billion per year' (National Institute for Health and Care Excellence 2015: 5). The nature of this burden grants physical health a high priority on the healthcare agenda. It is recognized that, although health is influenced by individual choice, government policy makers and other powerful groups in society also play a part in personal health choices (Lloyd 2007).

There are many national and local initiatives that contribute towards improving the physical health of individuals and communities (NHS England 2015). A well-publicized national drive is the 'Couch to 5k' project which encourages individuals to build themselves up over a period of five weeks to the fitness capability to undertake a 5k run (NHS Choices 2014a). There are supportive resources to facilitate this, including a print-out exercise schedule and the option of downloading a free app. This allows for maximum appeal across the lifespan; whilst the techno-logical aspect may engage the adolescent and emerging adult groups (discussed in Chapter 15), the paper version may suit those in later adulthood. The scheme also incorporates an understanding of differences in individual ability for, whilst all participants are united in the common goal of completing the 5k run, there is no set time limit within which the distance must be covered.

There are other similar schemes provided specifically for people who have longer term medical conditions which may change their needs and limit cap-abilities. An idea that has been evaluated in recent years is a scheme which uses dance to aid rehabilitation in patients with Parkinson's disease (Dreu *et al.* 2012). Parkinson's disease is a progressive degenerative movement disorder that predomi-nantly affects those in late adulthood. Community programs supported by charitable organizations have also been set up with the focus of facilitating enjoy-ment and alleviating some of the symptoms of this disease (Dance for Parkinson's UK 2015; Dance for PD 2015). These programs harness the power of play by introducing the spontaneity of dance, inspiring creativity and incorporating individual flexibility. The use of dance and drama as a play form is explored in detail in Chapter 11.

Physical health innovations have also sprung up at grass-roots level, encouraging families to seek alternative forms of leisure activity which boost physical activity levels. An example of this is the emergence of indoor trampoline parks which are gaining popularity both in the US and the UK (Bounce 2015). Adults are encouraged to participate in this playful activity with their children, encompassing a holistic approach to health and wellbeing across generations. These physical health strategies take their place within the wider context of new horizons to public health, community initiative and preventative medicine.

Emotional health

Emotional health is important for the achievement of all-round health and wellbeing in that it will influence an individual's motivation and capacity to make positive lifestyle choices (as discussed in Chapter 7). Emotional intelligence, self-expression and self-awareness contribute to a sense of fulfilment, build resilience and aid the development of coping strategies throughout life.

Art as a medium can be utilized to promote wellness in various areas of health-care provision and is a widely-accepted means of emotional expression. Art provides a therapeutic means of 'expressing difficult emotions' which are not 'prefrontal cortex stuff – it's gut stuff, it's heart stuff … so art therapy is a good non-verbal way for people to connect the head and the heart' (Berry, cited in Meyers 2014). Meyers (2014) states that 'the medical process is traumatising both physically and emotionally, and it can be hard for people to express that trauma verbally'. The role of art within healthcare is explored in detail in Chapters 12 and 13.

Grief is a universal emotion that can have a profound effect on our sense of wellbeing and grief work or grief counseling utilizes different means of providing an outlet for feelings of sadness and loss (as discussed in Chapter 8). Play has been incorporated into this form of therapy and art therapy is a commonly recognized method used by counselors to facilitate the emotional expression of grief (Humphrey and Zimpfer 2008). Art allows spontaneous expression of feelings that may otherwise be supressed and can be adapted for individuals with varying style preferences and at different stages of life (Meyers 2014). If grief and the accompanying emotions are not explored and processed then they can have a disabling effect on psychological and social functioning and quality of life at a later stage (Zisook and Shear 2009). It is therefore imperative that both professional and social networks understand the need to explore and manage emotional health at an early stage to prevent complications in later life.

A challenging area for the promotion of emotional health is where there is a pre-existing disability of emotional processing, as in the case of autism. Autism is a lifelong developmental disorder that affects interpersonal communication, social interaction and perception of the world. One initiative to improve the emotional expression, and therefore wellbeing, of people with autism is the playful use of music. This relies on improvisation and interaction between the participant and the therapist rather than a structured intervention and has been shown to facilitate emotional synchronicity, motivation and communication (Kim *et al.* 2009). Music as a spontaneous form of self-expression fits well with the concept of play as a freely chosen and freely motivated activity; this is discussed further in Chapter 9. Music can also be used as a therapeutic tool to facilitate engagement and participation for people with dementia and this is explored in Chapter 10.

It has long been recognized that emotional and physical health have a synergetic relationship; however emotional health by its nature is more difficult to define and describe and therefore can be more easily overlooked.

Social health

The attainment of positive health and wellbeing cannot be achieved by an individual in isolation; it relies on the maintenance of social health and community wellbeing. This sentiment has been adopted by the government as part of healthcare policy, with an increasing shift of focus towards the importance of community-centred public health and preventative medicine (NHS England 2015).

A popular means of integrating social health into the landscape of public health is via the utilization of patient support groups. These groups may take the form of face-to-face meetings or internet forums, thus allowing for the engagement of people with different social skills and preferences and varying technological abilities. Prominent examples of this are Epilepsy Action and Diabetes UK, with their focus on two conditions which affect people of all ages. These support networks encourage locality-based 'coffee and chat' groups, as well as fundraising and awareness campaigns. The work of organizations such as these demonstrate that relatively simple, community-driven, interventions can make a big difference –

such as providing cups of tea after treatment as a means of socialization and peer support. For example, a series of tweets discussed the use of china cups for cancer patients, who said the 'tea tasted better and made them feel special after chemo' (ESasaruNHS 2015). One of the best examples of a fundraising initiative which exploited the affinity between sustenance and social support was the world's biggest coffee morning, organized by Macmillian Cancer Support (2015) who raised over £25 million through this initiative in 2014.

These initiatives serve to empower members and forge supportive relationships that collectively promote the social health of the whole community. As with all the other aspects of health, policy facilitates public engagement and this is explored within Chapter 22. This has been mirrored internationally by the World Health Organization (WHO) which has collaborated with multiple countries to identify support groups for a wide range of health issues. Research has echoed the notion that peer support groups are a valuable tool to encourage successful self-management of disease. This is not confined to the urban developed population as illustrated by studies from rural communities in China which have documented positive health outcomes linked to patient support groups (Liu *et al.* 2012).

Another means of promoting social health is via the establishment of day services for older adults. These can offer an opportunity for those in late adulthood to build and maintain relationships, to develop social interaction and to avoid isolation. Day services can also facilitate access to physical, occupational or speech therapies. They also provide a setting within which the value of play and hobbies may be introduced to the older generation offering a diverse range of activities such as music, art, dance and pets. The friendships and social experiences built at these centers can act as the building blocks for emotional and social security as well as nourishing a healthy community spirit. In addition, the provision of day centers gives carers and relatives of older adults important respite opportunities, a benefit which is overwhelmingly supported by the literature (Fields *et al.* 2014).

Overall, social health is a part of a reciprocal relationship between the other aspects of health and wellbeing. Social health, relationships and community involvement can positively contribute to emotional and physical wellbeing.

Spiritual health

A further aspect of health and wellbeing is spiritual health, which is perhaps also the most subject to personal interpretation. Spiritual health is not a distinct entity and will have different meanings for different people. For some, spiritual health is addressed through adherence to organized religious principles and teachings, whilst for others it refers to a more personal journey of self-discovery, purpose and moral living (Reese and Meyers 2012). Mueller *et al.* (2001) report that most studies suggest that religious and spiritual involvement positively influence clinical outcomes. The concept of spiritual health is likely to fluctuate and evolve as an individual passes through the different stages and experiences of life, with some scholars advocating spiritual development as a 'vital process and resource in young

64 Rachel Bayliss and Jenni Etchells

people's developmental journey from birth through adolescence' (Roehlkepartain *et al.* 2005: 11).

During the closing stages of life, the importance of spiritual health and well-being assume a particular poignancy. The field of palliative care emphasizes the critical importance of giving due consideration to the spiritual beliefs and wishes of the dying person and their family. Dying with dignity is a widely-accepted ideal that embraces a recognition of an individual's needs and preferences. This concept is included in healthcare guidance aimed at care-givers involved in frontline palliative care (Together for Short Lives 2012). This is particularly relevant within oncology services where there is widespread recognition that spiritual care is valued, not only by the individual with cancer, but also by those involved in the care process (Phelps *et al.* 2012).

Spiritual health is traditionally propagated by community institutions which represent religious organizations and groups. Local churches, mosques, synagogues, temples and other establishments all run varied activity programs, with community outreach events and fundraisers. These activities bridge the age gap; as well as groups for children and families, many places offer separate men's, women's and older adults groups. These can contribute to spiritual health when a group of people who share similar beliefs and values can collectively affirm their spiritual direction and purpose. Play can be incorporated into this spiritual dimension, a specific example being 'Messy Church', an international phenomenon based on creativity, hospitality and celebration for all ages (Messy Church 2015). Featured activities include crafts, cooking, physical games and interactive resources. Play and having fun underpin these recreational opportunities as a way of bringing together individuals who share common values and beliefs. This can also be extended to the adult specific groups who can harness recreational activities such as games nights, day-trips and social dinners as a means of maintaining a collective spiritual identity through a play agenda.

Spirituality is a subjective and personal subject which resists generalized description or easy understanding. The link between spiritual health and a general experience of wellbeing is well documented in history, art and literature; the relationship between spirituality and wellness is further examined in Chapters 19 and 20.

Mental health

Mental health is an increasingly recognized issue worldwide; in the UK alone one in four British adults will experience a diagnosable mental health problem in the course of one year (Mental Health Foundation 2015). Mental health matters are not age-specific and transcend culture, nationality and gender.

A public initiative funded and launched by national bodies in 2008 is the *Speak Out* campaign (Time to Change 2008a). This is directed at encouraging creativity for people to open up and share their mental health experiences. The campaign focuses on writing music, directing plays and making films and offers people the

Health and wellbeing across the lifespan **65**

opportunity to use forms of play as an emotional outlet as well as increasing public awareness. Resources are aimed across the lifespan with a campaign toolkit for school and youth clubs, GP practices and community events (Time to Change 2008b). Projects such as these serve to encompass and weave together many of the different aspects of health.

Creativity as a means of emotional expression and building self-confidence can also be highlighted through the practice of art therapy in mental health. This encourages free self-expression via painting, drawing, modelling and collage (Meyers 2014). This intervention is also open to people of a wide range of capabilities as no previous experience or skill is necessary for participation. It can also be translated to a variety of different settings such as psychiatry, education, social services and work in prisons. A recent systematic review of the literature has demonstrated the positive effects of art therapy for patients with different clinical profiles (Uttley *et al.* 2015).

Play can also be used as a form of a preventative technique for managing stress. The prevalence of stress in the workplace is on the increase, with the 45–54 year old age group being most at risk (Health and Safety Executive 2014). Work-related stress impacts on the economic situation in terms of the number of working days lost as well as the potential personal and medical ramifications of untreated or unrecognized high stress levels. A number of businesses are now recognizing the benefits of play and recreation in the workplace to enhance mental health whilst contributing to a general creative atmosphere. An example of this is Google, whose employees rate their workplace to be one of the best in the world. Initiatives used include a Lego play-station, a ladder and slide to replace stairs, freely wandering pets and the opportunity for employers to scribble spontaneous ideas on the walls (New York Times 2013). Further discussion around the role of play within the workplace is documented within Chapter 21.

Mental health is a key component in the mosaic of holistic wellbeing, interacting synergistically with the other five aspects of health. Cognitive processing, psychological resilience and emotional self-awareness require equal attention to physical health throughout the lifespan. The role of play for promoting mental wellness is explored further in Chapter 8.

Environmental health

The term 'environmental health' includes considerations such as the quality of the external environment (air pollution, water), social housing conditions and nutrition. Due to the nature of this concept, direct control by the individual is often unachievable and external influences and policy can overwhelmingly govern this aspect of health (Barton and Grant 2006), yet the potential impact of environmental factors on health and wellbeing is well documented (Reese and Myers 2012). Play is a key feature of the environmental health scene.

International acknowledgement of the health benefits of proximity to natural green environments is gathering pace. These are considered to be beneficial to health through decreasing stress (thereby enhancing mental wellbeing) and by encouraging physical activity (Godbey 2009). The benefits of this can be enhanced further, when exercising outdoors is close to water (Cox 2012). 'Blue gym' research promotes the value of the natural water environment (also known as blue space) emphasising the restorative effect that this induces (White *et al.* 2010).

These natural landscapes can also serve as opportunities for the fruition of other aspects of health such as social interaction and building relationships through outdoor recreation and sport (Cox 2012) as well as the maintenance of physical and emotional health. In addition to conventional children's playgrounds, there is now an escalating commitment to providing outdoor gyms and adult playgrounds. These launched in the UK in 2007, drawing inspiration from Chinese governmental schemes which installed adult gym equipment in public parks (BBC News 2012). Projects such as these clearly highlight that play can be a beneficial route to health throughout the lifespan. By removing the financial and accessibility constraints of conventional gym membership, the public provision of outdoor gyms opens-up opportunities for individuals to partake in and enjoy the natural environment whilst improving their overall health and wellbeing. The informal nature of these adult outdoor gyms appeals to those with different levels of physical ability, allowing them to exercise control over their individual circumstances and exercise environment.

It is within the remit of environmental health to give consideration to differences in the perception of vulnerability to injury at different life stages. The safety of a proposed physical or leisure activity has been shown to be an important factor for an individual's participation. This is particularly evident in the older age group (50 years +) who are more likely to have physical ailments and poorer physiological reserve (City and Guilds 2008). This is acknowledged within qualifications for physical instructors who work with older people, and exercise regimes that cater for the biological effect of aging can be integrated into more recreational style activities and pastimes (City and Guilds 2008).

An additional consideration has been publicized by Evans and Sleap (2012) who established that the elderly population were more reluctant to engage in aquatic activities due to lack of confidence and the imagined physical hazards of slipping or falling at the poolside. The topic of body image also arose in this context as the interviewed population were concerned about their perceived body image. This is not just an issue for the elderly population and is cited as a cross-generational barrier to participation in physical exercise regimes. This has been acknowledged by Sport England whose research revealed that millions of women and girls cite a fear of judgement and prejudice as a factor in non-participation in sport. This may be contributing to a gender disparity between men and women's involvement in physical activity which interestingly is not mirrored to the same extent in other European countries (Sport England 2015). The widely publicized 'This Girl Can' UK campaign has stemmed from this research and focuses on getting women and girls more active whilst building their self-worth, self-esteem and encouraging challenge against stereotypical images of the perfect body (Sport England 2015).

Environmental health is the platform upon which other aspects of health stand. A healthy environment is fundamental to our overriding sense of wellbeing and is an important factor for consideration by policy makers responsible for setting and achieving global health targets.

Conclusion

The flexibility and adaptability of play is ideally suited to the multi-faceted notion of health and wellbeing. The interlinking and synergistic aspects discussed in this chapter are fluid across the lifespan and are flexible elements that change in line with changing needs and capabilities. Play in adult healthcare is an emerging concept that is only recently gaining ground. Play lends itself to a symbiotic relationship with health as both are concepts that are dynamic, subjective and require an understanding of individual differences, preferences and abilities.

References

Barton, H. and Grant, M. (2006) A health map for the local human habitat, *The Journal of the Royal Society for the Promotion of Health*, 126 (6): 252–253.

BBC News (2012) *The Rise of the Adult Playground*. Online. Available at www.bbc.co.uk/news/magazine-17818223 (accessed 10 July 2015).

BBC News (2015) *Airport Expansion: What Happens Next?* Online. Available at www.bbc.co.uk/news/uk-19570653 (accessed 10 July 2015).

Bounce (2015) *Bounce Indoor Trampoline Parks*, Online. Available at www.bouncegb.com/ (accessed 9 July 2015).

Bruce, T. and Meggit, C. (2005) *Child Care and Education*, 3rd ed., London: Hodder Arnold.

City and Guilds (2008) Level 3 NVQ in Instructing Physical Activity and Exercise (4834–4841, 4842, 4843, 4847): Standards and assessment requirements 500/3832/1, London: City and Guilds.

Cox, S. (2012) *Game of Life: How Sport and Recreation Can Make us Healthier, Happier and Richer,* London: Sport and Recreation Alliance.

Dance for Parkinson's UK (2015) *Welcome to the Dance for Parkinson's Network UK Website*, Online. Available at www.danceforparkinsonsuk.org/ (accessed 9 July 2015).

Dance for PD (2015) *Welcome to the Official Dance for PD Site,* Online. Available at http://danceforparkinsons.org/ (accessed 9 July 2015).

De Dreu, M., Van Der Wilk, A., Poppe, E., Kwakkel, G., and Van Wegen, E. (2012) Rehabilitation, exercise therapy and music in patients with Parkinson's disease: a meta-analysis of the effects of music-based movement therapy on walking ability, balance and quality of life, *Parkinsonism & Related Disorders*, 18 (1): 114–119.

@ESasaruNHS (2015) *Improving Care for All Can be Just Small Things: China Cups for Cancer Patients Said Tea Tasted Better and made them feel better after chemo*, 12 July Online. Available at https://twitter.com/Whoseshoes/status/620138595001704449 (accessed 12 July 2015).

Evans, A.B. and Sleap, M. (2012) 'You feel like people are looking at you and laughing': Older adults' perceptions of aquatic physical activity, *Journal of Aging Studies*, 26 (4): 515–526.

Fields, N., Anderson, K., and Dabelko-Schoeny, H. (2014) The Effectiveness of adult day services for older adults: a review of the literature from 2000 to 2011, *Journal of Applied Gerontology*, 33 (2): 130–163.

Godbey, G. (2009) *Outdoor Recreation, Health, and Wellness: Understanding and Enhancing the Relationship*, Online. Available at www.rff.org/documents/RFF-DP-09-21.pdf (accessed 12 July 2015).

Health and Safety Executive (2014) *Stress-related and Psychological Disorders in Great Britain 2014*, Health and Safety Executive.

Humphrey, G., and Zimpfer, D. (2008) *Counselling for Grief and Bereavement*, 2nd ed., London: Sage.

Kim, J., Wigram, T. and Gold, C. (2009) Emotional, motivational and interpersonal responsiveness of children with autism in improvisational music therapy, *Autism* 13 (4): 389–409.

Liu, S., Bi, A., Fu, D., Fu, H., Luo, W., Ma, X., and Zhuang, L. (2012) Effectiveness of using group visit model to support diabetes patient self-management in rural communities of Shanghai: a randomized controlled trial, *BMC Public Health*, 12, 1043. Online. Available at http://doi.org/10.1186/1471-2458-12-1043

Lloyd, C. (2007) Introduction, in: Lloyd, C., Handsley, S. Douglas, J., Earle, S. and Spurr, S. (eds.) *Policy and Practice in Promoting Public Health*. London: Sage.

Macmillan Cancer Support (2015) *World's Biggest Coffee Morning 25 Sept: Cakes Taste Better Together*, Online. Available at http://coffee.macmillan.org.uk/ (accessed 12 July 2015).

Mental Health Foundation (2015) *Mental Health Statistics*, Online. Available at www.mental-health.org.uk/help-information/mental-health-statistics/ (accessed 10 July 2015).

Messy Church (2015) *Messy Church*, Online. Available at www.messychurch.org.uk/ (accessed 9 July 2015).

Meyers, L. (2014) *In Search of Wellness*, Online. Available at http://ct.counseling.org/2014/02/in-search-of-wellness/ (accessed 10 July 2015).

Mueller, P., Plevak, D. and Rummans, T. (2001). Religious involvement, spirituality, and medicine: implications for clinical practice, *Mayo Clinic Proceedings*, 76 (12): 1225–1235.

National Institute for Health and Care Excellence (2015) *Physical Activity: Encouraging Activity in All People in Contact with the NHS*, London: NICE.

NHS Choices (2014a) *Couch to 5K: Week by Week*, Online. Available at www.nhs.uk/Livewell/c25k/Pages/couch-to-5k-plan.aspx (accessed 10 July 2015).

NHS Choices (2014b) *Five Steps to Mental Wellbeing*, Online. Available at www.nhs.uk/Conditions/stress-anxiety-depression/Pages/improve-mental-wellbeing.aspx (accessed 10 July 2015).

NHS England (2015) *A Guide to Community-centred Approaches for Health and Wellbeing*, London: Public Health England.

Nielsen, T.S. and Hansen, K.B. (2007) Do green areas affect health? Results from a Danish survey on the use of green areas and health indicators, *Health & Place* 13 (4): 839–850.

Phelps, A., Lauderdale, K., Alcorn, S., Dillinger, J., Balboni, M., Van Wert, M., Vanderweele, T. and Balboni, T. (2012) Addressing spirituality within the care of patients at the end of life: perspectives of patients with advanced cancer, oncologists, and oncology nurses, *Journal of Clinical Oncology*, 30 (20): 2538–2544.

Reese, R. and Myers, J. (2012) Ecowellness: the missing factor in holistic wellness models, *Journal of Counseling and Development*, 90 (3): 400–406.

Roehlkepartain, E., King, P., Wagener, L. and Benson, P. (2005) *The Handbook of Spiritual Development in Childhood and Adolescence*, London: Sage Publications.

Smith, K. and Akbar, S. (2012) Health-damaging air pollution: a matter of scale, in McGranahan, G. and Murray, F. (eds). *Air Pollution and Health in Rapidly Developing Countries*. London: Earthscan Publications Limited: 21–33.

Sport England (2015) *This Girl Can,* Online. Available at www.sportengland.org/our-work/national-work/this-girl-can/ (accessed 10 July 2015).

The National Institute for Play (2015) *Science and Human Play,* Online. Available at www.nifplay.org/science/overview/ (accessed 9 July 2015).

The New York Times (2013) *Looking for a Lesson in Google's Perks,* Online. Available at www.nytimes.com/2013/03/16/business/at-google-a-place-to-work-and-play.html ?_r=0 (accessed 10 July 2015).

Time to Change (2008a) *Speak Out!* Online. Available at www.time-to-change.org.uk/speakout (accessed July 10 2015).

Time to Change (2008b) *Guides and Toolkits.* Online. Available at www.time-to-change.org.uk/resources/guides-toolkits (accessed 10 July 2015).

Together for Short Lives (2012) *A Guide to End of Life Care. Care of Children and Young People before Death, at the Time of Death and After Death,* Bristol: Together for Short Lives.

Uttley, L., Stevenson, M., Scope, A., Rawdin, A. and Sutton, A. (2015) The clinical and cost effectiveness of group art therapy for people with non-psychotic mental health disorders: a systematic review and cost-effectiveness analysis. *BMC Psychiatry,* 7 (15): 151.

White, M., Smith, A., Humphryes, K., Pahl, S., Snelling, D. and Depledge, M. (2010) Blue space: the importance of water for preference, affect, and restorativeness ratings of natural and built scenes, *Journal of Environmental Psychology,* 30 (4): 482–493.

Zisook, S., and Shear, K. (2009). Grief and bereavement: what psychiatrists need to know, *World Psychiatry,* 8 (2): 67–74.

6

USING PLAY AS A MEANS TO WIDEN ACCESS TO HEALTH AND WELLBEING

Julia Whitaker and Claire Weldon

This chapter will explore how play may be used when individual differences make access to services problematic. It will discuss the use of play as a communication and therapeutic tool for adults who may have different needs, such as a learning difficulties, autism or dementia.

Introduction

We take for granted that the expectation of a healthy life is no longer the preserve of the young or the rich. Ethical healthcare practice demands 'the highest attainable standard of health as a fundamental right of every human being' (World Health Organization 2015). What this means in actuality, depends on how health is defined.

The World Health Organization (2003) defines health as 'a state of complete physical, mental and social wellbeing and not merely the absence of disease or infirmity' but this definition has not been amended since 1948. Huber *et al.* (2011) have critiqued this definition as no longer fit for purpose due to the rise in chronic health problems and they shift the emphasis towards the idea of health as represented by the capacity for adaptation and self-management in the face of social, physical, and emotional challenge. The holistic nature of health is discussed in more detail in Chapter 5. Healthful adaptation is a concept that applies as much to societies and their structures as it does to populations.

The inception of a National Health Service in 1948 made healthcare services in Britain accessible to all regardless of social or economic status; this remains a commonly held ideal, despite the changing tides of social and economic policy. A global economic recession and the accompanying austerity measures which have characterized the opening decades of the twenty-first century have highlighted the need for adaptation and change in the delivery of healthcare services, with greater emphasis being placed on prevention and early intervention. A growing awareness of the potential health-impact of lifestyle changes (such as improvements to diet and exercise levels) and of greater access to green spaces has paved the way for an exploration of an increasing range of alternative, low-cost, low-impact options for reducing health differentials in the population at large. These include options which traditionally reside in the fields of play and recreation.

According to the United Nations (2015), 'experience and scientific evidence show that regular participation in appropriate physical activity and sport provides people of both sexes and all ages and conditions, including persons with disabilities, with a wide range of physical, social and mental health benefits'. The National Leisure and Culture Forum also acknowledges that, 'there is a vital role for culture and leisure to play in improving the health and wellbeing of local communities' (Chief Cultural and Leisure Officers Association 2014). Outdoor play and recreation are further recognized as serving preventive and protective functions, in some cases in preference to medication: 'In addition, faced with rising costs of medication for some conditions such as Attention Disorder Hyperactivity Syndrome (ADHD), the use of green spaces might also be considered within the range of potential treatment options' (Faculty of Public Health and Natural England 2010).

A primary consideration in the discussion of access to health initiatives and the promotion of health and wellbeing throughout the lifespan, is the means by which health information is communicated to service-users and the strategies deployed to engage target groups. Health literacy as a prerequisite of good communication is covered in Chapter 14. The present chapter explores the role of play and playfulness as a communication and therapeutic tool with adults for whom access to services presents a particular challenge – including those with cognitive, social or sensory impairments. The second half of the chapter presents evidence from two contrasting wellbeing initiatives that are using play as a communication and engagement strategy to widen access to services and the attainment of health improvement outcomes.

The challenge of communication

Government statistics suggest that there are almost 11 million disabled individuals in the UK (gov.uk n.d.). This total includes 700,000 people – or more than 1 per cent of the UK population – identified as having autism (The National Autistic Society 2015a) and an estimated 850,000 people living with dementia in the UK in 2015 (Alzheimer's Society 2015).

The Equality Act 2010 (legislation.gov.uk n.d.) states that service providers have a duty to make reasonable adjustments to the delivery of services in order to accommodate the needs of the whole population, regardless of ability. The challenge for healthcare providers and practitioners is to identify the areas of difficulty specific to those with additional access and communication needs and to find effective and efficient means of addressing these areas of additional need.

The concept of 'capacity' is a significant consideration in any discussion of what constitutes the achievement of effective communication between the healthcare professional and the service-user. In order for an individual to play an active part in their engagement with services, they need to be in a position to participate in the healthcare interaction, to understand its implications and to communicate their thoughts and wishes with regard to outcomes. Even when an individual is deemed to lack capacity to make independent decisions regarding their healthcare options, the health professional has a moral duty to make a reasonable attempt to convey relevant information in an accessible manner and to find alternative ways to create and maintain a meaningful relationship.

It is widely accepted that communication involves much more than the verbal language used. Hogan and Stubbs (2003) re-state the popular opinion that at least two-thirds of the communication between individuals is non-verbal. Para-language (volume, pitch and tone), posture, gestures, environment and emotional tagging all have greater impact on the value attached to a communication than the words used. Health service-users with restricted expressive and/or receptive verbal language will be even more reliant on these non-verbal elements of an interaction. A report by the Scottish Executive in 2007 found that healthcare services in Scotland persistently failed to meet the needs of those with additional communication needs and that poor communication between healthcare staff and service-users was compromising diagnosis and effective treatment (Scottish Executive 2007).

Evidence suggests that a high proportion of those with hearing impairment, for example, have difficulty effectively accessing healthcare services and that their health is consequently poorer than that of other groups. 'Twenty per cent of the people who went alone had a problem knowing when it was their turn to see the GP, usually because they missed their name being called out' (Reeves *et al.* 2004). According to a study on 'deaf health' by Kyle *et al.* (2013), there were 'major concerns about the state of deaf people's health. Our health assessments carried out on a typical sample of deaf adults in the UK showed significantly higher rates than in the general population of obesity, and hypertension'. Whilst methods such as providing information in written form or using sign language interpretation can be helpful, hearing impaired service-users may still not fully understand the outcome of a consultation or have difficulty communicating questions and concerns, despite the availability of this additional support. According to Ringham (2012), '41% of respondents have left a health appointment feeling confused about their medical condition because they couldn't understand the sign language interpreter'.

The use of new technology (text-phone systems, email and social media) may be deployed to enable some patients to communicate their thoughts and questions without the need for an interpreter. This affords greater privacy as 'deaf people will determine whether or not to use an interpreter based on their decision on whether the matter will be confidential, private or even personal … if the content of that strays into the private or personal area, the deaf person will be very uncomfortable' (Kyle *et al.* 2013).

Interface with health services is widely associated with feelings of anxiety (Anxiety Care UK 2015). The surrender of control to professional experts, coupled with personal investment in high expectations, can be incapacitating. An awareness of one's own vulnerability and of the reality of personal mortality are widely experienced concomitants of a healthcare interaction or medical diagnosis, and anxiety can disempower even a normally confident communicator. When a patient has a pre-existing intellectual, sensory or social disability, the experience of anxiety and confusion can be overwhelming. Moyle (2008) comments that 'the hospital environment produces multiple and competing stimuli that can be unsettling for people who have impaired cognition'. It has been shown that people with dementia have identified psychological and emotional barriers that inhibit their ability to cope in unfamiliar settings, with over 66 per cent of 500 people surveyed citing a lack of confidence, as well as anxiety about becoming confused, as significant barriers to their participation (Green and Lakey 2013). These effects are likely to be increased when accessing healthcare services, leading to additional stress and vulnerability and a reluctance to engage with the help available. The nervousness characterized by so-called 'white coat syndrome' (Swan 2010) may result in false clinical readings and inaccurate symptom reporting with consequent time and cost implications due to repeated testing and ineffectual interventions.

There is an argument to be made that, in an era dominated by the use of electronic media, many different user groups may find the anonymity of virtual communication a preferable option. A study by Kummervold *et al.* (2002) found that a majority of those using online mental health forums found it easier to discuss personal problems online than face-to-face and almost half said that they discuss problems online that they would not raise in a face-to-face consultation. Tim Kelsey, National Director for Patients and Information in the National Health Service is quoted as saying,

> The fact that those most in need of NHS services are those least likely to have the skills they need to access online services is something that needs to be addressed urgently. The internet can be a powerful leveller in ensuring everyone can access the services that they need, but we need to invest in supporting those who don't have the skills.
>
> *(NHS England 2015)*

Staff awareness of the communication challenges faced by those with additional access needs is an essential precursor to the provision of services that are supportive of, and responsive to, individual differences. Continuity of care has been described as an essential feature of patient-centred healthcare practice in England. The National Institute for Health and Care Excellence (NICE 2012) state that, 'continuity and consistency of care and establishing trusting, empathetic and reliable relationships with competent and insightful healthcare professionals is key to patients receiving effective, appropriate care'. Generally, relationship continuity is highly valued by both patients and healthcare professionals and the evidence indicates that it leads to more satisfied patients and staff, reduced costs and better health outcomes (Freeman and Hughes 2010).

Pre-assessment visits are regularly offered to patients in advance of a planned hospital admission. These visits, designed with the aim of reducing the time spent in hospital by carrying-out certain clinical tests prior to admission, also serve as an introduction to the hospital environment and allow an opportunity for the patient to ask any questions they may have and to clarify what might be expected. Information is usually provided in a verbal or written format unsuited to those with sensory, intellectual or social impairments but the pre-assessment context is one in which creative alternatives to preparation for hospital and clinical interventions might reasonably be explored.

Using play as an alternative to reliance on verbal communication as a means of conveying health-related information to children and young people, is now considered to be the norm in many pediatric healthcare settings (National Association of Health Play Specialists 2012). It has been shown that many of the play-based strategies used in pediatric healthcare have potential or actual applicability with other user groups for whom a traditional oral approach is unhelpful or inadequate (Majzun 2011). When processes and procedures can be helpfully and successfully explained through a play-based intervention, co-operation is increased, as is the quality of the patient/health-giver experience, with consequent positive impact on healthcare outcomes. Play can be used to circumvent the thinking process by using feelings and behaviors as routes to mutual understanding. Health Play Specialists use a variety of tools to help prepare young patients for a hospital admission or course of treatment. Photo-books and the use of real medical equipment will usually convey more meaning than a descriptive account alone, as will environmental familiarization through sensory tours of specific departments of a hospital. These allow the patient to experience at first hand the sights, smells, sounds and feelings that go to make up the actual patient experience. There is now widespread availability of computer software (Diversionary Therapy Technologies 2015) to support the preparation process in addition to the traditionally used play props such as dolls and models.

Social Stories and Comic-strip Conversations are communication tools developed by Carol Gray (2010) in the 1990s to help people with autism to achieve an effective understanding of social situations and are increasingly used in the healthcare context for patients who experience difficulties with communication (Autism Speaks n.d.). The aim of Social Stories is to convey information about what to expect from a situation through the use of a process description of an event or activity. Comic-strip Conversations develop this idea in the form of a visual representation of a conversation and may include the things people might say as well as their intended meanings and emotional interpretations. The comic-strip format uses symbols and stick-figure drawings and can be customized to different contexts and specific areas of difficulty. Both of these strategies can be effective in communicating an understanding of the more complicated features of a social interaction, such as a healthcare consultation, which those with social or cognitive disabilities may find difficult to understand (The National Autistic Society 2015b).

Storyboards, a similar concept to Social Stories, are pictorial representations that provide the user with a detailed view of a process to be undertaken. At the Sussex Cancer Centre in the UK, these are being used for patients with dementia to describe and explain the course of a treatment journey. Storyboards may helpfully include images of the patient at each stage of a course of treatment in an attempt to personalize the experience and assist with sequencing. Complex clinical procedures can be made more manageable by breaking them down into their component parts and visual schedules such as Comic-strip Conversations, storyboards and picture cards can assist information-processing for those who have difficulty understanding verbal language or staying focused on a task through to its completion. Visual strategies can help to encourage independence as well as reducing the potential anxiety which arises from confusion and misunderstanding (Picture Exchange Communication System 2015).

There is a growing evidence base that shows how the nature of the healthcare environment can impact on the quality of the patient experience (Ulrich 2001). Lighting, sound and interior design can have significant effects on both the accessibility of the environment and the patient response to it and simple modifications can be relatively easily achieved. The use of contrasting colors to highlight key features facilitates spatial orientation and may help individuals to use the facilities more safely and easily (Boex n.d.). 'Good lighting can make the most of people's capabilities and help to compensate for poor eyesight; it can assist people in finding their way around both new and familiar spaces and help them to undertake specific tasks.' (Building Better Healthcare 2014). The implications of the design of the healthcare environment on healthcare outcomes is discussed in Chapter 18.

Two contrasting approaches to engagement and communication

There follow two examples of health and social care projects which have faced the challenge of effective engagement and communication with individuals with different access needs.

Orwell Arts (2015), part of the wider Garvald Edinburgh community and based on the teachings of Rudolf Steiner, uses the creative arts along with therapeutic participation in the core activities of daily living, to engage and enliven the wellbeing of individuals with learning difficulties. Combining an appreciation of the value of play-enriched interactions with the need to satisfy the outcome-driven demands of its funding partners, Garvald's social therapy approach (Garvald Edinburgh 2003) has shown that the two need not be mutually exclusive.

In contrast, Lego-based therapy is a systematic model for engaging and working with young people with autism, focusing on a specific skill set and utilizing existing enthusiasms as a point of both engagement and behavioral change.

Orwell Arts, Edinburgh

A humanistic paradigm of health is characterized by the notion that a healthy life may be regarded as a process of self-actualization, of being able to cope and adapt to different circumstances and to fulfil personal and group potential. Seedhouse (2001) describes health as 'the foundations of achievement' and an optimum state of health as being 'equivalent to the set of conditions that enables a person to work to fulfil her realistic chosen and biological potentials' (Seedhouse 2001: 61).

Social therapy is the term used to describe an approach to wellness which recognizes the social nature of experience and places value on the healing that takes place within a community context. The social therapy approach practiced by Garvald Edinburgh is a living example of a humanistic model which is also mindful of the spiritual aspect of humanity. Anthroposophy, the theoretical approach of Rudolf Steiner (1861–1925), and its practical application in the Camphill movement founded by Karl Konig (1902–1966), inform Garvald's holistic approach to living and working in community with people with learning disabilities. A central principle of its work is one of respect for the other person, regardless of ability or of any difficulties they may encounter in their social interactions. A recognition of the mutuality inherent in the relationship between staff and service-user is reflected in the use of the term 'member' to describe all those who make up the Garvald community (Garvald Edinburgh 2003). Garvald strives to equip its members to explore the choices and opportunities that make for a full and healthy life; at its heart is the belief that a healthy social environment is essential for all adults, in order that they might live productive, independent, and joyful lives.

The field of positive psychology continues to highlight the link between joyfulness and the corresponding benefits to physical and mental health (Seligman 2002). A joyful life has been described as 'an active embracing of the world' (Davidson *et al.* 2003) and the active co-creation of the physical, social and spiritual conditions within which community can thrive is both the art and the science underlying the Garvald approach.

Acton and Malathum (2000) found that sensory satisfaction and personal approval are key influences on our positive behavioral choices. In all of Garvald's projects, priority is given to the sensory quality of the social environment, with careful attention devoted to the use of color, design and ambience in order to create an aesthetically inspiring living and working space. The creative work of members is celebrated through its use to enhance and enliven the physical environment, whilst at the same time acknowledging the personal investment of individuals in a shared experience of community.

The Natural Environment White Paper (HM Government 2011) recognizes that 'a healthy, properly functioning natural environment' has positive implications for 'prospering communities and personal wellbeing'. Modern life distances many people from the natural sources of the materials and products which add quality and meaning to everyday life (Department of the Environment, Food and Rural Affairs 2011). Like other Steiner-inspired initiatives, Garvald strives to foster an

Using play as a means to widen access to health and wellbeing 77

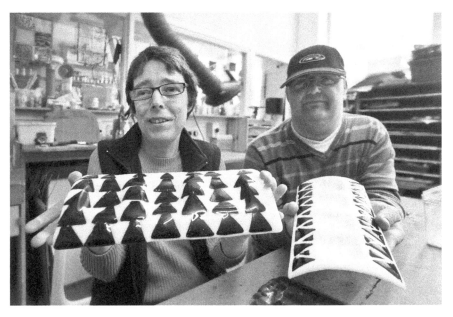

FIGURE 6.1 A feeling of joyfulness arises from the celebration of creative achievement

awareness and appreciation of these sources through the cultivation of a respectful attitude for the natural world; the use of natural materials in their craft projects; the recognition of the significance of good nutrition; and an appreciation of the cyclical nature of life, death and renewal.

Sternberg (2010) has examined the complex relationship between the sensory environment, the emotions and the immune system and makes the link between the health of the environment and personal health. A rich sensory experience can create a link between perceptions and evolving conceptions, revealing the true essence of things and unlocking creative channels to fulfilment (Day and Midbjer 2007). There is a tendency to underestimate the impact of the sensory environment on our sense of wellbeing. Rudolph Steiner enumerated and described twelve human senses (Steiner 1981) and, in an article in the New Scientist, Durie (2005) went even further by identifying a potential twenty-one, suggesting that sensory experience is a more complex process of interrelated perceptions than has previously been assumed.

Chapter 13 offers an insightful account of how the creative arts can be practised and understood as the embodiment of a lived experience of wellbeing. Working actively with the human senses to maximize the potential of its members, Garvald uses a range of sensory experiences as a means to enrich personal experience of life through the awakening of dormant powers of observation, awareness and creativity. Movement, balance, music, speech and listening encourage the development of a broad repertoire of communication options, and immersion in the social life of the

78 Julia Whitaker and Claire Weldon

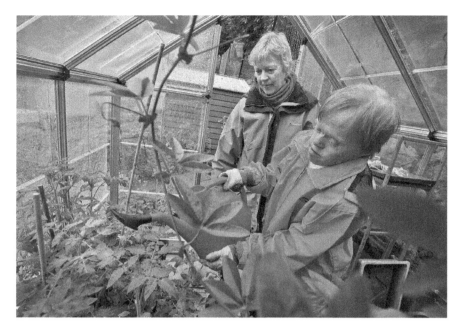

FIGURE 6.2 A respectful attitude for the natural world adds quality and meaning to everyday life

community supports the recognition and affirmation of human individuality. Through participation in art, craft, music, drama and social relationships, Garvald members are helped to find the means of both expressing and communicating their inner worlds and of finding their unique places in the outer world.

Creativity is relevant to all the activities of daily living and without it the daily necessities can become empty and meaningless. When everyday activities are invigorated by a playful attitude of curiosity and enthusiasm, they are endowed with both therapeutic value and a quality of satisfaction. Richman *et al.* (2005) have found that such attitudes of curiosity and hopefulness can also have protective benefits in term of physical health. Knutson (cited in Lemonick 2005) states that a significant component of happiness is having something to look forward to, an observation that is reflected in the following statement by Pam, a current member of the Garvald community:

> I've been at Garvald for thirty years, I absolutely love it! I've done pottery, weaving, the shop, painting, a variety of things, it's fun, it's entertaining, very entertaining. I like going on outings, all sorts of fun, variety is the spice of life, I've got loads of friends, I feel happy, cheerful, very cheerful, full of life and full of action. I like variety you see.
>
> *(Pam Craig 2015)*

The challenge for Garvald Edinburgh, and for other organizations taking a broad view of health and wellbeing, is to achieve correspondence between their holistic approach and the goal-oriented measures of effectiveness demanded by funding partners. Garvald's Social Charter (2003) concludes with an acknowledgement that it is possible for a social therapy project to work in a complementary and co-operative way with other agencies, without needing to compromise its own philosophical underpinning. This is manifest in Garvald's partnership working with the Scottish Government's *Talking Points* program (Cook and Miller 2012). This approach encourages and enables Garvald's members to identify their own personal health and social care outcomes and the help they might need to achieve them, demonstrating that creativity and community can be routes to measurable health improvements in the broadest sense.

Lego-based therapy: play to get well

Moor (2002: 17) states that 'Play and social development go hand in hand – one is a vehicle for the other. Underpinning play is interaction.' The popular Danish construction toy Lego has had widespread appeal among young and old alike since its appearance in 1930. Lego translates from the Danish as 'Play Well' (Whitworth 2009, cited in Andras 2012) but its contemporary use as a therapeutic medium adds a whole other layer of meaning – 'Play to Get Well'. Lego-based therapy (Le Goff 2014) originated in the USA in the 1990s as a means of connecting with children with Autistic Spectrum Disorders (ASD) and has since been adapted as a form of play therapy with young adults as a route to engagement with services, skill development and behavioral change.

Autistic Spectrum Disorder (ASD) is the term commonly used to refer to the group of disorders included in the grouping of 'pervasive developmental disorders' in the International Classification of Diseases (World Health Organization 1992) This social disability is 'characterized by qualitative abnormalities in reciprocal social interactions and in patterns of communication, and by a restricted, stereo-typed, repetitive repertoire of interests and activities' (The National Autistic Society 2015). Individuals with autism exhibit a 'triad of impairments' to social interaction, social communication and social imagination, with implications for the formation of social relationships and collaborative activities such as working as part of a group. These challenges to social communication and integration are fre-quently accompanied by the presence of repetitive or stereotyped behaviors and preoccupations, and a commonly held attraction to processes of a systematic, logical nature.

Lego, itself a highly systematic toy, has particular appeal to certain individuals with autism, the structured nature of the play activity providing both incentive to participation and play satisfaction. People on the autistic spectrum commonly have an appreciation of rule-based, mechanical play in association with highly developed spatial skills (Macintosh and Dissanayake 2006) which lend themselves to Lego construction. The communication style characteristic of those with ASD tends to be pragmatic and purposeful and an activity such as Lego, which derives from a shared interest, has been identified as an effective motivator for communication with others (Dissanyake cited in Kermond 2014). Although autism is often associated with children, it is not confined to childhood and 'children with autism will grow up to be adults with autism' (The National Autistic Society 2015a). This provides a challenge for future healthcare provision, particularly as 33 per cent of adults with autism 'are experiencing severe mental health problems' and 70 per cent of adults with autism report feelings of isolation, mainly due to a lack of support (The National Autistic Society 2015a). Lego is a construction toy with universal appeal and so lends itself to being used as an aid to social communication for both adults and children with ASD.

In 1990, clinical psychologist Daniel Le Goff observed that children with ASD and other similar social communication difficulties were naturally drawn to Lego over other toys and devised a structured methodology by which Lego is used to naturally reinforce socially appropriate behavior (Le Goff 2014). An original study by Owens and LeGoff (2007) discovered that, by allocating specific collaborative and interactive tasks within the context of a Lego-building activity, the resulting interaction promoted the development of new social skills such as shared focus, turn-taking, collaboration, verbal and non-verbal communication and conflict resolution. The shared experience of the Lego play resulted in a greater understanding of others' points of view, an atypical stance for those with ASD. Owens *et al.* (2008) went on to favourably compare Lego-therapy with both an alternative social education program and a control. The subjects of Owens' study engaged with the Lego-therapy because they enjoyed it, with a corresponding improvement in social skills – but it was the enjoyment that was both the motivator and the reward. Lego-therapy has shown how joint focus and role definition might be transferrable to other social settings to exploit naturally playful tendencies to a therapeutic end. For example:

> You can even use the same approach to bake a cake – splitting up the roles, joint focus, etc. But having said that, Lego is extremely versatile. You can be creative but within certain boundaries. There are themes to suit different interests, and then there's the behind the scenes stuff – online clubs to join, video games, stop motion films to be made in groups. It gives children with autism a topic to discuss with peers that is socially acceptable and of interest to others – at least some others!'
>
> *(Gina Gomez cited in Sutton 2012)*

The potential of Lego play has found additional application in both the worlds of business (Lego Serious Play 2015) and clinical research. An experiment carried out by the Lego Learning Institute (Gauntlett *et al.* 2011) suggested that collective building processes may lead to stronger heart-rate synchronization among participants, and greater activity in the social areas of the brain. Norton *et al.* (2011) found that when individuals invest personal effort to create or produce something ('the IKEA effect'), they invest it with more positive attributes and feel a greater emotional attachment to it. Psychologists are re-discovering what children have always known: that the intrinsic qualities of play promote feelings of satisfaction and wellbeing, and that freedom, sociability and physical activity are the crucial components of meaningful play experience (Play England 2008).

Conclusion

Whilst Garvald's holistic approach is concerned with the development of the whole person, Lego-based therapy is designed to address a particular skill set – yet these two conceptually contrasting approaches share a common component: an appreciation of the value of play. At Orwell Arts, members engage with a chosen activity because it has a natural appeal, which is then reinforced and enriched through the social experience in which it is embedded. Lego-based therapy is a playful learning approach which is also based around a shared attraction to a specific set of activities. Both offer an insight into how play is a method of communication in itself, as well as a means to the acquisition of life and health enhancing competencies.

References

Acton, G.J. and Malathum, P. (2000) Basic need status and health-promoting self-care behavior in adults. *Western Journal of Nursing Research*, 22 (7): 796–811.

Alzheimer's Society (2015) *Statistics*, Online. Available at www.alzheimers.org.uk/statistics (accessed 10 April 2015).

Andras, M. (2012) The value of Lego® Therapy in promoting social interaction in primary-aged children with autism, *Good autism practice*, 26 September 2012 Online. Available at www.aettraininghubs.org.uk/wp-content/uploads/2014/06/Lego-therapy-paper.pdf (accessed 14 December 2015).

Anxiety Care UK (2015) *Overcoming Medical Phobias,* Online. Available at www.anxiety care.org.uk/docs/medical.asp (accessed 16 October 2015).

Autism Speaks (n.d.) *A Parent's Guide to Blood Draws for Children with Autism,* Online. Available at www.autismspeaks.org/sites/default/files/documents/atn/blood-draw-parent.pdf (accessed 23 October 2015).

Boex (n.d.) *Dementia Ward*, Online. Available at www.boex.co.uk/project/dementia-ward-design/ (accessed 23 October 2015).

Building Better Healthcare (2014) *How small design interventions can improve the lives of dementia sufferers,* Online. Available at www.buildingbetterhealthcare.co.uk/technical/article_page/How_small_design_interventions_can_improve_the_lives_of_dementia_suf ferers/99727 (accessed 28 October 2015).

Chief Cultural and Leisure Officers Association (2014) *The Role of Culture and Leisure in Improving Health and Wellbeing,* Ipswich: Chief Cultural and Leisure Officers Association on behalf of National Leisure and Culture Forum.

Cook, A. and Miller, E. (2012) *Talking Points: Personal Outcomes Approach,* Edinburgh: Joint Improvement Team Scotland.

Craig, Pam (n.d.) personal communication.

Davidson, R., Kabat-Zinn, J., Schumacher, J., Rosenkranz, M., Muller, D., Santorelli, S.F., Urbanowski, F., Harrington, A., Bonus, K. and Sheridan, J.F. (2003) Alterations in brain and immune function produced by mindfulness meditation, *Psychosomatic Medicine,* 65 (4): 564–570.

Day, C. and Midbjer, A. (2007) *Environment and Children: Passive Lessons from the Everyday Environment,* London: Routledge.

Department of the Environment, Food and Rural Affairs (2011) *The Natural Choice: securing the value of nature' by Secretary of State for Environment, Food and Rural Affairs,* London: DEFRA.

Diversionary Therapy Technologies (2015) *Diversionary Therapy Technologies: Ditto,* Online. Available at http://dtt.net.au/ (accessed 23 October 2015).

Durie, B. (2005) Senses Special: Doors of Perception, *New Scientist,* 26 January 2005 Online. Available at www.newscientist.com/article/mg18524841.600-senses-special-doors-of-perception.html (accessed 20 May 2015).

Faculty of Public Health and Natural England (2010) *Great Outdoors: How Our Natural Health Service Uses Green Space To Improve Wellbeing: Briefing Statement,* London: Faculty of Public Health and Natural England.

Freeman, G. and Hughes, J. (2010) *Continuity of Care and Patient Experience,* London: The King's Fund.

Garvald Edinburgh (2003) *Principles of Social Therapy as a Basis for Our Work: a Charter for Quality.* Online. Available at www.garvaldedinburgh.org.uk/wp-content/.../Social-Therapy-Charter.do (accessed 16 October 2015).

Gauntlett, D., Ackermann, E., Whitebread, D., Wolbers, T. and Weckstrom, C. (2011) *The Future of Play: Defining the role and value of play in the 21st century,* Billund: LEGO Institute.

Gov.uk (n.d.) *Disability Prevalence Statistics 2011/2012,* Online. Available at www.gov.uk/government/uploads/system/uploads/attachment_data/file/321594/disability-prevalence.pdf. (accessed 10 April 2015).

Gray, C. (2010) *The New Social Stories Book,* Arlington TX: Future Horizons.

Green and Lakey (2013) *Building Dementia-friendly Communities: A Priority for Everyone,* London: Alzheimer's Society.

HM Government (2011) *The Natural Choice: Securing the Value of Nature.* Norwich: The Stationery Office.

Hogan, K. and Stubbs, R. (2003) *Can't Get Through. Eight Barriers to Communication.* Gretna, LA: Pelican.

Huber, M., Knottnerus, J. A., Green, L., Horst, H., van der Jadad, A. R. and Kromhout D., Leonard, B., Lorig, K., Loureiro, M.I., van der Meer, J.W., Schnabel, P., Smith, R., van Weel, C. and Smid, H. (2011) How should we define health? *The British Medical Journal,* 343: d4163.

Kermond, C. (2014) *Fairfield Lego Club Inside the Brick Helps Children with Autism to Build Bridges,* Online. Available at www.essentialkids.com.au/development-advice/special-needs/fairfield-lego-club-inside-the-brick-helps-children-with-autism-to-build-bridges-20140224-33c4g (accessed 25 October 2015).

Kummervold, P. E., Gammon, D., Bergvik, S., Johnsen, J-AK., Hasvold, T. and Rosenvinge, J. H. (2002) Social support in a wired world: use of online mental health forums in Norway. *Nordic Journal of Psychiatry,* 56 (1): 59–65.

Kyle, J., Sutherland, H., Allsop, L., Ridd, M. and Emond, A. (2013) *Deaf Health. Analysis of the Current Health and Access to Health Care of Deaf People in the UK. Executive Summary, Deaf Health: A UK Collaborative Study into the Health of Deaf People,* Bristol: Centre for Deaf Studies and School of Social and Community Medicine at University of Bristol and Deaf Studies Trust.

Using play as a means to widen access to health and wellbeing **83**

legislation.gov.uk (n.d.) *Equality Act (2010),* Online. Available at www.legislation.gov.uk/ukpga/2010/15/contents (accessed 14 December 2015).

Le Goff, D. (2014) *LEGO-based Therapy,* London: Jessica Kingsley.

Lemonick, M. D. (2005) Health: The Biology of Joy. *Time Magazine,* Sunday 09 January 2005 Online. Available at www. time.com (accessed 22 February 2016).

Macintosh, K. and Dissanayake, C. (2006) Social skills and problem behaviours in school aged children with high-functioning autism and Asperger's disorder, *Journal of Autism and Developmental Disorders,* 36 (8): 1065–1076.

Majzun, R. (2011) Coloring outside the lines: what pediatric hospitals can teach adult hospitals, *Pediatric Nursing,* 37 (4): 210–211.

Moor, J (2002) *Playing, Laughing and Learning with Children on the Autistic Spectrum: A practical Resource of Play Ideas for Parents and Carers,* London: Jessica Kingsley.

Moyle, W., Olorenshaw, R., Wallis, M. and Borbasi, S. (2008) Best practice for the management of older people with dementia in the acute care setting: a review of the literature. *International Journal of Older People Nursing,* 3 (2): 121–130.

National Association of Health Play Specialists (2012) National Association of Health Play Specialists, Online. Available at www.nahps.org.uk/ (accessed 23 October 2015).

National Autistic Society (The) (2015a) *Myths, Facts and Statistics,* Online. Available at www.autism.org.uk/about/what-is/myths-facts-stats.aspx (accessed 14 December 2015).

National Autistic Society (The) (2015b) *Social Stories and Comic Strip Conversations,* Online. Available at www.autism.org.uk/living-with-autism/strategies-and-approaches/social-stories-and-comic-strip-conversations.aspx (accessed 23 October 2015).

NHS Choices (2015) *Consent to treatment – Capacity,* Online. Available at www.nhs.uk/Conditions/Consent-to-treatment/Pages/Capacity.aspx. (accessed 10 April 2015).

NHS England (2015) *Up to 100,000 People use the Internet to Improve their Health,* Online. Available at www.england.nhs.uk/2013/03/13/internet-health/ (accessed 16 October 2015).

National Institute for Health and Care Excellence (2012) *Patient Experience in Adult NHS Services: Improving the Experience of Care for People Using Adult NHS Services,* Online. Available at www.nice.org.uk/guidance/cg138/chapter/guidance (accessed 16 October 2015).

Norton, M.I., Mochon, D. and Ariely, D. (2011) The IKEA effect: when labor leads to love. *Journal of Consumer Psychology,* 22 (3): 453–460.

Owens, G., Granader, Y., Humphrey, A. and Baron- Cohen, S. (2008) LEGO therapy and the social use of language programme: an evaluation of two social skills Interventions for children with high functioning autism and Asperger syndrome, *Journal of Autism Developmental Disorders,* 38 (10): 1944–1957.

Owens, G. and LeGoff, D. (2007) *A Manual for the Implementation of Lego- Based Social Development Therapy for Children with Autism Spectrum Disorders.*

Picture Exchange Communication System. Online. Available at www.pecsusa.com/pecs.php (accessed 23 October 2015).

Play England (2008) *Fun and Freedom. What Children Say about Play in a Sample of Play Strategy Consultations.* Online. Available at www.playengland.org.uk/media/120429/fun-freedom-11-million-fair-play.pdf (accessed 3 June 2015).

Reeves, D., Kokoruwe, B., Dobbins, J. and Newton, V. (2004) *Access to Health Services for Deaf People,* Manchester: National Primary Care Research and Development Centre.

Richman, L.S., Kubzansky, L., Maselko, J., Kawachi, I., Choo, P. and Bauer, M. (2005) Positive emotion and health: going beyond the negative, *Health Psychology,* 24 (4): 422–429.

Ringham, L. (2012) *Access all Areas? A Report into the Experiences of People with Hearing Loss When Accessing Healthcare,* London: Action on Hearing Loss.

Scottish Executive (2007) *Communication Support Needs: a Review of the Literature,* Online. Available at www.qmu.ac.uk/casl/pubs/communication_support_needs_lit_review_2007.pdf (accessed 20 May 2015).

Seedhouse, D. (2001) *Health: The Foundations for Achievement,* Chichester: Wiley.

Seligman, M. (2012) *Authentic Happiness: Using the New Positive Psychology to Realize your Potential for Lasting Fulfilment,* New York: Free Press.

Steiner, R. (1981) Man's twelve senses in their relation to imagination, inspiration, intuition. *Anthroposophical Review,*3 (2): 1981 (UK). Online. Available at www.waldorflibrary.org/images/stories/articles/twelvesenses.pdf (accessed 14 December 2015).

Sternberg, E. (2010) *Healing Spaces: The Science of Place and Well-Being,* Cambridge MA: Belknap Press.

Sutton, J. (2012) *When Psychologists Become Builders,* Online. Available at https://thepsychologist.bps.org.uk/volume-25/edition-8/when-psychologists-become-builders (accessed 20 May 2015).

Swan, N. (2010). *Health Minutes – Hypertension,* Online. Available at www.youtube.com/watch (accessed 16 October 2015).

Ulrich, R.S. (2001) Effects of healthcare environmental design on medical outcomes, *Design and Health: Proceedings of the Second International Conference on Health and Design.* Stockholm, Sweden: Svensk Byggtjanst: 49–59.

United Nations (2015) *Sport and Health. Preventing Disease and Promoting Health,* Online. Available at www.un.org/wcm/webdav/site/sport/shared/sport/SDP%20IWG/Chapter 2_SportandHealth.pdf (accessed 10 April 2015).

World Health Organization (1992) *International Classification of Diseases,* 10th ed., Geneva: WHO.

World Health Organization (2003) *WHO Definition of Health,* Online. Available at www.who.int/about/definition/en/print.html (accessed 10 April 2015).

World Health Organization (2015) *The Right to Health. Fact Sheet 323,* Online. Available at www.who.int/mediacentre/factsheets/fs323/en/ (accessed 10 April 2015).

7

LIFESTYLE TRENDS AND THEIR IMPACT ON HEALTH

Claire Weldon, Denise Baylis and Alison Tonkin

This chapter will examine current lifestyle concerns arising from the increasingly sedentary patterns of behavior which have led to chronic health conditions such as obesity, type 2 diabetes and coronary heart disease. Concerns relating to sexual health across the age range are explored, along with substance abuse and the increasing problem of alcohol consumption. The chapter concludes by exploring a variety of play and recreational activities that can help to develop, maintain or recover health and wellbeing. This is neatly summarized by Biller (2002: 11) who states that: – 'whatever your age, regular participation in playful pursuits increase the likelihood of health, vigour and happiness'.

Introduction

According to The Kings Fund (2015), around 15 million people in England have a long-term health condition or chronic disease. These are defined as conditions that currently have no cure and are managed using medication or other forms of treatment (The Kings Fund 2015). The most common long-term conditions include hypertension, depression and asthma, as well as musculoskeletal conditions (Department of Health Long Term Conditions Team 2012).

The prevalence of long-term conditions varies with age and socio-economic status; older people and those belonging to the more deprived groups are more likely to be at risk. Chronic illness is known to follow the social gradient (Marmot 2010) with people in the lower socio-economic classes having a 60 per cent higher chance of prevalence than their richer counterparts, and that disease is also likely to be more than 30 per cent more severe (The Kings Fund 2015). Play and recreation can offer a flexible and cost-effective strategy to counter the adverse effects of modern day living and, as stated by Stitchlinks (2015a) 'there is something vitally important about being actively creative as opposed to being a

86 Claire Weldon, Denise Baylis and Alison Tonkin

passive recipient of a destructive force you feel you have no control over, such as stress, depression or pain'.

Chronic health conditions and illnesses

Some of the most common conditions will be briefly described, with suggested play-based strategies that may help to address the rising tide of lifestyle-related illness and disease in the early part of the twenty-first century.

Obesity

Obesity is known to 'impair health' and levels of obesity have been rising in the UK since the 1980s (WHO 2015). It is estimated that approximately 40 per cent of the UK population will be obese by 2030, with an estimated excess spend of £1.9 billion in healthcare costs (Patterson *et al.* 2014). Obesity leads to a wide range of medical problems and not only has an impact on the individual but on society as a whole, due to the social and financial pressures associated with the condition. The causes of obesity are multi-factorial, including genetics, how the body metabolizes energy, and lifestyle, leading to health effects such as high blood pressure, diabetes, heart disease, joint problems, sleep apnoea, a variety of cancers, metabolic syndrome and psychosocial problems (Stanford Health Care 2015).

According to Biller (2002: 9) 'whatever your genetic endowment and previous experiences … regardless of your age, gender or predispositions, you can play your way into better shape'. Biller (2002) suggests there are five 'interrelated and inter-acting' steps that can enhance the overall quality of life, which pay particular attention to physical activity and healthier eating patterns. These are:

1 Appreciating your biological identity
2 Understanding your personal potential
3 Enjoying your exercise experience
4 Improving your physical appearance
5 Maximizing your healthy lifestyle (Biller 2002: 10).

Biller (2002) promotes the value of finding enjoyable exercise patterns that suit the individual, which will improve physical functioning and help to ward off debilitating chronic illness. Advocating the 'combination of vigorous play and nutritious eating in disease prevention and longevity' Biller (2002: 10) suggests that 'continuing wellness involves the lifelong pursuit of playful, healthful activity'.

Diabetes

The increased incidence of diabetes is now a global health issue, with 382 million people who are now thought to have the condition (Diabetes.co.uk 2015a) and the

UK is following the global upward trend. There are approximately 3.2 million people in the UK living with diabetes, of which 90 per cent have type 2 diabetes which is directly linked to diet and lifestyle (Diabetes.co.uk 2015a) It is estimated that 7 million people could be at risk of developing diabetes and that, if these trends continue, 5 million people in the UK will have diabetes by 2025 (Diabetes UK 2013). According to Diabetes UK (2015a) type 2 diabetes usually appears in people over the age of 40 and is treated with a combination of a healthy balanced diet, increased physical activity and the use of medication, if required. There is an indication of problematic management of the condition in older people living in residential care as 'older people in care homes are often more likely to be under-weight than overweight and there is a high rate of undernutrition' (Diabetes UK, 2015b) which can be caused by irregular eating patterns, the side effects of medication and dehydration.

Sport and physical activity are considered important to the maintenance of a healthy lifestyle, but, in the case of diabetes, this can be problematic, especially for people with type 1 diabetes (Diabetes.co.uk 2015b). Monitoring blood-glucose levels is an essential part of the self-management process for people with type 1 diabetes, and testing may be required before, during and after exercise (Diabetes.co.uk 2015b). Despite the practical challenges of repeated blood-glucose monitoring, the health benefits of exercise can be significant, with enhanced physical fitness, reduced risk of cardiovascular disease and increased social and emotional wellbeing (Hornsby and Chetlin 2005). For those with type 2 diabetes, the need for physical exercise is similar to that for the general population (Hornsby and Chetlin 2005), and is considered essential for managing the condition.

Strokes

According to the Stroke Association (2013), every year approximately 152,000 people in the UK will suffer a stroke (or cerebrovascular accident), a serious medical condition caused by the interruption of the blood supply to the brain, usually because a blood vessel bursts or is blocked by a clot. Strokes are one of the main causes of severe disability among adults with 1.2 million stroke survivors living in the UK, a third of whom are dependent on others to help with everyday activities (Stroke Association 2013).

Play-based strategies can be particularly effective for people who have suffered strokes and, in the U.S., recreational therapists are considered essential members of the stroke management team. Shearing (2014) states that 'recreational therapy helps stroke survivors return to their favourite pre-stroke activities, whether it's hiking, playing board games, or cooking', which contributes to the rebuilding of physical and psychological skills. Mramor (cited in Shearing 2014) suggests that whilst physical therapy is good for assessing muscle function, recreational therapy focuses on what those muscles may be used for i.e. playing cards, fishing, or whatever the person finds enjoyable. Mramor (cited Shearing 2014) states that 'because

88 Claire Weldon, Denise Baylis and Alison Tonkin

recreation is wellness oriented, we focus on what is possible and what can be attained through active involvement'. Ultimately, involvement in 'purposeful and meaningful activities' will hasten recovery and make life more enjoyable (Shearing 2014).

Coronary heart disease (CHD)

Seventy-three thousand people die each year in the UK from CHD, a narrowing of the small blood vessels that supply blood and oxygen to the heart, making it the UK's biggest killer (BBC Science 2013). 23,000 of the deaths from CHD are of those under the age of 75. Death rates from CHD are higher in the north of England and Scotland, and lowest in the South. More men than women die from CHD and approximately 2.3 million people in the UK are living with this serious medical condition (British Heart Foundation 2015).

Physical exercise that is performed regularly is advocated as a means of reducing the risk factors associated with coronary heart disease. Halhuber and Halhuber (1983: 110) explain that 'as blood pressure is lowered and weight loss is made easier, the fat levels are also normalized'. However, the main message from Halhuber and Halhuber (1983) is addressed to those who have suffered a heart attack, the message being that exercise must be fun. For these patients, the benefits of exercise are as much psychological as physical, particularly in relation to self-confidence. Prevailing fears after a heart attack call for a sensitive approach and the need to ensure that any exercise undertaken is for fun, rather than competition, is a serious message that demands attention: 'patients who tend to be over-achievers must be made aware of the playful nature of exercise, because they should not be forcing themselves, or gritting the teeth to get exercising done' (Halhuber and Halhuber 1983: 110).

Dementia

The number of people with dementia is increasing worldwide, with countries such as China, India and Sub-Saharan Africa predicted to see an increase in the number of cases diagnosed (Alzheimer's Research UK 2015b). In Europe, it is estimated that by 2050 there will be 21 million people with dementia, which represents a rise from 11 million in 2013. In the UK, 1.3 per cent of the UK population have dementia, equating to 850,000 people (Alzheimer's Research UK 2015a). However, diagnosis rates are hugely variable with less than half of those living with dementia having a confirmed diagnosis (Alzheimer's Research UK 2015c). Alzheimer's Research UK (2015c) supports research into the causes and prevention of dementia, stating that 'there is growing evidence indicating that certain medical conditions – such as high blood pressure, diabetes and obesity – may increase the risk of dementia, whereas a healthy lifestyle may reduce the risk'.

Play and playfulness have much to offer as preventative strategies against dementia. Smith *et al.* (2015) describe the six pillars of Alzheimer's prevention, all of which are within the individual's sphere of influence:

1 Regular exercise
2 Healthy diet
3 Mental stimulation
4 Quality sleep
5 Stress management
6 An active social life

Mental stimulation provides plenty of scope for play, with activities such as enjoying puzzles, riddles, crosswords, strategy games, board games and card games to name just a few … and the benefits will be enhanced if done as a social activity with other people (Smith *et al.* 2015).

Lifestyle factors detrimental to health

This next section looks at specific lifestyle factors that have serious implications for the health of the individual.

Alcohol

According to Alcohol Concern (2015), more than '9 million people in England drink more than the recommended daily limits' of alcohol, with 34 per cent of men and 28 per cent of women drinking more than the recommended levels. There are also variations according to age, with older people drinking more frequently than younger people, although 'younger people tend to drink more heavily on a single occasion than older people' (Alcohol Concern 2015). Wadd *et al.* (2011) warn that 'the UK may be on the cusp of an epidemic of alcohol-related harm amongst older people', with an estimated 1.4 million people over the age of 65 currently exceeding recommended drinking limits. Between 2002 and 2010 there was a marked increase in alcohol-related hospital admissions across all age groups, but the increase was greatest for older people: for men aged 65 and over, admissions rose by 136 per cent, and for women in this age group by 132 per cent. In 2010, there were almost half a million alcohol-related admissions for those aged 65 and over, meaning that they accounted for 44 per cent of overall admissions, despite comprising just 17 per cent of the population.

Alcohol abuse problems have been categorized as either of 'early-onset' or 'late-onset'. It has been estimated that two-thirds of older people with alcohol problems fall into the 'early-onset' category – people who have a long history of alcohol misuse. Alcohol problems among those in the 'late-onset' category may begin as a result of a stressful life event such as retirement, marital breakdown, bereavement, social isolation or loneliness (DrugScope n.d.).

Physical problems associated with alcohol use include coronary heart disease, hypertension and strokes; gastrointestinal problems; liver problems, including cirrhosis, and cancer of the liver, oesophagus and colon. Mental health problems such as depression and cognitive impairment, which are common in older people, may also be linked to alcohol misuse. Substance abuse can also be associated with falls in the elderly and may exacerbate incontinence problems (Royal College of Psychiatrists 2011).

Wadd *et al.* (2011 cited in DrugScope n.d.) identify a range of professional attitudes that can hinder access to help. These include a lack of awareness of potential problems amongst the older age-group, an inability to identify the signs and symptoms of alcohol problems, which can be mistaken for age-related behavior changes, embarrassment about discussing potential problems with an older person, or thinking that the individual should not be deprived of their 'last pleasure in life' or are too old to change their behavior.

The importance of reducing alcohol intake is highlighted on the NHS Change4Life website which suggests:

> If you cut out a couple of large glasses of wine a week, that could be more than £400 a year you've got to spend on other things. Why not save up and treat yourself? You could get a manicure with a friend, see some sport with your mates, or even treat the family to a meal out.
>
> *(Change 4 Life 2015)*

The increase in alcohol consumption by women is a particular cause for concern, and Ian Ball 'was asked to come up with a short animation aimed at middle-aged habitual drinkers… like Brenda!' (Albinal 2009a). Using humor to convey a serious health message, the video shows how a few units of alcohol consumed every day soon add-up, and highlights some of the health conditions that can arise as a result of excessive alcohol consumption. In a short three-minute video, information is presented in a fun and engaging way, using 'Brenda's booze-o-meter to tot up the units of alcohol consumed, ending with a note of caution – humans do not have a "liver liberator" and therefore, minimising "detrimental drinking" means we need to be "sensible when we're on the sauce"' (Albinal 2009b).

Substance misuse

The 2014/15 Crime Survey for England and Wales shows that young people are the most likely to take illegal drugs, with 19.8 per cent of 20 to 24 years olds taking drugs compared to 2.4 per cent of 55 to 59 year olds (Home Office 2015). In the last year, approximately 8.6 per cent of adults between 16 and 59 are reported to have taken an illegal drug with 2.2 per cent of adults classed as frequent drug users (Home Office 2015).

In a 2011 report entitled *Our Invisible Addicts*, The Royal College of Psychiatrists (2011) highlighted that 'the proportion of older people in the population is increasing rapidly, as is the number of older people with substance use problems'. It is estimated that in Europe the number of older people with substance use problems or requiring treatment for substance misuse will more than double between 2001 and 2020 (European Monitoring Centre for Drugs and Drug Addiction 2008).

A National Treatment Agency (2011) report *Addiction to Medicines* highlighted that in 2009–10, 16 per cent (32,510) of people using drug treatment services reported addiction problems related to the use of prescribed and/or 'Over-the-Counter' medications. Two per cent of this group reported this as their primary problem and 14 per cent reported it as a problem that they have in addition to a dependency on illicit drugs (National Treatment Agency 2011). The Royal College of Psychiatrists has noted that, whilst older men are at greater risk of developing alcohol and illicit substance use problems than older women, 'older women have a higher risk of developing problems related to the misuse of prescribed and over-the-counter medications' (Royal College of Psychiatrists 2011). This is exacerbated 'because of physiological changes associated with aging, older people are at increased risk of adverse physical effects of substance misuse, even at relatively modest levels of intake' (Wadd *et al.* 2011).

Faulkner (1991, cited Keesmaat n.d.) suggests that 'Alcohol/drug addiction is a leisure disease and a disease of leisure! People pay for the feeling because they don't know how to get it for free. That is, they don't know how to play in a manner that produces the desired feeling'. Keesmaat (n.d.) proposes that leisure is also the way to a healthy recovery, providing a context for re-establishing family bonds and having fun at the same time. Therapeutic recreation in the early stages of recovery, especially in the form of social interaction, can provide a support mechanism at a difficult time. Combining a program of physical activity with recreational activity and purposefully-filled leisure time 'aids the development of a healthy recovery by addressing the individual's physical, social, emotional and spiritual needs – by addressing the whole person' (Keesmaat n.d.).

Sexual health

The present population of over 50s includes the 'baby boom' generation who grew up in a time of great social change. Feminism, civil rights and more liberal attitudes towards sex have characterized societal change over the past 50 years and the introduction of the contraceptive pill in the 1960s gave women the freedom to control their own fertility.

According to Lee and Nazroo (2015), older people are continuing to enjoy active sex lives well into their late seventies and eighties. Fifty-four per cent of men and almost 31 per cent of women over the age of 70 reported that they were still sexually active.

However, there appears to be a relatively low level of awareness of the risk of sexually-transmitted infections (STIs), including HIV, with the majority of older people reporting having received little information on sexually transmitted disease and HIV. However, a 'collaborative study, reported in 2008 … showed an increasing rate of sexual infections in people aged over 45 years in the West Midlands…'

(NHS South-West and Department of Health 2010) with men and women between the ages of 55 to 59 significantly more likely to be affected by an STI than others across the age group (Royal College of Nursing 2010).

The increase of STIs may reflect social attitudes that assume older people are relatively sexually inactive, resulting in this group being deprived of relevant information. Research by Olowokure *et al.* (2008, cited in Royal College of Nursing 2010) has found that 'current public health policies do not adequately cater for older people' (Royal College of Nursing 2010) with national and local health promotion campaigns appearing to focus on young people aged between 16 and 24 years.

Studies carried out by the University of Manchester have shown that older people seeking advice on sexual health problems are most likely to see their general practitioner. However, many older people do not pursue advice, either because they believe their symptoms are due to normal ageing or because of embarrassment (Age UK 2015). Many health professionals may not be aware of older people's sexual health needs, or may be reluctant to discuss this topic. Caroline Abrahams, Charity Director at Age UK, (cited in Lee and Nazroo 2015) reflects:

> The fact this is the first time that people over 80 years old have been included in this kind of research highlights how often the public health needs of older people, including sexual health, are ignored or overlooked. With an ageing population it is important that providers of sexual health services understand the needs of older people in both clinical settings and when developing information and advice.

Chapter 14 looks specifically at the role of play linked to health literacy and refers to a range of strategies that could be applied for the provision of information relating to sexual health. The sensitive nature of this topic, particularly for older people who may regard discussing sexual matters as embarrassing (Age UK 2015), means that a playful approach to conveying health messages of a personal nature may represent an alternative means of engaging the older generation.

Block *et al.* (2015) provide advice for the enjoyment of sex as people age, especially for those over 50 years of age. They stress the importance of interpersonal communication which may be facilitated through play and playfulness. Block *et al.* (2015) suggest using 'humor, gentle teasing, and even tickling to lighten the mood ... whatever it takes to have fun. With the issues you may be feeling physically or emotionally, play may be the ticket to help you both relax'.

Promoting play as a lifestyle trend

Thinking about play in the context of adult healthcare challenges the popular notion of play as an exclusively childhood pursuit. Adults may claim to be 'too busy' to play and the elderly might think themselves 'too old' to be playing games. However, play is already taken seriously when it refers to a sporting or recreational activity or participation in an interest or hobby. It follows that play can be used as

Lifestyle trends and their impact on health **93**

a way to address serious health issues, whilst remaining fun and both mentally and physically engaging.

Sporting activities

It is no longer the case that participation in sporting activities is reserved for the fit and healthy. It is recognized that there is a need for a wider variety of opportunities for individuals to participate in exercise, such as seated exercise, yoga and Pilates for the older age group.

Bowls and golfing are activities that are typically associated with older people but there have emerged many other novel ideas for staying fit and active into later adulthood. Health-walking and outdoor gyms join gardening and some domestic activities (such as vacuuming) as ways of incorporating physical activity into the daily routine. Many sports have been made more accessible, such as 'walking football' which enables individuals to participate in an alternative form of the game. Walking football clubs are increasing in popularity with over 400 clubs in the UK: 'The game is rapidly expanding, giving thousands of participants much valued health & social benefits' (Walking Football United n.d.).

Exercise referral schemes to promote physical activity

The National Institute for Health and Care Excellence (NICE) produces evidence-based information for health care, public health and social-care professionals. NICE have made recommendations for exercise referral schemes to promote physical activity for people aged 19 years and older. The guidelines focus on 'exercise referral schemes that try to increase physical activity among people who are inactive or sedentary and are otherwise healthy or who have an existing health condition or other risk factors for disease' (National Institute for Health and Care Excellence 2014). Exercise referral schemes usually operate as a partnership between a Clinical Commissioning Group and local leisure services. A health professional will refer a patient to an appropriately qualified fitness professional who will assess and plan a personalized program of physical exercise.

Play as relaxation

There are many opportunities for people of all ages to participate in play-based activities as a means of relaxation, with the potential for a secondary positive impact on both mental and physical health. Play and recreational opportunities also enable individuals to become involved and engaged in their local communities, to meet new people and to make friends. Leisure activities not generally associated with health, but which also carry benefits for health and wellbeing, include: bingo, bridge clubs, arts-and-crafts, cooking, computing classes, drama groups and community choirs. Many of these also perform a social function and groups such as book clubs, sewing bees and luncheon clubs all serve to combat the problems

94 Claire Weldon, Denise Baylis and Alison Tonkin

associated with social isolation. Pitkala *et al.* (2009) conducted a study into the 'Effects of psychosocial group rehabilitation on health, use of health care services, and mortality of older persons suffering from loneliness' and showed that the deteriorating health effects of loneliness may be reversed by intervention which socially activates lonely, elderly individuals (Pitkala *et al.* 2009). Betts Adams' *et al.* (2011, cited in Age UK 2011) state that a

> critical review of the literature on social and leisure activity and wellbeing in later life identified rigorous studies that validate and refine the activity theory of ageing. This theory assumes that there is a positive relationship between activity and life satisfaction; and that wellbeing is promoted by higher levels of participation in social and leisure activities, and by role replacement (e.g. at retirement).

Knitting

Perhaps one of the most vital recreational activities with a global following is knitting (Craft Yarn Council 2015). Knitting provides 'a 'whole-person' approach to wellbeing and health care so encourages variety, curiosity, exploration, creativity, laughter and a lot of fun!' (Stitchlinks 2015b). Just as the word *play* is sometimes seen as a barrier to its therapeutic potential, the word *knitting* can be an obstacle when it comes to promoting this form of handwork as a creative, therapeutic activity which has the potential to complement long-term treatments and which can lead to enhanced self-management of chronic health conditions (Stitchlinks 2015a). Knitting has multiple benefits and can be used to 'deliberately improve your wellbeing' while bringing about 'physiological, neurological, psychological, behavioral and social changes' (Stitchlinks 2015a). Knitting is portable and, as such, can be used in a variety of situations and places. Stitchlinks (2015a) are actively involved in generating an evidence base to demonstrate the efficacy of knitting as a therapeutic tool, which has been used in the NHS since 2006 (Stitchlinks 2015b). Stitchlinks (2015a) have produced a visual representation of the complex benefits of knitting called the *Knitting Equation*. It features fun, play and exploration along with meditation, relaxation and self-soothing, which has a calming effect that is beneficial to emotional wellbeing. 'Enjoyment of solitude' is also identified; the joy of knitting as an individual activity can be an appealing factor for many people. Meredith Keeton is 32 years of age and obliged to stay at home due to her rheumatoid arthritis. Keeton (cited in Craft Yarn Council 2015) refers to the isolation that is a consequence of her condition and states that 'knitting gives me something productive to do with my time. It's definitely good stress relief and helps keep my anxiety in check'. Stitchlinks (2015a) also note that knitting equates to 'Fun/play with others', and the social aspect of knitting as part of a group is recognized to be particularly beneficial to some people.

Men's sheds

The health and wellbeing needs specific to men are not well recognized within the community, and men themselves are less likely to recognize the detrimental effects of social isolation (Howard 2014). Loneliness is a major health concern which can 'disrupt sleep, raise blood pressure, lower immunity, increase depression, lower overall subjective wellbeing and increase the stress hormone cortisol' (Perry 2014). 'Men's Sheds' have emerged as a relatively simple solution to the problem of social isolation among men. According to the Irish Men's Sheds Association (2014) 'A Men's Shed is a dedicated, friendly and welcoming meeting place where men come together and undertake a variety of mutually agreed activities … to enhance or maintain the well-being of the participating men'. Men's sheds started to appear in South Australia in the 1990s and have developed since then 'through a growing awareness in Australia of the characteristics and potential benefits of personal men's sheds' (Golding *et al.* 2007). The value of these sheds for different sub-groups of the population is now well recognized, particularly for older men in care settings as well as for ex-military men. The Men's Shed movement has become established internationally and by May 2015 there were 1,416 Men's Sheds open globally: 933 across all states and territories of Australia, 57 in New Zealand, 273 across the Island of Ireland (including 16 in Northern Ireland), with 148 others elsewhere in the UK (including England, Scotland and Wales and five in Canada (Golding 2015). Although mainly accessed by older men, Men's Sheds are also open to women and young people, and irrespective of the activities undertaken, the shed 'is not a building … but the network of relationships between the members' (UK Men's Sheds Association 2015).

Social networking

Social networking via the internet has dramatically increased in recent years and is no longer the preserve of the young. Free training is available through libraries and local colleges to help the uninitiated to discover different ways of using the new technologies. It is not always easy to find groups or activities to join, especially if an individual lacks confidence. Social networking offers an alternative way for individuals to communicate with others and, whilst it does not replace actually meeting-up with people in person, it can help to reduce social isolation. Online dating enables older people to meet partners or friends and Facetime or Skype can help them to maintain contact with others and to stay up-to-date with family and friends. This topic is covered in more detail in Chapter 15.

Conclusion

Given the stated benefits of play for health and wellbeing, opportunities for play and recreation activities should be widely available and accessible to all. Play-based recreational activities are of potential value to all individuals, regardless of age,

96 Claire Weldon, Denise Baylis and Alison Tonkin

gender, background or ability as part of their attempts to improve, maintain or recover their health and wellbeing. The challenge for health and social care providers is to reach those in greatest need, affording all the possibility of enjoying life whilst staying well. This ambition is summarized by Ward-Wimmer (2003: 4) who states:

> Play can increase our self-esteem. It invites access to states of well-being and calm as well as silliness and joy. When relaxed in play, we often have an increased capacity for empathy and intimacy. Play is affirming.

References

Age UK (2015) *Sexual Health*, Online. Available at www.ageuk.org.uk/health-wellbeing/keeping-your-body-healthy/sexual-health/ (accessed 15 December 2015).

Age UK (2011) *Effectiveness of Day Services: Summary of Research Evidence*, London: Age UK.

Albinal (2009a) *Ian Ball – Brenda's Poisonous Pastime*, Online. Available at www.thelittlechimpsociety.com/2009/09/ian-ball-brendas-poisonous-pastime/ (accessed 14 December 2015).

Albinal (2009b) *Brenda's Poisonous Pastime*, Online. Available at https://vimeo.com/6377634 (available 14 December 2015).

Alcohol Concern (2015) *Statistics on alcohol*, Online. Available at www.alcoholconcern.org.uk/help-and-advice/statistics-on-alcohol/ (accessed 22 February 2016).

Alzheimer's Research UK (2015a) *10 Things You Need to Know about Prevalence*, Online. Available at www.alzheimersresearchuk.org/about-dementia/facts-stats/10-things-you-need-to-know-about-prevalence/ (accessed: 21 July 2015).

Alzheimer's Research UK (2015b) *10 Things You Need to Know about Dementia* Online. Available at www.alzheimersresearchuk.org/about-dementia/facts-stats/10-things-you-need-to-know-about-dementia/ (accessed 26 October 2015).

Alzheimer's Research UK (2015c) *Prevention*, Online. Available at www.alzheimers.org.uk/site/scripts/documents_info.php?documentID=183 (accessed 28 October 2015).

BBC Science (2013) *What Causes Coronary Heart Disease?* Online. Available at www.bbc.co.uk/science/0/21686950 (accessed 14 December 2015).

Biller, H. (2002) *Creative Fitness: Applying Health Psychology and Exercise Science to Everyday Life*, London: Greenwood Publishing Group.

Block, J., Smith, M. and Segal, J. (2015) *Better Sex as You Age*, Online. Available at www.helpguide.org/articles/aging-well/better-sex-as-you-age.htm (accessed 15 December 2015).

British Heart Foundation (2015) *BHF Headline Statistics*, Online. Available at www.bhf.org.uk/research/heart-statistics (accessed 20 July 2015).

Change4Life (2015) *Benefits of Drinking Less Alcohol*, Online. Available at www.nhs.uk/change4life/pages/benefits-drinking-less-alcohol.aspx#feelgood (accessed 26 September 2015).

Craft Yarn Council (2015) *The Truth About Knitting and Crochet… They are Good for You!* Online. Available at www.craftyarncouncil.com/health-therapeutic (accessed 15 December 2015).

Department of Health Long Term Conditions Team (2012) *Long Term Conditions Compendium of Information*, 3rd ed., Leeds: Department of Health.

Diabetes UK (2013) *State of the Nation 2013 England,* London: Diabetes UK.Diabetes.co.uk (2015a) *Diabetes Prevalence,* Online. Available at www.diabetes.co.uk/diabetes-prevalence.html (accessed 14 December 2015).

Diabetes.co.uk (2015b) *Sport Tips for Diabetics,* Online. Available at www.diabetes.co.uk/sport-tips-for-diabetics.html (accessed 14 December 2015).

Diabetes UK (2015a) *What is Type 2 Diabetes?* Online. Available at www.diabetes.org.uk/Guide-to-diabetes/What-is-diabetes/What-is-Type-2-Diabetes/ (accessed 30 October 2015).

Diabetes UK (2015b) *Older People and Diabetes,* Online. Available at www.diabetes.org.uk/Guide-to-diabetes/Older-people-and-diabetes/ (accessed 30 October 2015).

DrugScope (n.d.) *It's About Time: Tackling Substance Misuse in Older People* London: DrugScope

Golding, B. (2015) *Men's Sheds,* Online. Available at http://barrygoanna.com/mens-sheds/ (accessed 15 December 2015).

Golding, B., Brown, M., Foley, A., Harvey, J. and Gleeson, L. (2007) *Men's Shed's in Australia: Learning through Community Contexts,* Online. Available at http://library.bsl.org.au/jspui/bitstream/1/5114/1/GoldingB_Mens-sheds-in-Australia-Learning-through-community-contexts_2007.pdf (accessed 28 October 2015).

Halhuber, C. and Halhuber, M. (1983) *Speaking of Heart Attacks,* New Delhi: Sterling Publishers Ltd.

Home Office (2015) *Drug Misuse: Findings from the 2014/15 Crime Survey for England and Wales,* 2nd ed.London: Home Office.

Hornsby, W.G. and Chetlin, R.D. (2005) Management of competitive athletes with diabetes, *Diabetes Spectrum,* 18 (2): 102–107.

Howard, E. (2014) Mental Health: 'If I didn't come to the shed, I'd be alone, watching TV', *The Guardian,* 7 October 2014, Online. Available at www.theguardian.com (accessed 15 December 2015).

Irish Men's Sheds Association (2014) *What is a Men's Shed?* Online. Available at http://mens sheds.ie/2010/10/16/welcome-to-the-irish-mens-sheds-associations-website/ (accessed 27 October 2015).

Keesmaat, S. (n.d.) *How Does Therapeutic Recreation Apply in the Treatment of Addictions?* Online. Available at http://lin.ca/sites/default/files/attachments/sp001077.pdf (accessed 15 December 2015).

Lee, D. and Nazroo, J. (2015) *Love and Intimacy in Later Life: Study Reveals Active Sex Lives of Over-70s,* Online. Available at www.manchester.ac.uk/discover/news/article/?id=13745 (accessed 27 October 2015).

Marmot, M. (2010) *Fair Society, Healthy Lives,* The Marmot Review.

NHS South-West and Department of Health (2010) *Achieving Age Equality in Health and Social Care: NHS Practice Guide,* London: Department of Health.

National Institute for Health and Care Excellence (2014) *Physical Activity: Exercise Referral Schemes,* Online. Available at www.nice.org.uk/guidance/ph54 (accessed 26 December 2015).

National Treatment Agency (2011) *Addiction to Medicine: An Investigation into the Configuration and Commissioning of Treatment Services to Support Those who Develop Problems with Prescription-only or Over-the-counter Medicine,* London: National Treatment Agency.

Patterson, L., Kee, F., Hughes, C. and O'Reilly, D. (2014) The relationship between BMI and the prescription of anti-obesity medication according to social factors: a population cross sectional study, *BMC Public Health,* 14: 87.

Perry, P. (2014) Loneliness is killing us – we must start treating this disease, *The Guardian,* 17 February 2014, Online. Available at www.theguardian.com (accessed 15 December 2015).

Pitkala, K.H., Routasolo, P., Kautiainen, H. and Tilvis, R.S. (2009) Effects of psychosocial group rehabilitation on health, use of health care services, and mortality of older persons suffering from loneliness: a randomised, controlled trial, *Journal of Gerontology: Medical Sciences*, 64A (7): 792–800.

Royal College of Nursing (2010) *STI's – Age No Barrier (Resolution)*, Online. Available at rcn.org.uk/newsevents/congress/2010/congress_2010_resolutions_and_matters_for_dis cussion/19._stis_-_age_no_barrier (accessed 27 October 2015).

Royal College of Psychiatrists (2011) *Our Invisible addicts*, London: Royal College of Psychiatrists.

Shearing, E. (2014) *Recreational Therapy: Play Your Way to Recovery*, Online. Available at www.strokesmart.org/new?id=257 (accessed 14 December 2015).

Smith, M., Robinson, L. and Segal, J. (2015) *Alzheimer's and Dementia Prevention*, Online. Available at www.helpguide.org/articles/alzheimers-dementia/alzheimers-and-dementia-prevention.htm (accessed 14 December 2015).

Stanford Health Care (2015) *Obesity*, Online. Available at https://stanfordhealthcare.org/medical-conditions/healthy-living/obesity.html (accessed 14 December 2015).

Stitchlinks (2015a) *Where Are We Now?* Online. Available at http://stitchlinks.com/research.html (accessed 15 December 2015).

Stitchlinks (2015b) Welcome to the Home of Therapeutic Knitting since 2005. Online. Available at http://stitchlinks.com/ (accessed 15 December 2015).

Stroke Association (2013) *State of the Nation: Stroke Statistics.* London: Stroke Association.

The King's Fund (2015) *Long-term Conditions and Multi-morbidity*, Online. Available at www.kingsfund.org.uk/time-to-think-differently/trends/disease-and-disability/long-term-conditions-multi-morbidity (accessed 14 December 2015).

UK Men's Sheds Association (2015) *What is a Men's Shed?* Online. Available at http://menssheds.org.uk/what-is-a-mens-shed/ (accessed 15 December 2015).

Wadd, S., Lapworth, K., Sullivan, M. and Forrester, D. (2011) *Working with Older Drinkers 2010,* Online. Available at http://alcoholresearchuk.org/downloads/finalReports/FinalReport_0085 (accessed 26 October 2015).

Walking Football United (n.d.) *The Growth of Walking Football,* Online. Available at www.walkingfootballunited.co.uk/ (accessed 09 September 2015).

Ward-Wimmer, D. (2003) Introduction: The Healing Potential of Adults at Play, In: Schaefer, C.E. (ed.) *Play therapy with adults*, Hoboken, NJ: John Wiley and Sons: 1–11.

World Health Organization (WHO) (2015) *Obesity and Overweight*, Online. Available at www.who.int/mediacentre/factsheets/fs311/en/ (accessed 26 October 2015).

8

PLAYING FOR MENTAL WELLNESS

Julia Whitaker and Alison Tonkin

Play concepts have a major contribution to make to the mental health and emotional wellness of individuals. Play as a route to resilience will be exemplified with reference to contemporary projects designed to promote mental wellness from the UK and the wider international community.

Introduction

Play has a major contribution to make to the mental wellness and emotional wellbeing of individuals. However, framing the benefits of play within the complex and often contradictory mental health arena means that the value of play is not always recognized. According to the Mental Health Foundation (n.d.) 'Our mental health is about how we think and feel, our outlook on life and how we are able to cope with life's ups and downs. It's an essential part of our health. Some people prefer to call mental health 'emotional health' or 'wellbeing' and it's just as important as good physical health'. This chapter will explore how the medical categorization of mental illness has contributed to an over-reliance on pharmacological treatments, and what this may mean for our collective wellbeing. It will also explore how play can provide and support viable, relatively inexpensive, alternative treatment options and how play can promote and support mental wellness and psychological healing throughout the lifespan.

The mind-state of the nation

Every year, one in every four people in the UK will experience a mental health problem (Mind 2013a). Almost 10 per cent of UK adults report feelings of anxiety and depression, whilst 3 per cent experience some form of post-traumatic stress. Statistics suggest that 17 per cent of people have nurtured suicidal thoughts, whilst three in every hundred have self-harmed (Mind 2013a). It is likely that we all work alongside someone who is mentally unwell – whether we realize it or not (Time to Change 2008) – and it is encouraging to note that our attitudes as a nation are becoming more tolerant, with 76 per cent of people saying they would be willing to work with someone who has a mental illness (TNS BMRB 2014). UK prevalence data closely matches that from the US where 18.5 per cent of adults were diagnosed with a mental illness in 2013 (National Institute of Mental Health 2015). Mental health and wellbeing are global health priorities with vast cost implications for the economy, political and social stability (Harnois and Gabriel 2002).

The latest available figures for British households were gathered as part of the National Wellbeing Measures in 2012–2013 through the General Health Questionnaire (Office for National Statistics 2015). The figures for *psychosocial health* are significant because they provide evidence of self-reporting linked to subjective measures of wellbeing as opposed to medical diagnosis.

Respondents were asked 12 questions linked to their recent feelings and the responses were quantified and placed on a scale from 0–12. If respondents had a score of four or more, this was interpreted as an indication that the person had a mild to moderate illness, such as anxiety or depression (Office for National Statistics 2015). The percentages in Tables 8.1, 8.2 and 8.3 suggest that people's responses vary according to geographic region, age and gender.

Witchen *et al.* (2011) found that rates of depression among women across Europe have doubled since the 1970s, pinpointing a rise during the 1980s and 1990s, with a levelling-off in recent times. Bebbington *et al.* (2011) concurred that the occurrence of mental illness in England has remained stable over the past 20 years, reporting that, '[the] finding of stable rates contradicts popular media stories of a relentlessly rising tide of mental illness'. This is supported by longitudinal data

TABLE 8.1 Variation according to region (Office for National Statistics 2015)

Region	(%)
England	18.4
North East	18.6
North West	19.3
Yorkshire and the Humber	19.4
East Midlands	18.5
West Midlands	19.4
East of England	17.0
London	19.9
South East	17.4
South West	16.4
Wales	19.2
Scotland	17.0
Northern Ireland	16.9

TABLE 8.2 Variation according to age (Office for National Statistics)

Age (years)	(%)
16–24	20.8
25–44	19.5
45–54	21.5
55–64	17.8
65–74	11.9
75 and over	14.8

presented as part of the 2012–2013 National Wellbeing Measures (Office for National Statistics 2015) which does indeed show a reduction in the overall incidence of feelings associated with anxiety and depression.

Whilst the overall rate of mental illness appears to have levelled off over the past 20 years, Berthoud (2011) provides data suggesting that the rate of mental illness among working age people is more than a third higher at the start of the twenty-first century than it was in the 1970s. This invites us to question whether there is an underlying reason why people are more likely to experience (or report) mental health problems nowadays than they did 50 years ago. One possible explanation is that there is less stigma attached to mental illness than in the past – although this is culturally determined and refuted by many (Davey 2013). It may be that, in the Western world at least, people are more likely to present to health services with symptoms of mental distress and that the helping professions are more likely to recognize signs of mental illness than in the past, due to advancing sophistication in the measuring of psychiatric and related psychological conditions (Brugha *et al.* 2004). Or we may ask whether life in the early twenty-first century poses greater psychological challenges than in earlier times?

One hypothesis is that life in the twenty-first century is characterized – at least in the West – by an expectation of happiness and fulfilment, as demonstrated in many surveys of wellbeing, which explicitly ask questions such as 'How happy do you feel on a scale of 0–10?' (Rutledge *et al.* 2014). According to Wilson-Mulnix and Mulnix (2015) happiness appears to be regarded as a social achievement, suggesting that 'perhaps the function of a nation is to ensure the happiness of its citizens' (Wilson-Mulnix and Mulnix 2015: 261). This fits with Aristotle's original framing of politics as a practical science that should facilitate the happiness of citizens through good governance (Miller 2011). This notion of health as happiness is explored in more detail in Chapter 22.

TABLE 8.3 Variation according to gender (Office for National Statistics 2015)

Gender	(%)
Male	14.8
Female	21.5

TABLE 8.4 Longitudinal incidence of feelings associated with anxiety and depression (Office for National Statistics 2015)

Year	(%)
2002	20.0
2003	19.3
2004	19.3
2005	20.6
2006	19.5
2007	20.5
2008	18.0
2009/10	20.0
2010/11	18.7
2011/12	18.3
2012/13	18.3

Exploring mental health and the impact of cultural relativism

Mental wellbeing has often been linked to the concept of happiness. For example, Glasser (cited Buck 2013) provides the following working definition of good mental and emotional health:

> Generally, you are happy and are more than willing to help an unhappy family member, friend, or colleague to feel better. You lead a mostly tension-free life, laugh a lot, and rarely suffer from the aches and pains that so many people accept as an unavoidable part of living ... Finally, even in difficult situations when you are unhappy – no one can be happy all the time – you'll know why you are unhappy and attempt to do something about it.

The World Health Organization (2014) describes mental health as a state of wellbeing and a positive dimension of health, defining mental health as 'a state of well-being in which every individual realizes his or her own potential, can cope with the normal stresses of life, can work productively and fruitfully, and is able to make a contribution to her or his community' (World Health Organization 2014).

The counter-definition of 'mental illness', and the associated statistical recording of its prevalence, are widely attributed to the publication in 1952 of the Diagnostic and Statistical Manual of Mental Disorders (DSM), now in its fifth revision (American Psychiatric Association 2013), which represented the first attempt to standardize the diagnosis of mental ill-health.

The resultant categorization or classification of mental disorder, which underpins the DSM, hangs on the concept of 'abnormality' (Pomerantz 2014). One of the problems with the notion of abnormality – either in terms of deviation from a common perception of optimum mental health, or deviation from social norms or of statistical infrequency – is the fact that none of the diagnostic criteria used in the DSM adequately accommodates cultural variations. Cultural relativism supports the view that beliefs about what constitutes abnormality differ between cultures and their sub-groups. Thoughts and behaviors regarded as abnormal in one culture may be deemed perfectly acceptable in another, and one of the reasons that definitions of acceptability/abnormality vary between cultures is that there are real differences in the way that people understand, express and respond to mental experiences. However, Pomerantz (2014) also points out that just because a certain behavior is valued, accepted and considered 'normative' within a particular culture, it does not necessarily follow that it is 'conducive to healthy psychological functioning'.

Many non-Western cultures recognize an integration of internal emotional experiences and their physiological parallels, and may focus more on the physical than the psychological features of a complaint. Traditional Chinese Medicine, for example, perceives mental health disorders in terms of a disruption in the flow of vital energy, or *Qi*, through the body, which can disrupt the immune system or lead to symptoms of pain, sleep disturbance, headaches, gastric and hormonal irregularities. Treatment of these physiological features is seen as key to the restoration of mental equilibrium (British Acupuncture Association 2015). This approach to the maintenance and restoration of wellbeing is discussed in more detail in Chapter 17.

Whilst some cultures value displays of emotion, others emphasize containment, resulting in contrasting interpretations of emotional demonstrativeness. Parkes *et al.* (2003) examined the cultural variations in mourning rituals and behavior and the extent to which emotional expression is deemed acceptable or 'abnormal'. Wikan (1988) found that women in Bali were strongly discouraged from crying, whilst in Egypt women were considered abnormal if they did not engage in demonstrative displays of weeping, underlining the significance of cultural tagging.

Some cultures emphasize the religious or spiritual aspects of mental illness and might look for a religious rather than a medical solution to a psychological problem (Ngoma *et al.* 2003). A religiously-induced hypnotic state is considered a valued spiritual experience among certain fundamentalist Christian groups, whilst other faith traditions would regard the same behavior as symptomatic of psychological distress or disturbance. Many cultures have a more fluid view of the self and of reality than we do in the West. For example, a Native American who hears the voice of a recently deceased family member would view this as a perfectly normal experience (Ojibwa 2014), whereas in contemporary Western societies such an event might be interpreted as an example of auditory hallucination.

Among some communities, seeking help from a mental health practitioner is still seen as a sign of weakness or shame (Abdullah and Brown 2011) with consequent lower reporting rates of symptoms of mental distress. Others believe that problems should be managed within the family context and consider it disrespectful to discuss personal and family problems with a stranger (Paul and Nadkani 2014). Again, this affects patterns of reporting and potential responsiveness to external intervention. Such cultural variations are essential considerations for the healthcare practitioner intent on engaging communities in health prevention and treatment initiatives. This becomes even more significant now that attitudes towards mental health are seen to be changing. For example, in England there has been a rise of 6 per cent (since 2008) to 89 per cent (in 2013) in the number of people surveyed who state that society should be far more tolerant toward people with a mental illness. Seventy-seven per cent of those surveyed also feel that, wherever possible, mental health services should be 'provided through community-based facilities' (TNS BMRB: 4).

Contrasting approaches to treating mental health conditions

Cultural relativism calls into question the validity of the DSM, although the medical model remains the most widely used diagnostic measure of mental ill-health. The range of symptoms categorized as indicative of mental disorder in the current edition, DSM-5 (American Psychiatric Association 2013), now includes mood states and behaviors which might, in other historical, social and cultural contexts, define common ('normal') responses to adversity. What was once described as 'sadness' or 'eccentricity' has now acquired a medical interpretation with value implications for both the subject and the societal response to it:

> With the DSM5, patients worried about having a medical illness will often be diagnosed with somatic symptom disorder, normal grief will be misidentified as major depressive disorder, the forgetfulness of old age will be confused with mild neurocognitive disorder, temper tantrums will be labelled disruptive mood dysregulation disorder, overeating will become binge eating disorder, and the already overused diagnosis of attention–deficit disorder will be even easier to apply.
>
> *(Frances 2013)*

This so-called 'diagnostic over-expansion' (Frances 2013; Wakefield 2013) has widespread implications for how societies perceive and respond to psychological deviation from what they perceive as 'the norm'. When a thought pattern or behavior is interpreted as a symptom of a mental disorder, a play-based intervention might understandably be perceived as inadequate or inappropriate. However, when the same psychological features are re-framed within a socio-cultural context, alternative treatment options – including play – can reasonably be considered as part of a holistic therapeutic strategy.

Since the discovery of psychotropic drugs for treating bi-polar disorder in the 1950s, prescribed medication has been widely used to treat psychosis, depression, and anxiety. Data from different parts of the world indicate an increase in the prescribing of drugs used for mental disorders, particularly antidepressants and antipsychotics. Ilyas and Moncreiff (2012) have reported that the prescription of psycho-pharmaceuticals to treat mental illness has risen exponentially over the past 20 years, with antidepressant prescriptions increasing by an average of 10 per cent annually between 1998 and 2010.

In addition to concerns about over-diagnosis and treatment, the increase in long-term prescribing for people with depression is potentially unhelpful – it may suggest that commonly prescribed drugs encourage dependency, or that they are not regularly reviewed. Improving Access to Psychological Therapies (IAPT) supports the front-line NHS in implementing National Institute for Health and Clinical Excellence (NICE) guidelines for people suffering from depression and anxiety disorders. It was created to 'offer patients routine front-line treatment, combined, where appropriate with medication which traditionally had been the only treatment available' (Improving Access to Psychological Therapies 2015). However, this does not seem to have had the expected impact on prescription rates, and drug treatment remains the treatment of choice for most diagnosed cases of mental illness (Ilyas and Moncreiff 2012).

Therefore, it is not surprising that the treatment of mental health conditions (which is taken to include dementia) is the largest single area of expenditure in England for the NHS at £11.48 billion in 2012/13 (Nuffield Trust 2015).

Big Pharma (a pseudonym for the global pharmaceutical industry) has an incontrovertible influence on how we both perceive and treat mental illness. Professional connections and a potential conflict of interests between the pharmaceutical industry and those responsible for the diagnostic protocols have been widely reported: it is notable that 69 per cent of the DSM-5 Task Force (the group that revised the DSM in 2013) had direct links to the pharmaceutical industry (Cosgrove and Krimsky 2012).

There is no doubt that the development of psycho-pharmaceutical treatments has positively transformed the lives of many people who would otherwise be incapacitated by their psychological symptoms. One obvious benefit of the availability of effective symptom control is the dismantling of the long-term institutionalization of those diagnosed with mental disorders. Psychological problems can present insurmountable obstacles to personal fulfilment and social participation, the impact of which is represented in Maslow's theory of a 'hierarchy of needs' (1943) and explored in Chapter 2. This model recognizes that it is the potency of personal needs which dictates behavioral motivations. If a person is suffering from a mental health issue which directly threatens their feelings of safety and security, then 'all other needs may become simply non-existent or be pushed into the background' (Maslow 1943:373).

An alternative to the categorization associated with the DSM is a 'dimensional approach' to the diagnosis of mental health (Haslam 2003). Rather than placing people into diagnostic *categories*, the dimensional model places people along *dimensions* of behavior and personality and the diagnostic focus shifts from the presence or absence of a problem to the degree to which a particular characteristic is present. This re-directs the concept of mental states as being either 'normal' or 'abnormal', towards the idea of a continuum of mental wellness which individuals traverse throughout the course of a lifetime and in response to life-stage transitions and experiences and consequently allows for a more flexible consideration of a whole raft of preventive and restorative options.

There are instances in a person's life (following a loss or relationship breakdown, for example) when a downturn in mood might be regarded as appropriately adaptive. The depressed or elated mood states may be accepted as integral to the human condition, and the associated temporary variations in behavior and cognition may be considered as 'normal' stress reactions to challenge or adversity. Conversely, momentary happiness can also be considered a conscious emotional state and, as such, 'core to the ebb and flow of human mental experience' (Rutledge *et al.* 2014: 12255).

Drawing on the work of Gould (1996), Sutton-Smith notes that successful biological and social evolution, rather than being dependent on pre-determined adaptations, requires '[a] set of characteristics usually devalued in our culture: sloppiness, broad potential, quirkiness, unpredictability, and above all, massive redundancy. The key is flexibility, not admirable precision' (Gould 1996: 44; cited in Sutton-Smith 1997: 221) These are the very characteristics of play and perhaps key to its function in developing mental resilience in the face of challenge and change. Applying a dimensional approach, allows the sorrow of bereavement, the mood swings of adolescence or the bleakness of 'empty nest' syndrome to be understood and tackled as universal life challenges, which can be anticipated or alleviated through lifestyle interventions.

Examples of adaptive practices include rituals such as the Jewish tradition of the mourners' *Kaddish* following bereavement, or the Chinese tradition of *zuo yue zi,* the month-long period of confinement of a new mother, both of which have evolved as protective and supportive strategies for accommodating and alleviating occasions of anticipated psychological vulnerability. Chapter 19 will explore more fully the significance of rituals and festivals for personal and social health and wellbeing.

A dimensional approach to mental illness/wellness allows for a fuller discussion of non-pharmacological responses to psychological disturbance or distress, including responses which represent extensions or re-interpretations of naturally occurring activities and pursuits – many of them with play or playfulness at their heart (Robinson *et al.* 2014).

Increasing knowledge of brain function, and of the distinct neural circuits responsible for different emotional experiences, offers a new understanding of the psychological problems that arise when these circuits malfunction and presents a different focus to treatment options (Rutledge *et al.* 2014). *Neuroplasticity*, the idea that 'the brain can change itself' (Doidge 2007) in response to mental experience, is perhaps the most important development in our understanding of the human mind since the aforementioned discovery of psycho-pharmaceuticals during the postwar period. Changes in thought patterns, in combination with motor activity, have been shown to alter brain circuitry and neurochemical activity (Kandel 2012) in ways that can alleviate even long-standing psychological symptoms. This can be patently demonstrated through the practice of therapeutic knitting, which gives 'immediate, multisensory feedback which will stimulate positive thoughts, behaviors and emotional responses' (Corkhill 2014).

The concept of neuroplasticity gives credence to the body-mind connection which has long been central to traditional Eastern medicine and which is a fundamental component of yoga, tai-chi and other meditative practices. Furthermore, the active participation of the 'patient' in these practices alters the whole dynamic of healing, endowing the individual with a shared sense of responsibility for their own healing, rather being merely a passive recipient of professional expertise (Corkhill 2014).

A study by Weich *et al.* (2011) makes the interesting differentiation between mental *wellness* and mental *wellbeing*. This study distinguished the hedonic (happiness and satisfaction with life) aspects and the eudemonic (optimum social functioning) aspects of wellbeing and found that associations with mental wellbeing were relatively independent of symptoms of mental illness. A sense of wellbeing can be maintained, even in the presence of mental distress or disturbance.

The recognition and treatment of mental ill-health is not diminished by considerations of playfulness as a complementary approach which has a unique role in maintaining and enhancing feelings of wellbeing independently of mental health status. It is a reasonable proposition that play completes the healing process, giving meaning and purpose to recovery and serving as a psychological mantle during periods of challenge and change.

A case in point is the emergence of a new market dedicated to the production of therapeutic coloring books for adults. In 2014, this was described somewhat flippantly in an article in the *Guardian* which reported that, in France, sales of coloring books aimed at adults had reached over 350,000 copies, exceeding sales of cookery books (Bromwich 2014). The article included a statement to the effect that adults who were 'coloring in' were 'regressing to the mental age of seven' (Bromwich 2014). Compare this coverage to an article by Williams (2015) a year later, in the same newspaper, which highlighted the virtues of this hugely popular leisure activity as a means of reducing anxiety and stress. Williams suggests that therapeutic coloring is 'a crossover with mindfulness and also with mantras: activities in which the brain is engaged just enough to stop it whirring, but not so much that the concentration is draining'. Experimental studies by Curry and Kasser (2005) and van der Vennet and Serice (2012) have shown that it is not only the act of coloring that can have a therapeutic effect but that the effect is also influenced by the choice of subject to be colored. Results suggest that coloring a mandala reduces anxiety to a greater extent than simply coloring a plaid design or coloring on blank paper, with the implication that structured coloring of a geometric pattern may induce a meditative state that benefits individuals suffering from anxiety.

Adult coloring has become a global phenomenon with Amazon reporting that adult coloring books equate to five of its 'Top Ten' non-fiction sales, whilst in Brazil the figure is six out of every ten non-fiction books (Williams 2015). Furedi (2015) offers a cautionary note and suggests that adult coloring books 'resonate with the zeitgeist, which communicates the idea that we live in a uniquely stressed-out, anxious world'. Furedi laments 'the infantilization of the therapeutic imagination' and the marketing of relaxation in a way that reflects the nostalgia of childhood.

However, the real insight comes from 100 comments made by people in response to Furedi's article and the wider debate around what constitutes 'time to relax'. These clearly demonstrate the significant differences in opinion regarding the 'usefulness' of how time is spent. The majority of respondents suggest 'doing something just because it brings you joy is the best relaxation there is' (Sparks 13, cited Furedi 2015) and perhaps the most encouraging comment is made by Foxy (cited Furedi 2015) who simply states:

> If someone is in need of therapy then the best medicine is to do something for others. It almost doesn't matter what, just the action of helping someone else is what is needed. There is time for reflection in most tasks, from gardening to cooking, but we are social animals and defined by what we do for others. The happiest and most fulfilled are not those who have turned away from the world, but rather those who have engaged with it and tried to make it a better place.

Enhancing mental wellness for all

The inter-related nature of the factors affecting mental capacity was captured in 2008 by the Foresight Project. This project was designed to explore how the best possible mental development and mental wellbeing could be achieved for everyone in the UK (gov.uk 2008). The final project report was intended for policy-makers, professionals, and researchers interested in mental capital and wellbeing and, whilst it focused on the UK, it was promoted as being 'relevant to other interested countries' (Foresight Mental Capital and Wellbeing Project 2008b).

A series of systems maps were produced as part of the project (Foresight Mental Capital and Wellbeing Project 2008a), including a valuable conceptual overview of how mental capacity varies throughout the lifespan. The final report identified 'five ways to mental wellbeing', described in Table 8.5, which it hoped would become as familiar and widely used as the concept of 'five a day' aimed at boosting the consumption of fruit and vegetables as part of a healthy diet (Foresight Mental Capital and Wellbeing Project 2008b).

Play-based strategies feature heavily among the activities identified in Table 8.5 and some of these have already been described within Chapter 1 (NHS Choices 2014). The potential benefit of physical play, for example, is encompassed in a statement by the Mental Health Foundation: 'Physical activity can be as effective as antidepressant medication in treating mild to moderate depression, which is why exercise therapy is available on prescription in many areas' (Mental Health Foundation n.d.: 41). Acknowledging the holistic nature of health and the 'influence by association' of play and playfulness on all aspects of health, the following example of a current project accessed by people with identified mental health issues shows how enhancing mental capacity can be beneficial to health, not only for the individual but for society as a whole.

TABLE 8.5 'Five ways to mental wellbeing' (quoted from Foresight Mental Capital and Wellbeing Project 2008b)

Way	Description
Connect ...	With the people around you. With family, friends, colleagues and neighbours. At home, work, school or in your local community. Think of these as the cornerstones of your life and invest time in developing them. Building these connections will support and enrich you every day.
Be active ...	Go for a walk or run. Step outside. Cycle. Play a game. Garden. Dance. Exercising makes you feel good. Most importantly, discover a physical activity you enjoy and that suits your level of mobility and fitness.
Take notice ...	Be curious. Catch sight of the beautiful. Remark on the unusual. Notice the changing seasons. Savour the moment, whether you are walking to work, eating lunch or talking to friends. Be aware of the world around you and what you are feeling. Reflecting on your experiences will help you appreciate what matters to you.
Keep learning ...	Try something new. Rediscover an old interest. Sign up for that course. Take on a different responsibility at work. Repair a bike. Learn to play a musical instrument or how to cook your favourite food. Set a challenge you enjoy achieving. Learning new things will make you more confident as well as being fun.
Give ...	Do something nice for a friend, or a stranger. Thank someone. Smile. Volunteer your time. Join a community group. Look out, as well as in. Seeing yourself, and your happiness, as linked to the wider community can be incredibly rewarding and creates connections with the people around you.

In 2007, the mental health charity Mind (2007) recognized the potential of the natural outdoor world as part of a new green agenda. The *Ecominds* initiative was designed to provide an alternative, non-pharmacological treatment option for people with mental health issues. Between 2009–2013, 'over 12,000 people used the projects to look after their mental health by doing gardening, farming, food growing, exercise, art and craft, or environmental conservation work – supported by trained professionals' (Mind 2013b). As a form of social prescribing, the *Ecominds* project has shown positive social health benefits, promoting participants' resilience, the building of relationships, confidence and self-esteem as well as the acquisition of new vocational skills (Maughan 2014). However, despite the actual and potential health benefits of these projects, some have been suspended regardless of available evidence supporting their effectiveness (Maughan 2014). It would appear that an inability to demonstrate direct cost savings at a time of serious financial constraints within the NHS means that alternative methods such as eco-therapy will not be pursued, to the detriment of society as a whole. This denies the fact that they could 'bridge the gap between reducing environmental and economic costs of services while improving quality of care' (Maughan 2014).

Eco-therapy is an example of a structured mental health enterprise, but health-promotion initiatives that advocate the benefits of simple activities like a walk in the park, sharing time with friends and family, or trying out a new hobby or game, can all contribute to mental wellbeing.

There is a clearly established geographical link between economic wellbeing and mental health. Mitchell *et al.* (2015) found compelling evidence that access to green or recreational space has a greater impact on reports of mental wellbeing than any of five other neighbourhood factors. The mental health divide between those living in wealth and those living in poverty is reduced by 40 per cent for those with access to green spaces, giving legitimacy to the status of 'a walk in the park' as a mood stabilizer.

The Mobility, Mood and Place (2015) project will build on the evidence for the link between mood and environment, mapping the social and dynamic context of place in order to better understand how the settings in which we live, work and play impact on our mood and behavior.

The Mental Health Foundation (n.d.) has produced a publication for people in later life who are approaching retirement or who have recently retired from work, which offers ten practical ways to stay mentally well in later life. It suggests play-related strategies to achieve each of these protective factors, challenging the perception that mental health problems are an inevitable feature of growing older (Table 8.6). It is interesting to note how these dovetail into the 'five ways to mental wellbeing' in Table 8.5.

TABLE 8.6 Ten practical ways to stay mentally well (adapted from the Mental Health Foundation n.d.)

Practical way	Suggested activities
1. Be prepared for change	This should include making time for your own interests… for example trying a new activity such as dancing the tango or learning new skills like using the internet. Opportunities to volunteer are also advocated, particularly helping out in a charitable organization or a conservation project.
2. Talk about problems and concerns	'Conversations don't have to be all about the difficulties. Tell each other about the enjoyable events too!' The value of a chat over a cup of tea features in several chapters in this book!
3. Ask for help	This is where the third sector really comes into its own … for example Age UK can offer support with staying physically active as well as learning new skills that can be used to stay in contact with others such as Skype or Facetime.
4. Think ahead and have a plan	Addressing potential worries and planning how to maintain things such as physical health through staying active can boost confidence and self-esteem as well as maintaining positive mental wellness.

TABLE 8.6 Continued.

Practical way	Suggested activities
5. Care for others	Caring for others is seen as a positive means of maintaining strong relationships and is particularly good for promoting inter-generational relations i.e. looking after grandchildren or elderly parents or relatives also provides opportunities for sharing recreational pastimes and hobbies together.
6. Keep in touch	Friendships are seen as one of the most important factors for maintaining good emotional health … although this can sometimes be hard work and requires time and effort. Playing games on a regular basis can provide a routine which is easier to maintain.
7. Be active and sleep well	Physical activity is known to enhance feelings of self-worth, confidence and self-esteem and this is even better if it is something you enjoy. This also applies to keeping mentally active, through activities such as playing games, like chess, card games and bingo, all of which are social activities. Likewise, getting a good night's sleep is really important and using relaxation techniques to optimize readiness for sleep can enhance the body's natural reparation mechanisms.
8. Eat and drink sensibly	Sharing food and drink is a very social experience and this can be a good way to maintain friendships.
9. Do things you enjoy	This can be a social experience or pastimes and hobbies that are done by ourselves. Meaningful activities are essential for good emotional wellbeing and if hobbies are combined with helping others, then they hold added value i.e. charities such as Knitting for Africa or Loving Hands which has members all over the UK making items such as fiddle mats or baby clothes for charity.
10. Relax and have a break	This can be things that you enjoy such as doing a crossword or reading a book to a regular weekly trip to an art gallery or the park. As long as it is something you enjoy …

Perhaps the true role of play and playfulness in the mental health arena lies in the development and maintenance of positive mental wellness for the significant majority of people. There is a general perception that mental ill-health is on the increase, which is not borne out by the statistics. Whilst some people's lives are made unbearable by serious mental health problems, most of us get through life's ups-and-downs without being incapacitated by unwanted psychological symptoms. The General Health Questionnaire in 2012/13 found that 81.7 per cent of people surveyed, did not have indicators of anxiety or depression (Office for National Statistics 2015). The challenge for healthcare providers and practitioners is to recognize and resource the protective features of play and playfulness such that they can be promoted and supported for everyone from the start of life to its conclusion.

References

Abdullah, T. and Brown, T.L. (2011) Mental illness stigma and ethno-cultural beliefs, values, and norms: an integrative review, *Clinical Psychology Review*, 31: 934–948.

American Psychiatric Association (2013) *Diagnostic and Statistical Manual of Mental Disorders (DSM-5)*, American Psychiatric Association.

Bebbington, N., McManus, P., Brugha, S., Jenkins, T.R., and Meltzer H. (2011) Age and birth cohort differences in the prevalence of common mental disorder in England: the National Psychiatric Morbidity Surveys, 1993–2007, *British Journal of Psychiatry*, 198: 479–484.

Berthoud, R. (2011) *Trends in the Employment of Disabled People in Britain*, London: Institute for Social and Economic Research.

British Acupuncture Association (2015) *How Does Acupuncture Work?* Online. Available at www.acupuncture.org.uk/public-content/public-faqs/3827-how-does-acupuncture-work.html (accessed 1 October 2015).

Bromwich, K. (2014) Why colouring-in books are the new therapy. *The Guardian,* 29 June 2014 Online. Available at www.theguardian.com (accessed 5 October 2015).

Brugha, T.S., Bebbington, P.E., Singleton, N., Melzer, D., Jenkins, R., Lewis, G. Farrell, M., Bhugra, D., Lee, A. and Howard Meltzer (2004) Trends in service use and treatment for mental disorders in adults throughout Great Britain, *British Journal of Psychiatry,* 185, 378–384.

Buck, N. (2013) *Mental Health and Happiness.* Online. Available at www.psychologytoday. com/blog/peaceful-parenting/201308/mental-health-and-happiness-2 (accessed 1 October 2015).

Corkhill, B. (2014) *Knit for Health and Wellness: How to Knit a Flexible Mind and More...*, [Kindle version]. Available at http://amazon.co.uk (accessed 1 October 2015).

Cosgrove, L. and Krimsky, S. (2012) A comparison of DSM-IV and DSM-5 panel members' financial associations with industry: a pernicious problem persists, *PLoS Medicine*, 9 (3): e1001190.

Curry, N. A. and Kasser, T. (2005) Can coloring mandalas reduce anxiety? *Art Therapy, 22 (2)*: 81–85.

Davey, G. (2013) Mental health and stigma: mental health symptoms are still viewed as threatening and uncomfortable, *Graham CL Davey Blog.* 20 August 2013. Online. Available at www.psychologytoday.com/blog/why-we-worry/201308/mental-health-stigma (accessed 27 September 2015).

Doidge, N. (2007) *The Brain that Changes Itself.* London: Penguin.

Frances, A. (2013) *DSM-5 and Psychiatric Diagnosis Inflation.* Available at www.thepoison-review.com/2013/05/21/dsm-5-and-psychiatric-diagnosis-inflation/ (accessed 20 November 2015).

Foresight Mental Capital and Wellbeing Project (2008a) *Systems Maps*, London: The Government Office for Science.

Foresight Mental Capital and Wellbeing Project (2008b) *Final Project Report*, London: The Government Office for Science.

Furedi, F. (2015) Hey, Grown-ups: Put down the colouring pens! *Sp!ked,* 31 August 2015 Online. Available at www.spiked-online.com (accessed 5 October 2015).

Gould, S.J. (1996) *Full House: The Spread of Excellence from Plato to Darwin*. New York: Crown Pubs.

gov.uk (2008) *Collection: Mental Capital and Wellbeing*, Online. Available at www.gov.uk/government/collections/mental-capital-and-wellbeing (accessed 1 October 2015).

Harnois, G. and Gabriel, P. (2002) *Mental Health and Work: Impact, Issues and Good Practices*, Geneva: World Health Organization and the International Labour Organization.

Haslam, N. (2003) Categorical versus dimensional models of mental disorder: the taxometric evidence. *Australian and New Zealand Journal of Psychiatry*, 37 (6): 696–704.

Ilyas, S. and Moncreiff, J. (2012) Trends in prescriptions and costs of drugs for mental disorders in England, 1998–2010, *British Journal of Psychiatry*, 200 (5): 393–398.

Improving Access to Psychological Therapies (2015) *About Us*, Online. Available at www.iapt.nhs.uk/about-iapt/ (accessed 1 October 2015).

Kandel, E. (2012) *Principles of Neuroscience*, 5th ed., New York: McGraw Hill.

Maslow, A. (1943) A theory of human motivation, *Psychological Review*, 50 (4): 370–396.

Maughan, D. (2014) *Social Prescribing: A Pathway to Sustainability*, Online. Available at http://sustainablehealthcare.org.uk/mental-health-susnet/blog/2014/05/social-prescribing-pathway-sustainability (accessed 1 October 2015).

Mental Health Foundation (n.d.) *How to Look after Your Mental Health in Later Life*, London: Mental Health Foundation.

Miller, F. (2011) *Aristotle's Political Theory*, Online. Available at http://plato.stanford.edu/cgi-bin/encyclopedia/archinfo.cgi?entry=aristotle-politics (accessed 1 August 2015).

Mind (2007) *Ecotherapy: The Green Agenda for Mental Health*, Online. Available at www.mind.org.uk/media/273470/ecotherapy.pdf (accessed 6 December 2015).

Mind (2013a) *Mental Health Facts and Statistics*, Online. Available at www.mind.org.uk/information-support/types-of-mental-health-problems/statistics-and-facts-about-mental-health/how-common-are-mental-health-problems/ (accessed 29 September 2015).

Mind (2013b) *Ecominds*, Online. Available at www.mind.org.uk/ecominds (accessed 1 October 2015).

Mitchell, R.J., Richardson, E.A., Shortt, N.K. and Pearce, J.R. (2015) Neighborhood environments and socioeconomic inequalities in mental well-being, *American Journal of Preventive Medicine*, 49 (1): 80–84.

Mobility, Mood and Place (2015) *Mobility, Mood and Place: A Lifelong Health and Wellbeing funded research project*, Online. Available at https://sites.eca.ed.ac.uk/mmp/ (accessed 6 December 2015).

National Institute of Mental Health (2015) *Any Mental Illness (AMI) Among Adults*, Online. Available at www.nimh.nih.gov/health/statistics/prevalence/any-mental-illness-ami-among-adults.shtml (accessed 29 September 2015).

Ngoma, M.C., Prince, M. and Mann, A. (2003) Common mental disorders among those attending primary health clinics and traditional healers in urban Tanzania, *British Journal Psychiatry*, 183: 349–355.

NHS Choices (2014) *Five Steps to Mental Wellbeing – Stress, Anxiety and Depression*, Online. Available at www.nhs.uk/conditions/stress-anxiety-depression/pages/improve-mental-wellbeing.aspx (accessed 3 November 2014).

Nuffield Trust (2015) *NHS Spending on the Top Three Disease Categories in England*, Online. Available at www.nuffieldtrust.org.uk/data-and-charts/nhs-spending-top-three-disease-categories-england (accessed 1 October 2015).

Office for National Statistics (2015) *Measuring National Well-being: Domains and Measures, September 2015: Percentage with Some Evidence Indicating Depression or Anxiety*, Online. Available at domainsandmeasuresseptember2015_tcm77-417949.xls (accessed 1 October 2015).

Ojibwa (2014) *Traditional Native Concepts of Death*, Online. Available at http://nativeameri-cannetroots.net/diary/1726 (accessed 1 October 2015).

Panksepp, J. (2002) ADHD and the neural consequences of play and joy: a framing essay, *Consciousness and Emotion*, 3 (1): 1–6.

Parkes, C., Laungani, P. and Young, W. (eds.) (2003) *Death and Bereavement across Cultures*, London: Routledge.

Pomerantz, A. (2014) *Clinical Psychology: Science, Practice, and Culture*, 3rd ed., *DSM-5 Update*. London: Sage.

Robinson, L., Smith, M. and Segal, J. (2014) *Why Play Matters for Adults*. Online. Available: www.helpguide.org/life/creative_play_fun¬¬_games.htm. (accessed 1 October 2015).

Rutledge, R., Skandali, N., Dayan, P. and Dolan, R. (2014) A computational and neural model of momentary subjective wellbeing, *Proceedings of the National Academy of Sciences USA*, 111 (33): 12252–12257.

Paul, S. and Nadkani, V.V. (2014) A qualitative study on family acceptance, stigma and discrimination of persons with schizophrenia in an Indian metropolis, *International Social Work*, Online. Available at http://isw.sagepub.com/content/early/2014/10/07/0020872814547436 (accessed 6 December 2015).

Sutton-Smith, B. (1997) *The Ambiguity of Play*, Cambridge, MA: Harvard University Press.

Time to Change (2008) *Stigma Shout Service user and carer experiences of stigma and discrimination*, London: Time to Change.

Time to change (2008) *Mental Health Statistics, Facts and Myths*, Online. Available at www.time-to-change.org.uk/mental-health-statistics-facts (accessed 29 September 2008).

TNS BMRB (2014) *Attitudes to Mental Illness 2013 Research Report*, TNS BMRB.

Van der Vennet, R. and Serice, S. (2012) Can coloring mandalas reduce anxiety? A replication study, *Art Therapy*, 29 (2): 87–92.

Wade, J. (2015) *How to be Happy: The Health Squad*, Online. Available at www.bromfordlab.com/labblog/2015/5/22/bromfordsquads-health (accessed 1 October 2015).

Wakefield, J. C. (2013) DSM-5: An overview of changes and controversies. *Clinical Social Work Journal*, 41: 139–154.

Weich, S., Brugha, T., King, M., McManus, S., Bebbington, P., Jenkins, R., Cooper, C., McBride, O. and Stewart-Brown, S. (2011) Mental well-being and mental illness: findings from the Adult Psychiatric Morbidity Survey for England 2007, *The British Journal of Psychiatry*, 199 (1): 23–28.

Wikan, U. (1988) Bereavement and loss in two Muslim communities: Egypt and Bali compared, *Social Sciences and Medicine*, 27 (5):451–460.

Williams, Z. (2015) Adult colouring-in books: the latest weapon against stress and anxiety, *The Guardian*, 26 June 2015. Online. Available at www.theguardian.com (accessed 5 October 2015).

Wilson-Mulnix, J. and Mulnix, M.J. (2015) *Happy Lives, Good Lives: A Philosophical Examination*, Toronto: Broadview Press.

Witchen (2011) The size and burden of mental disorders and other disorders of the brain in Europe 2010. *European Neuropsychpharmacology*, 201: 655–679.

World Health Organization (2014) *Mental Health: A State of Well-being*, Online. Available at www.who.int/features/factfiles/mental_health/en/ (accessed: 27 September 2015).

9

MUSIC AS MEDICINE

Rachel Bayliss

This chapter will explore the many positive benefits that music has to offer. Music offers enjoyment and pleasure in its own right, which contribute to positive health and emotional wellness across the lifespan, both at participatory and spectator levels. As Browne (1864) suggests, 'there is or may be hidden life within, which may be reached by harmony'.

Introduction

That music itself may be a medicinal agent is not a new sentiment. Music and medicine have been inextricably linked as twinned arts since ancient times and the echoes of this are seen in the modern professions of music therapy and healthcare play specialism. Stories and case studies emerge from the shadows of the past and from the dark labyrinths of medical history of music being used as a prescriptive adjunct to healthcare, as a form of therapy and as a means of engaging people who might otherwise have struggled to integrate themselves into health and social services. The universal and ageless entity of music decorates the research pages of healthcare and healthcare play specialism and enriches medical experiences contributing to a deeper sense of health and wellbeing across the lifespan.

Historical context

Ancient beginnings

The historical context sets the backdrop, the tapestry from which the entities of music therapy and play specialism are woven. Early musings of musical medicine took root in the fertile soils of philosophy, mathematics and medicine cultivated by the Ancient Greeks. Greek Medicine centred on the concept of balance, harmony and a body in equilibrium. Music was identified as a means of restoring imbalance to neutrality. In Greek mythology, the god Apollo presided over medicine but his divine remit extended into the world of music and in most depictions he is shown as holding a lyre in his hand as shown in Figure 9.1. This has been heralded by many as a symbolic interrelation of these two disciplines (Alvin 1975).

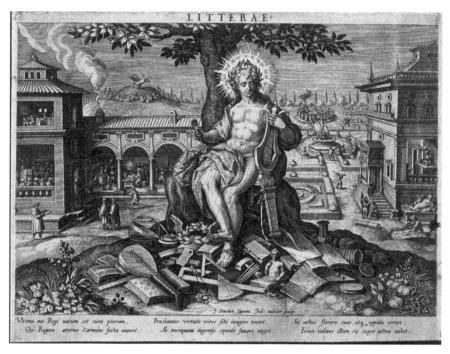

FIGURE 9.1 Apollo, God of literature, plays his harp; a town goes about its rituals (van der Straet 1594, produced courtesy of the Wellcome Library under Creative Commons Licence CC BY 4.0)

Several of the Greek heavyweight thinkers were also proponents of music as a means of medicine. A specific example is uncovered in the writings of Aristotle, the renowned Greek philosopher, who stipulated that music had the power to imprint feelings on the soul and thereby its melodies could be akin to medicines (Aristotle 350 BC, cited in West 2001). In this respect, the Ancient Greeks could be seen as leaving the blueprints of music as medicine upon which later centuries could build.

Continuing musical evolution

The musical tradition was sculpted by a transition through many different eras, cultures and nationalities. The rich legacy inherited from the ancients was built upon and evolved into a multi-faceted scientific art. The stepping stones of the Greek tradition were mirrored in the attitudes of Roman civilization and the practices of healing music continued to reverberate through the streets of Rome just as they had done through Athens. In this period, the self-fashioned epitome of Hippocratic medicine was Galen. As a physician, he appreciated that music could have a profound influence on a person's 'ethos' and therefore health; he prescribed songs to alleviate perceived imbalance in the body's equilibrium (West cited in Horden 2001). Another archetypal physician in this age was Celsus and he too heralded music as a beneficial agent to wellbeing and described case studies of its use in mental illness (Celsus 1 BC, cited in West 2001). Long after the demise of the Roman Empire, these notions of music as medicine were kept alive, continually receiving impetus from many a contrasting culture and era.

Those inclined to excavate the writings of the early religious traditions will find that etched beneath the stones of spiritualism there lies a delicate web of musical healing. Biblical accounts found in the Old Testament can be viewed as reinforcing the concept of music as a medicine for the mind. One such example is with the story of David and Saul, described as 'David took a harp, and played with his hand; so Saul was refreshed, and was well' (I Samuel 16 v 23 as cited in New International Version (NIV) Bible 2011). This idea is reciprocated within the historical Islamic tradition. Ibn Hindu, an Islamic poet and physician of the tenth century postulated that 'the science of music belongs to the medical art' (Hindu as cited in Burnett 2000). The symbiotic relationship between music and medicine is invoked here; music is depicted as the *science* with medicine as the *art*. This practice was extended into the wider landscape of Arabic medicine. This used musical modes known as 'maqamat' (a paralleled form of the musical scale); certain 'maqam' were used in order to incite specific emotional effects to combat particular illnesses (Burnett 2000). The hallmark historical physician of Arabic medicine, Avicenna, published his 'Canons of Medicine' which encapsulated notions of musical medicine with suggestions of 'agreeable music' to soothe and incline people to sleep (Avicenna 1020 AD cited in Licht 1946). As well as the international dimension to musical medicine, this highlights the important interrelation between the different aspects of health (as discussed in Chapter 5) as spiritual wellbeing is closely connected to achieving overall health across the lifespan.

The awakenings of evidence for musical medicine

During the Renaissance, discussions of music as a form of medicine were re-ignited. At this time, attitudes to both music and medicine were changing; new discoveries were unearthed, foundations of ancient assumptions were being shaken and the emerging secular art of musical medicine was freeing itself from the shackles of previous theory. Further to this, a real blossoming of music as a medical entity began to materialize in eighteenth century. This was a dawning horizon for the visionary music therapists.

118 Rachel Bayliss

One of the first academic scholarly treatises to be published on the subject of musical medicine was written in 1749 by Brocklesby, English physician to the famous lexicographer Dr Samuel Johnson. His work surveyed the anecdotal evidence of music as medicine before stepping into new territory. By writing with strong scientific undertones and furnishing his pages with case studies the result was a glittering piece of music therapy writing that, in many ways, was a forerunner to various modern tenets of musical therapy. One of his cases described a gentleman who had suffered with depression following the death of two of his sons. After all other remedies had been exhausted, a violin was tried and this was identified as the turning point for his pathway back to wellbeing (Brocklesby 1749). Intertwining these case-based examples was a landmark development that served to bolster the authenticity of music as medicine by harnessing an evidence-based dimension to its practice.

The journey of musical medicine further unfolds later in the nineteenth century, within the epoch of history known as the 'asylum era'. This was a time where real engravings of change were cementing, both within musical medicine and in attitudes towards psychiatric illness in general. The previous 'museums of madness' (Scull 1993) dotted across the country were brought together in a national infrastructure and the asylum came to a national consciousness and organization. Music was increasingly recognized as having an inherent quality to unlock something within the tainted mind and bring the grey darkness of depression into the colors of recovery. Reports emerged of musical instruments being used as a means of emotional release, sung participation was encouraged and professionals were employed to play music to individuals residing within the asylums (Hunter and Macalpine 2013). The literature from this period is brimming with examples of similar practice: case reports of stringed instruments used in the treatment of depression (Knight 1827), asylum concerts and patients being encouraged to participate and play instruments as a means of therapy (MacKenzie 1992). Medical journals started to sit up and take notice and there was a growing realization that music was a valuable medium to serve as an expressive emotional outlet; a means of communication for crying minds whose pains could not be articulated through words.

This brief and limited snapshot through history merely provides a glimpse of the journey of musical medicine through the centuries and is intended only to scratch the surface. This international, extended heritage has resulted in musical medicine being a reflective kaleidoscope of different traditions with inputs distilled from contrasting civilisations, religions, cultures and nations.

Music across the lifespan and in specific situations

Music can resonate with each of the six aspects of health as identified by Bruce and Meggitt (2005) and discussed earlier in Chapter 5. It can beneficially influence wellbeing across the lifespan and forms a natural alliance with play both through spontaneous participation and the improvisation born from creative melody. Music

Music as medicine **119**

has been analysed and utilized in a variety of different healthcare settings across the age range and is a promising area for further development.

It has been speculated that music can affect the human mind from in utero right up until death. The much publicized and debated 'Mozart effect' (i.e. that listening to selected pieces of Mozart's music may enhance brain functions) has been researched from the womb through to the elderly. A recent quantitative Italian study found a positive correlation between Mozart's music and activation of neurological circuits involved in cognitive functions (Verrusio *et al.* 2015). More extensive research is needed but it is a potentially exciting finding that listening to music at spectator level can augment cognitive processing. This effect of music on the mind is by no means limited to adult life and research has demonstrated that our brains, even in the earliest stages of life, are susceptible to music. A research paper published in America demonstrated that as early as the postnatal hours, neonatal brains are sensitive to changes in musical key, dissonance and consonance (Perani *et al.* 2010).

This idea that music can exert a powerful influence on wellbeing has been incorporated into practical schemes of musical therapy which have been initiated at local, national and international levels. Preti and Boyce-Tillman (2015) have undertaken research to evaluate the multi-arts project 'Elevate: using the arts to uplift people in hospital'. This program, delivered by ArtCare for Salisbury District Hospital in England, is focused primarily on older patients (Preti and Boyce-Tillman 2015). The Elevate program appears to be effective on a number of levels, not only for the patients themselves, but also for the staff and the artists involved. The medium of singing was used to promote socialization among patients who subsequently reported experiencing 'physical, cognitive, social and emotional benefits' (Preti and Boyce-Tillman 2015: 34). One of the most effective and enjoyable elements of the project were the monthly concert performances. These concerts were performed by 'world class musicians' across various locations in the hospital. For the patients,

> the Elevate concert series exposed some of the patients to new instruments and new music repertoires, pushing their cultural boundaries and stimulating their memories; The concerts also enabled the patients and their caregivers to share a special and very different time together in the hospital and to build a positive memory of the hospital as a culturally conducive environment.
>
> *(Preti and Boyce-Tillman 2015: 6)*

The musicians also performed in the staff canteen on the day of the concert so that staff could also enjoy the performance during their lunchbreak. The concerts generated a relaxing ambience which was seen to facilitate the work of staff and led to the development of a music system that could be used to play background music throughout the day (Preti and Boyce-Tillman 2015). Another popular element of the Elevate program was the monthly tea-party entitled 'Everything stops for tea'. A professional dancer, in vintage 1950s garb, would serve 'tea and cakes on bone china to patients' to live musical accompaniment (Preti and Boyce-Tillman 2015: 9). These musical interludes appeared to have a longer lasting effect on the wards, particularly for staff who were often heard to hum or sing a familiar tune whilst attending to a patient's personal care or as a means of distraction during the performance of nursing tasks (Preti and Boyce-Tillman 2015).

The playful possibilities of music as a healthcare intervention are gaining increasing credibility.

It is important to recognize that music as a means of medicine is a cross-cultural, international concept. The appreciation of music as a potential medical agent is one that is not confined to first world developed countries. Music has a longstanding and vibrant relationship with the African tradition. The history of the African holistic approach to health is peppered with religious ideology, shrine ceremonies and musical healing. More recently, an experimental study published in South Africa concluded that traditional Djembe drumming may improve overall cardiovascular health via the coupled benefits of physical exertion (with the drumming technique) and the emotional value of the decreased stress and anxiety levels (Smith *et al.* 2014). In a wide range of contexts across the world, music is gaining recognition for its positive health and social benefits.

Music has also been utilized in specific medical situations as a facilitator of the recovery process. The intricate and elusive nature of the relationship between music and the human mind has posed many questions to researchers and practitioners alike and has been shown to have a dramatic impact on therapeutic interventions. Dr Oliver Sacks, a renowned practising neurologist and musician in New York, has published several books detailing his observations on individuals afflicted by various illnesses where music has steered the rehabilitation journey. He describes a gentleman known as 'Clive' who had been an eminent musician before contracting encephalitis (an infection of the substance of the brain) that sadly resulted in a profound amnesia leaving him with a memory span of only a few seconds. After the re-introduction of music to his life, the entire picture of his recovery was changed and he demonstrated a surprising ability to remember musical pieces he once knew despite not knowing his personal past. Sacks also observed that he was able to 'improvise, joke and play with any piece of music' (Sacks 2008: 212). This had a domino effect on his social skills, conversational ability and overall emotional wellbeing (Sacks 2008).

This therapeutic inspiration of music has been reflected in cases of other acquired brain injuries such as trauma and stroke. Music therapy with stroke patients has shown that musical guided intonation can enhance speech ability. It has been elicited, through functional MRI studies, that music activates particular locations within the right brain hemisphere (as distinct from the conventional speech centers in the left) which may explain the phenomenon whereby stroke patients can initially sing sentences but not speak them verbally. Extending this process, it is thought that music can therefore help to rebuild speech pathways by igniting the linguistic potential of the right side of the brain to compensate for the left-sided stroke damage (Norton *et al.* 2009; Odezmir *et al.* 2006). Musical benefits also encompass physical health in this dimension. A Cochrane review in 2010 concluded that Rhythmic Auditory Stimulation (RAS), a musical cuing technique to aid training of movement, may improve gait parameters in those with acquired brain injuries (Bradt *et al.* 2010).

Musical play has also found its place in dementia care. Dementia is fast becoming a global health explosion with over 44 million people worldwide thus diagnosed (Alzheimer's Disease International 2015) and healthcare provision and policy have needed to realign themselves with growing demands. Music has been uncovered as a communicative method of evoking response, engaging participation and inviting social interaction. When the cognitive faculties are damaged, communication can be facilitated through music; singing familiar songs serves to ignite the surviving self and bring alive retained familiarity. Just as we respond to music from the early hours of life (Perani *et al.* 2010), it is understood that our primitive response to music is preserved even in advanced dementia and can provide a lifeline of precious anchorage to the previous self (Sacks 2009; Cowles *et al.* 2003). This notion has been developed by Alzheimer's UK who have instigated 'Singing for the Brain', a simple vocal musical scheme set up for the purpose of bringing together people with dementia and their carers by stimulating fun and play through songs (Alzheimer's UK 2015). This concept further links in with the wider practice of reminiscence therapy. This uses reminders and tangible prompts of past activities, events and experiences to provide valuable grounding links to memories, identity and a sense of self which can be easily lost as dementia takes hold. This has been shown to be of significance in improving cognition, mood and behavioral function of those with dementia (Woods *et al.* 2005). A more detailed insight into music and its role in dementia care is explored in Chapter 10.

Musical medicine is also branching-out into less conventional and newer areas of implementation across the world, such as within the field of anaesthetics. The calming nature of music has been analysed as an adjunct to analgesia in the operative setting. A Chinese research group promisingly found that music exerted a positive impact on decreasing anxiety, stress and postoperative pain in a group of elderly patients (Wang *et al.* 2014). Additionally, evidence has also signalled that music may be of value even for the sickest patients. A Cochrane review of international studies looking at the value of listening to music for mechanically ventilated patients on intensive care units, demonstrated that music not only served to alleviate anxiety but that it was observed to consistently decrease respiratory rate and blood pressure and therefore augment conventional sedatives and analgesics (Bradt and Dileo 2014).

Overall, this limited exploration into the literature and evidence for music as medicine is flourishing with examples of music being utilized in a wide variety of settings and healthcare systems worldwide. However, promising early research needs to be extended and although musical play is finding its feet as a medical entity, there is still a long way to go.

122 Rachel Bayliss

Conclusion

Music inherently emits a cohesive beauty that transcends lifespan, culture, inequality and international differences. It can go hand in hand with play as it naturally overflows with opportunities for spontaneity, improvisation, learning and enjoyment. This notion of music as a tool within medicine and health play specialism has crystallized from a rich tradition of elements mixed together in the cauldrons of theory and observation that have simmered through history as the centuries have rolled on into the light of modernity.

The art of music can be analysed and dressed in the cloak of science but, as yet, science does not have the power to fully understand it; perhaps therein lies music's beautiful paradox. The carefully calculated mathematical and quantifiable notes of music can exert such a powerful immeasurable effect on the human mind and reach into crevices that have not yet been mapped by medicine and perhaps never will be.

References

Alvin, J. (1975) *Music Therapy,* London: Hutchinson.
Alzheimer's Disease International (2015) *Dementia Statistics,* Online. Available at www.alz. co.uk/research/statistics (accessed 21 July 2015).
Alzheimer's UK (2015) *Singing for the Brain,* Online. Available at www.alzheimers.org.uk/ site/scripts/documents_info.php?documentID=760 (accessed 21 July 2015).
Bradt, J. and Dilco, C. (2014) Music interventions for mechanically ventilated patients, *Cochrane Database of Systematic Reviews*. Online. Available at http://onlinelibrary.wiley. com/doi/10.1111/jebm.12143/pdf (accessed 11 December 2015).
Bradt, J., Magee, W.L., Dileo, C., Wheeler, B.L. and McGilloway, E. (2010) Music therapy for acquired brain injury, *Cochrane Database of Systematic Reviews*. Online. Available at http://onlinelibrary.wiley.com/doi/10.1002/14651858.CD006787.pub2/full (accessed 11 December 2015).
Brocklesby, R. (1749) *Reflexions on Antient and Modern Musick: with the Application to the Cure of Diseases,* London: Cooper (accessible at the Wellcome Trust Library, London).
Browne, R. (1864) *Medicine Musica: Or, a Mechanical Essay on the Effects of Singing, Musick, and Dancing, on Human Bodies,* Gale ECCO, Print Editions.
Bruce, T. and Meggit, C. (2005) *Child Care and Education,* 3rd ed., London: Hodder Arnold.
Burnett, C (2000). Spiritual medicine: music and healing in Islam and its influence in Western medicine, in Gouk, P. (ed.), *Musical Healing in Cultural Contexts,* London: Ashgate: 84–101.
Cowles, A., Beatty, W., Nixon, S.J, Lutz, L.J., Paulk, J., Paulk, K. and Ross E.D. (2003) Musical skill in dementia: a violinist presumed to have Alzheimer's disease learns to play a new song, *Neurocase* 9(6): 493–503.
Horden, P. (2001) *Music in Medicine: The History of Music Therapy since Antiquity,* London: Ashgate.
Hunter, R. and Macalpine, I (2013). *Three Hundred Years of Psychiatry,* Montana: Literary Licensing Company LLC.
Knight, P. (1827) *Observations on the Causes, Symptoms and Treatment of Derangement of the Mind, Founded on an Extensive Moral and Medical Practice in the Treatment of Lunatics,* London: Longman.

Licht, S. (1946) *Music in Medicine.* Boston: New England Conservatory of Music.

MacKenzie, C (1992) *Psychiatry for the Rich: A History of the Ticehurst Private Asylum 1792–1917,* New York: Routledge.

New International Version (NIV) Bible (2011) *NIV Student Bible,* Grand Rapids, MI: Zondervan.

Norton, A., Zipse, L., Marchina, S. and Schlaug, G. (2009) Melodic intonation therapy. Shared insights on how it is done and why it might help, *Annals of the New York Academy of Sciences,* 1169: 431–436.

Ozdemir, E., Norton, A. and Schlaugh, G. (2006) Shared and distinct neural correlates of singing and speaking. *Neuroimage,* 33: 628–635.

Perani, D., Saccuman, M., Scifo, P., Spada, D., Andreolli, G., Rovelli, R., Baldoli, C. and Koelsch, S. (2010) Functional specializations for music processing in the human newborn brain, *Proceedings of the National Academy of Sciences of America – PNAS),* 107 (10): 4758–4763.

Preti, C. and Boyce-Tillman, J. (2015) *Elevate: Using the Arts to Uplift People in Hospital,* Salisbury: ArtCare.

Sacks, O. (2008) *Musicophilia,* Oxford: Picador.

Scull, A. (1993) *The Most Solitary of Afflictions: Madness and Society in Britain 1700–1900,* New Haven, CT: Yale: University Press.

Smith C., Viljoen, J.T., and McGeachie, L. (2014) African drumming: a holistic approach to reducing stress and improving health? *Journal of Cardiovascular Medicine (Hagerstown),* 15(6): 441–446.

Verussio W,. Ettorre, E., Vicenzini, E., Vanacores, N., Cacciafesta, M and Mecareli, O. (2015) The Mozart effect: a quantitative EEG study, *Consciousness and Cognition,* 35: 150–155.

Wang, Y., Dong, Y. and Li, Y. (2014) Perioperative psychological and music interventions in elderly patients undergoing spinal anaesthesia: effect on anxiety, heart rate variability, and postoperative pain, *Yonsei Medical Journal,* 55 (4): 1101–1105.

Wellcome Images Collection. Apollo plays his harp, a town goes about its rituals. IVC collection reference 7790, Online. Available at http://wellcomeimages.org/indexplus/page/Home.html. (accessed 20 July 2015).

West, M. (2001) Music therapy in antiquity, in Horden, P. (ed.), *Music in Medicine: The History of Music Therapy since Antiquity,* Farnham: Ashgate: 72–97.

van der Straet, J. (1594) Apollo, god of literature, plays his harp; a town goes about its rituals, [Photograph]. Wellcome Library, London. IVC collection reference 7790. Online. Available at http://wellcomeimages.org/indexplus/page/Home.html (accessed 20 July 2015). Copyrighted work available under Creative Commons Attribution only licence CC BY 4.0 http://creativecommons.org/licenses/by/4.0/

Woods, B., Spector, A., Jones, C., Orrel, M. and Davies, S. (2005) Reminiscence therapy for dementia, *Cochrane Database of Systematic Reviews.* Online. Available at http://online library.wiley.com/doi/10.1002/14651858.CD001120.pub2/pdf (accessed 11 December 2015).

10
THE GAME OF CHAMBER MUSIC IN DEMENTIA MUSIC THERAPY

Emilie Capulet

To complement Rachel Bayliss's overview of music and medicine in the previous chapter, this chapter provides an example of how a series of classical chamber music workshops were used to facilitate the creativity, spontaneity and playfulness of a small group of people with early-onset dementia, by creating a shared 'space of play' and contributing to the promotion of their wellbeing through music.

Introduction

Dementia affects an estimated 46.8 million people worldwide, a figure which may grow exponentially in the coming years as the world's population ages (Alzheimer's Disease International 2015). It is not a disease as such, but a clinical syndrome defined by a collection of symptoms (Dening and Sandilyan 2015) which have broadly been characterized by Aldridge (2005) as being 'dialogic-degenerative'. The clinical features of dementia include, amongst other symptoms, memory and language impairments, as well as a decline in cognitive functions, often leading to a break-down in communication, social isolation, anxiety, compulsive behaviors and/ or depression. Finding a way to enhance the quality of life of people with dementia whilst stimulating their cognitive functions is gradually becoming a significant concern for healthcare providers, as no drug treatment has yet been found to cure dementia. As Zeilig (2015: 13) has argued, 'it is crucial to recognize that "dementia" represents more than a medical condition and that the wider social, cultural and political context also influences the ways in which people live with this diagnosis'.

Music is increasingly seen to have an essential non-pharmacological therapeutic role within healthcare. As Thaut (2005: 115) has argued,

> brain research involving music has shown that music has a distinct influence on the brain by stimulating physiologically complex cognitive, affective, and

Chamber music in dementia therapy **125**

sensorimotor processes. [...] This is a very critical step in the historical understanding of music in therapy and medicine.

Relying on a wide array of musical activities to engage the patients on cognitive, emotional, behavioral and physiological levels, music therapy (understood here as the use of music in therapy) has also recently started to take into account the patients' socio-cultural background, musical culture and institutional setting, in order to tailor the musical sessions to the individual needs and circumstances of the participants (Ruud 2010). Musical activities, as well as potentially stimulating patients' cognitive functions, also help to re-initiate dialogue and communication, and ultimately re-establish, if only briefly, a sense of shared (musical) experience and personal identity, therefore playing a significant role in dementia healthcare (Aldridge 2005; Ridder 2005). Although there is clear need for further clinical research into the cognitive effects of music for people with dementia, it does appear that non-pharmacological interventions such as group music interventions potentially relieve some of the dementia-related anxiety (Ing-Randolph *et al.* 2015). Recent research in music therapy has shown that, although passive or 'receptive' music therapy which solely involves listening to music, can be useful as a tool to help stimulate memory and reduce stress (Simmons-Stern *et al.* 2010), Sakamoto *et al.* (2013: 783) have argued, in a promising study of the effects of music therapy on severe dementia cases, that it is the actual act of playing/singing music, or *active* music therapy, which helps to 'directly stimulate cognitive and emotional function in individuals with cognitive reserve', thus concluding that 'interactive music intervention can provide a useful and effective caregiving tool' (Sakamoto *et al.* 2013: 782).

Arts4Dementia, jointly with the English Chamber Orchestra Ensemble (ECO Ensemble) and the London College of Music (LCM), University of West London (UWL), developed a series of classical chamber music workshops involving musicians of different backgrounds, age and musical abilities. Over eight weeks, the participants, which included four musicians in the initial stages of early-onset dementia, six undergraduate and postgraduate students on the LCM BMus (Hons) or MMus degree courses in music performance, and six professional orchestral musicians, took part in collaborative chamber music sessions. The participants with dementia had all regularly played an instrument during their lives and had a certain degree of technical musical skills which allowed them to actively participate in the chamber music workshops. Whilst not all participants with dementia were present every week, the core group of students and professional musicians maintained a sense of group cohesion and continuity between sessions. The relatively small number of participants with dementia at each given session (often a ratio of six to one or six to two) meant that they were integrated in the group as musicians rather than people with dementia. Participants with dementia noticed this, commenting:

They are professionals and they want to interact with me, and I towards them, so I think it will be a great match.

126 Emilie Capulet

> I liked the passion with which they're blending me in. I really do.

> It was good. I like the informality of it, the comradeship of it. I felt part of it straight away.

> I loved the players' attitude. They were so inviting. We had a very interactive session. I wouldn't have missed it for the world. There's nothing like live music.

As the musicians with dementia were still in the early phase of the condition, they were quite conscious of the limitations it imposed on them. Most of the participating student musicians, as well as some of the professional musicians, had a limited experience of dementia but they all participated in a dementia awareness training day to help them understand the syndrome. Although there was a tacit understanding during the sessions that participants were there to share a musical experience which went beyond individual circumstances, the sheer conviviality of the sessions opened up a space for dialogue. This was always freely initiated by the musicians with dementia, who shared insights into their condition, how it affects their lives, and the meaning music holds for them. The fact that music played such an important role in the lives of the people with dementia, opened up the students' eyes (and ears) as to how music is more than just about playing the notes, but is truly meaningful to a wide range of people. Student participants thus reflected after the sessions:

> I felt satisfaction in knowing how much the workshops meant to some of the participants and was helping them find new strategies and musical ideas for their dementia.

> Most of all [the workshops] made me realize the effect of music in medical kind of terms. How it helps people in their daily struggles.

> I started to have the belief that the music is worth more than I thought before, which motivates me.

> By working with people with dementia, I started to seek more honest and truly good ways of musical expression in playing.

The musicians with dementia were very honest in sharing their difficulties but as this took place within the learning context of the university, with the participating students also facing technical challenges during the sessions, this put the dementia-related challenges into a more neutral perspective. Whilst the learning process was not, originally, part of the rationale behind the sessions, one of the participants with dementia remarkably summed up this up:

Chamber music in dementia therapy **127**

The thing about this is that it is educational, but there's no pressure. When he got me to lead, I had to develop a technique of conducting with my instrument. I'd never played with stringed instruments. It's expanded my musical experiences. It was that relaxed that I was able to say I'll give it a go. There wouldn't be any criticism if it wasn't right. It puts it back to pure enjoyment of music and no pressure. While you're playing, whatever else is happening in your life that takes second place because you were there in the moment.

As one student remarked, the 'English Chamber Orchestra members made us like improvise and transpose on spot, something that violinists never do often'. This in turn, led the musician with dementia to say that:

The interaction today was very good, the way they tried to see the challenges that exist for me. They all then started transposing and they could see the difficulties even when they haven't got a cognitive impairment. They were challenged though as much as I was being challenged. Everything was on a level playing field as they tried to feel my difficulties.

The distinctive features of the music workshops was the intergenerational nature of the sessions, the focus on active musical playing, and the participation of musicians in the early stages of early-onset dementia, thus illustrating what Hartogh *et al.* (2014: 6) describes as an 'absolutely essential exchange between the generations [which] suggests an intergenerational orientation that opens up a lot of opportunities for musical encounters'. Significantly though, it was this concept of a 'level playing field' which became central to the success of these chamber music workshops.

Unlike one-to-one instrumental tuition, listening activities or conducted musical ensembles where a facilitator, usually a professional musician, positions him/herself as an expert to be followed, chamber music is an activity which puts everybody on the same creative footing in what could be described as a non-hierarchical community of music-making. Mark Making's 'The Arts in Dementia Care' research project, based at the University for the Arts (London), has similarly highlighted 'the ability for the arts to unite groups of people who are otherwise disparate in generation, gender, occupation and physical or mental health' (cited in Zeilig 2015). As one LCM student participant said, the workshops

Enabled me to think of working in the future in more different environments and made me think I have the possibility and ability to work with a wider variety of people.

Shepherd and Wicke (1997 cited in Hara 2011: 38) have argued that 'music is not an object, a "thing", but a set of processes that inevitably involves people. Music is an inherently social process'. Being in such close contact with a variety of

128 Emilie Capulet

musicians highlighted the social relevance of musical performance. Often, this social process can be forgotten by younger musicians, who often spend much of their time practising alone. Rooted in a long pedagogical tradition initiated by William James (1907) and John Dewey (1938), the idea of connecting students to the realities of society has been the subject of discussion for over a century. Dewey (1907) argued that it is critical that educational strategies include what has been called 'experiential learning'. More recently, Boyer (1990: 21) argues that 'what we urgently need today is a more inclusive view of what it means to be a scholar – a recognition that knowledge is acquired through research, through synthesis, through practice and through teaching'. He asks the question 'can social problems themselves define an agenda for scholarly investigation?' (Boyer 1990: 21). As Deeley (2015) has argued, this has yet to be regularly embedded within the higher education culture in the UK. The above mentioned workshops went beyond experiential learning methodologies to align themselves with what is called the community-based service-learning approach to pedagogy. Service learning has been defined by Jacoby (1996) as a form of experiential education in which students engage in activities that address human and community needs together with structured opportunities intentionally designed to promote student learning and development. Reflection and reciprocity are key concepts of service learning. It is tied up with notions of voluntarism and citizenship. It also fosters a reciprocal and symbiotic relationship between Institutions of Higher Education and the local and wider community. It makes our curriculum more meaningful for the students as it challenges them to think critically about how they can address the welfare needs of society as a whole. Our workshops brought the social context into sharp focus as students had to adapt to playing in new circumstances, as exemplified in the following quotes:

> Working with people with dementia means to learn how to interact with people in different circumstances. It is always relevant for me to be challenged into something new and understand the wider world.

> It took me to the stage that I played the music and used my skill directly to the people and not for the sake of music itself. So the quality of playing had to be somehow more directly interactive.

Chamber music players are undeniably finely attuned to the inherently collaborative, creative and communicative nature of their musical practice. Playing without a conductor, these musicians are especially attentive to each other's creative processes through acute listening, shared musical and physical gestures, a sense of common purpose and, importantly, that vital degree of spontaneity, playfulness and musical repartee which, more than anything else, brings to life the music being performed. Though it would seem that the rules of musical performance are clearly embedded within the score itself, the notes on the page are but the starting point for a spirited performance whose 'meaning is always constituting itself anew'

(Adorno 1981: 144). In *The Letter and the Spirit*, Ralph Vaughan Williams humorously declared that:

> Heard music has the same relation to the printed notes as a railway journey has to a time table. But the printed notes are no more music than the map is the country which it represents or the time table the journey which it indicates.
>
> *(1920/1987: 124)*

Musical performance is a paradox resulting from the inescapable discrepancy which exists between the composer's musical vision as imperfectly notated in the score and the musician's physical execution of what is thus imperfectly notated. Chamber music in particular allows scope for musicians to explore what Ingarden (1989: 90) has termed *Unbestimmtheitsstellen* or places of indeterminacy. Chamber musicians have to spontaneously follow their personal musical sensibility, competitively taking the lead in turn, in order to shape and direct the musical journey, instigating a musical dialogue with their partners. Although they cannot break the fundamental rules of the musical game as set by the score's notated rhythms, pitches and dynamics, musicians are certainly able (if not, at times, implicitly expected to) to bend these rules in performance, heightening what Adorno (1981: 144) describes as the 'tension between the composition's essence and its sensuous appearance'. Speaking in similar terms about the writing process, Roland Barthes has argued that the 'space' of tension between text and reader is in fact a space of *play* which allows for the 'possibility of a dialectic of desire, the unpredictability of pleasure: that the dice may not be cast, that the game isn't over' (1973: 11). In the original French text, the verb *jouer* (to play) is given the noun *le jeu* (the game), allowing Barthes a play with words here.

Similarly, in the case of music we could argue that it is the space of performance, between score and musician, that is a space of play. With language, and arguably, with music also, 'we are playing with an exceptional object [...]: immutably structured and yet infinitely renewed: rather like a game of chess' (Barthes 1973: 82). Thus, paradoxically, the game of chamber music is at once predictable (in its score) and unpredictable (in its execution). It is a collaborative act of interpretation, but it is shaped by individual responses to the music. It is inventive but also repetitive. It is creative and yet its outcome is pre-determined by the score.

Though chamber music immerses the musicians into a space of shared creativity, it is the fact that it leads the participants to interact with each other in a meaningful and stimulating way which turns it into a stimulating game. Indeed, though the musical piece is determined by the musical notes on the page, the musical game is played on another level altogether: without a leader, the players are required to make a decision concerning how to interpret the score on an individual basis, although each decision affects how, in turn, the other players respond. This echoes Gilles' definition of a game as:

130 Emilie Capulet

> A social interactive decision situation … The decision makers are called the players within that game. Each player is assumed to have control over at least one decision moment in the course of the game. At each decision moment under her control, a player selects from a well-described set of multiple actions.
>
> *(Gilles 2010: 1)*

Building on Winnicott's (1971) concept of the 'transitional' space in a child's early development – an imaginary world of play where the child can be creative, original, authentic and true to its self, Kenny (1989) speaks of the musical 'space' in music therapy as being a space of play, or in her terms, a 'field of play': 'the Field of Play … is about imagination, consciousness, presence, attitude, and being. The Field of Play is all about conditions in the space, the primary one being … *being*' (Kenny 2014). Though all musical activities immerse the participants, to a certain degree, in an act of musical re-creation which takes place in that moment of 'being', not all participatory musical activities are as close to being a 'space of play', as is chamber music. Kenny (2014) has furthermore argued that what defines the 'being' within the 'field of play' is a sense of 'connection to all living things', echoing Tajfel and Turner's (1986 cited in Mapes 2004: 149) assertion that 'a significant part of our individual identity is derived from group membership'. Being connected is a concept which touches the very essence of chamber music – it is what chamber music is about.

When considered within the framework of McCallum and Boletsis's (2013) SG4D taxonomy of serious dementia games, our chamber music sessions fulfilled all three game category criteria at once: they had the potential to stimulate the cognitive functions of the players, encouraged physical activity and coordination through playing an instrument, and encouraged players to communicate with their musical partners. Engaging all four health user/player types, in terms of game types, chamber music corresponds primarily to the preventative and/or rehabilitative types although, in the case of our workshops, it also touched on the educative type, as it was a learning experience for all participants. What was particularly striking was the fact that the participants with early-onset dementia were quite keen and honest about sharing their experience of dementia and how it had affected their musical skills. As one student remarked: 'Listening and learning from the participants was a very valuable experience – how they try to overcome their dementia with dignity'. Another felt that 'their life stories and musical experiences are very inspirational and I learnt a great deal about music through them such as N's Indian instruments'.

The workshops thus created a 'space of play', and triggered enhanced communication between participants through what Hessenberg and Schmid (2013) calls the 'unifying gesture of music', whilst also breaking down any social barriers between the participants (Hessenberg and Schmid 2013). Playing a range of instruments, including tenor horn, violin, cello, double-bass, Indian accordion, flute, saxophone and piano, the group of musicians shaped, in turn, the different interpretations and approaches to the music being performed in a creative and innovative ways. During the sessions, the group explored different ways of playing music together, including familiar chamber music repertoire and/or improvisation. They also spent quite a lot of time talking about their instruments, comparing them and trying them out. There was no obligation to take part in the actual playing. Some participants with dementia preferred to sit and listen before gaining the confidence to actively take part. As one of the carers said:

> I notice that J played the piano the first week, then conducting last week but this week he was content to watch. I don't know if it's the decline. I know he's fully engaged.

One participant brought his father's sitar to some of the sessions. Although he couldn't play the instrument himself, as he was an Indian accordion player, he got the string players of the group to try it out with a degree of success. To help demarcate the opening and ending of the sessions one particular piece, a Passion Chorale by J.S. Bach, was chosen as a 'theme tune' albeit played differently at each session. In this 'space of play', the score's *Unbestimmtheitstellen,* allowed musicians to play with dynamics, articulation, pitch and tempo through leading gestures, thus initiating a dynamic musical dialogue. Each musician spontaneously or voluntarily took the lead in deciding how to play it, the others following suit (or not!). Often, the players with dementia would use metaphors to describe the musical effect they were hearing. On playing the Bach pizzicato, one participant exclaimed: 'Sounds like sparkling shower of drops, like a water sprite'. Each performance reflected the participants' mood and personality. As one of the professional musicians said: 'personality comes through in the music, that's why it's interesting to us to work with someone else'. One of the participants with dementia remarked about conducting the ensemble:

> I'm conducting – the way musicians communicate – that's why conductors have personality – they are playing to my whims, my style, but it will develop, I guarantee it.

Emphasis is often put in music therapy on choosing music which is familiar (and thus more meaningful) to the individual participants. Even Ruud (2010: 57) has argued:

> How we experience music and how music will affect us will depend on our musical background, the influence of the music we have chosen, and the particular situation in which we experience the music. In other words, in such a contextual understanding, the music, the person, and the situation work together in a relational or mutual relation where changes in any of these components will change the meaning produced.

132 Emilie Capulet

This is particularly the case in dementia care where patients have been known to respond more readily to tunes known from childhood which are very often some of the last musical memories to be recalled (Clair: 1996; Jensen *et al.* 2004; Baird and Samson 2009). However, more than the familiarity of the music being played, the strength of active group music therapy lies in an understanding of how group dynamics may foster individual creativity. One particular aim of the sessions was to compose a new piece for the ensemble derived from the exotic sounds of the Indian harmonium which one of the participants with dementia played:

> We started a new piece – my piece – and they accompanied it very well and we're going to improve on it. So we have work to do. I tremendously enjoyed it – can you imagine being part of that. I want to see it develop into a performance level.

The exchange below, between the professional players (P and J) and the Indian accordion player (N) shows how collaborative the sessions were as they built this new composition together:

N: My idea is that it should be really sweet with the idea that you would all blend in with it. Let me play it and see how it goes and if you want we can make some changes.

(Plays a phrase.)

P: What sort of character would you like in the accompaniment … still or with a rhythm?
N: More … at the end, and then aggressive, kind of… (*Demonstrates on the Indian accordion*)
J: (*Tries it out in turn on the violin*) It can be quite spikey and still work out with your tune. We'll start with the accompaniment, then you can play and we'll adjust. Now we've got an initial feel, we'll get going and you join in with your tune.
N: My thoughts were that I'd start, then you join in. I would do it and you would complement it. There'd be portions where you would take over, then I'd join in.

(All improvise together.)

N: I'm amazed that you managed to blend in'
J: That was you as the main voice.
N: East and West I guess.

Composing something new for the ensemble allowed the musicians to link the sessions together, giving a meaning to the whole process and culminated in a performance of the piece by the ensemble at the Arts 4 Dementia Best Practice Symposium 2015 at the Wigmore Hall in April 2015.

Although these workshops were not conducted with any research outcomes in mind and did not have the rigour of a scientific study, they still shed light on how chamber music can override social and emotional barriers. The experiential outcome of the workshops was a positive one for all participants, in that they highlighted the underlying sense of 'play' which was achieved through sharing musical practice. More research is needed to ascertain if there are any long-term cognitive benefits, but there were undoubtedly short-term emotional benefits, as exemplified by the comments and feedback given by the people with dementia. Above all, the sessions were characterized by the fact that, not only were all the musicians seriously engaged in making music, facing many challenges in the process, they were also immersed in a game and as such, 'had nothing to lose' by getting into the (musical) spirit of the sessions. As one of the participants with dementia commented:

'I'm having a lot of fun here. I'm loving this'.

References

Adorno, T. (1981) *Prisms,* Cambridge, MA: MIT Press.

Aldridge, C. (2005). Dialogic-degenerative diseases and health as a performed aesthetic, in Aldridge, C. (ed.), *Music Therapy and Neurological Rehabilitation: Performing Health,* London: Jessica Kingsley: 39–60.

Alzheimer's Disease International (2015) *Dementia Statistics,* Online. Available at www.alz.co.uk/research/statistics (accessed 13 December 2015).

Baird, A. and Samson, S. (2009) Memory for music in Alzheimer's disease: unforgettable? *Neuropsychology Review,* 19: 85–101.

Barthes, R. (1973) *Le plaisir du texte,* Paris: Editions du Seuil.

Boyer, E. (1990) *Scholarship Reconsidered: Priorities of the Professoriate,* San Francisco: Jossey-Bass.

Clair, A. (1996). *Therapeutic Uses of Music with Older Adults,* Baltimore, MD: Health Professions Press.

Deeley, S. J. (2015) *Critical Perspectives on Service-Learning in Higher Education,* Basingstoke: Palgrave-Macmillan.

Dening, T. and Sandilyan M. (2015) Dementia: definitions and types, *Nursing Standard,* 29 (37): 37–42.

Dewey, J. (1938/1998) *Experience and Education,* Indiana: Kappa Delta Pi.

Gilles, R. (2010) *The Cooperative Game Theory of Networks and Hierarchies,* London: Springer.

Hara, M. (2011) Music in dementia care: increased understanding through mixed research methods, *Music and Arts in Action,* 3 (2): 34–58.

Hartogh, T., Kehrer, E. and Wickel, H. (2014). Music geragogics – making music with the elderly, in Sagrillo, D. and Ferring, D. (eds), *Music (Education) from the Cradle to the Grave,* Weikersheim: Margraf Publishers: 69–84.

Hessenberg, C. and Schmid, W. (2013) 'Sounding bridges – an intergenerational music therapy group with persons with dementia and children and adolescents in psychiatric care, *Voices: A World Forum for Music Therapy,* 13 (2), Online. Available at https://normt.uib. no/index.php/voices/article/view/692/599 (accessed 13 December 2015).

Ing-Randolph, A., Phillips, L. and Williams, A. (2015) Group music interventions for dementia-associated anxiety: a systematic review, *International Journal of Nursing Studies,* 52 (11): 1775–1784.

Ingarden, R. (1989) *Ontology of the Work of Art*, Athens, OH: Ohio University Press.

Jacoby, B. (1996) *Service-learning in Higher Education*, San Francisco, CA: Jossey-Bass Publishers.

James, W. (1907/1991) *Pragmatism*, Buffalo, NY: Prometheus.

Jensen, U., Lewsi, B., Tranel, D. and Adolphs, R. (2004) 'Emotion enhances long-term declarative memory' [Abstract 203.9], *Proceedings of the Society for Neuroscience*. 203–209.

Mapes, N. (2004) Memory groups: facilitating open dialogue between persons with dementia, in Jones, G. and Miesen, B. (eds), *Care-Giving in Dementia: Research and Applications*, vol. 3. Hove: Brunner-Routledge: 138–154.

Kenny, C. (1989) *The Field of Play: A Guide for the Theory and Practice of Music Therapy*, Atascadero, CA: Ridgeview Publishing Company.

Kenny, C. (2014) The field of play: an ecology of being in music therapy, *Voices: A World Forum for Music Therapy*, 14 (1) Online. Available at https://voices.no/index.php/voices/article/view/737/626 (accessed 13 December 2015).

McCallum, S. and Boletsis, C. (2013) A taxonomy of serious games for dementia. *Games for Health: Proceedings of the 3rd European Conference on Gaming and Playful Interaction in Health Care*, New York: Springer: 219–232.

Ridder, H. M. (2005) An Overview of Therapeutic Initiatives when Working with People Suffering from Dementia, In: Aldridge, C. (ed.), *Music Therapy and Neurological Rehabilitation: Performing Health*, London: Jessica Kingsley: 61–82.

Ruud, E. (2010). *Music Therapy: A Perspective from the Humanities*. Gilsum, NH: Barcelona Publishers.

Sakamoto, M., Ando, H. and Tsutou, A. (2013) Comparing the effects of different individualized music interventions for elderly individuals with severe dementia, *International Psychogeriatrics*, 25 (5): 775–784.

Schmidt Peters, J. (2000) *Music Therapy: An Introduction* 2nd ed., Springfield, IL: Charles C. Thomas Publisher.

Simmons-Stern, N., Budson, A. and Ally, B. (2010) Music as a memory enhancer in patients with Alzheimer's disease, *Neuropsychologia*, 48 (10): 3164–3167.

Thaut, M. (2005) *Rhythm, Music, and the Brain: Scientific Foundations and Clinical Applications*, New York: Routledge.

Vaughan Williams, R. (1920/1987) *National Music and Other Essays*, Oxford: Oxford University Press.

Winnicott, D. (2005) *Playing and Reality*, Abingdon: Routledge.

Zeilig, H. (2015) What do we mean when we talk about dementia? Exploring cultural representations of 'dementia', *Working with Older People*, 19 (1): 12–20.

11

DRAMA, DANCE AND PLAY

Creative play as therapy

Leanne Grundy

This chapter covers the application of dance and drama as tools for personal and group expression. These areas of the expressive arts are increasingly being used to explore personal relationships and social situations, with the aim of facilitating the development of self-esteem and personal self-awareness. In the healthcare context, dance and drama are particularly effective within the realms of mental health and wellbeing and for working with people with learning disabilities.

Introduction

When exploring the etymology of the word 'play', the suggested derivation from the Old English *pleg(i)an* 'to exercise' and *plega* 'brisk movement' (Huizinga 1950) clearly reflects the active notion of play as applied in the practices of drama and dance. The processes of drama and dance for what Bach (1950) terms *'fantasy release'*, are forms of physical play that are enjoyed by adults across cultures, both as a means of expression and for physical and emotional release. In essence 'there is a dynamic congruency between emotions and movement' (Sheets-Johnstone 2010: 1). Thus the terms 'play', and 'dance' and 'drama' cannot be considered as mutually exclusive; as Myers (cited in Brooks 2007 :124) states 'Play... [is the]... symbolic language of self-expression', a central tenet to the processes of both art forms.

It is important to understand that both drama and dance perform two distinct functions: first, that of art forms in their own right, and second, as tools for therapeutic action. At the most simplistic level, this may be seen in the intrinsic joy people experience when participating in the creation of theatre for others, or in social dancing. At a therapeutic level (in dance and drama therapy), movement, role play, metaphor and projection are regarded as essential to the creation of the emotional distance required for the therapeutic process to occur. In both instances,

136 Leanne Grundy

drama and dance can lead to personal development, whether emotional, physical or cognitive. Chasen (2011: 22) states: 'The joyous, exhilarating and intriguing and liberating feeling of fun prompts a desire to engage in and sustain play, the foundation of human development'.

The notion of play is central to the creation of drama in the most literal sense, through the use of role play which enables us to step into the shoes of others; to explore the world, whether imagined or real; and to make sense of the moral and ethical questions that arise through seeing the world through another's eyes and in new ways. The notion of play in drama is about discovery – of the self and of the wider world. It also allows the participant to explore their innermost desires with impunity, with the critical emotional distance provided by playing the 'other'. In essence this means that 'in the role of another person, they can act the way they want rather than the way they are expected to act' (Stern 1980: 84).

These are processes that come quite naturally to children, who actively adopt role play within their games (whether synthesising their understanding of adult roles in games of 'Mummies and Daddies' or 'Doctors and Patients', or in more fantasy play), allowing them to process and formulate an understanding of the world in which they live: – 'Creative expression. ... resolve(s) situations, and allow(s) for new possibilities' (Praglin n.d.: 2006). However, this style of play does not come naturally in adult life. As Langley (2006: 19) states, 'the capacity to play is a natural feature of childhood ... as the capacity for play develops ... other art forms become involved'. The child has not yet been inhibited by culturally proscribed values and modes of behavior that so often govern the adult world.

The intention of this chapter is to explore how drama and dance allow us to transcend these cultural constraints and to play with the childlike abandon.

The power of drama as play

'Drama as play' empowers the individual, or the collective, to articulate fantasies and to become something 'other', to inhabit other worlds. In essence, dramatic play is a transformative experience stemming from the notion of ritual. As Huizinga (1950: 9) identifies; 'there is no formal difference between play and ritual'. The correlation between play and ritual, each with its own codes, rules, sequential order and repetition of action and gesture, can also be recognized in the forms of dance or drama: by definition, there is an implicit correlation between these creative ritualistic activities and play. As Plato stated:

> 'Life must be lived as play, playing certain games, making sacrifices, singing and dancing, and then a man will be able to propitiate the gods, and defend himself against his enemies, and win in the contest' (cited in Salen and Zimmerman 2006: 152).

It is no surprise that dance and drama are used within festivals as a means of artistic expression and this is discussed in Chapter 19.

Although the notion of what makes 'good' drama is to an extent a subjective one, 'good' drama (in the Aristotelian sense) is that which evokes an emotional response from the watcher. This 'good' drama and its exploration of the human condition is based on tension or conflict, inherent traits of human relationships and interaction. Participation in dramatic activity allows us to flex our psychological muscles in a 'safe' environment where the critical emotional distance between action and reality allows for the exploration of possibilities; for trial responses; and for the exploration of the 'what if'. As Stern (1980: 81) observes, play within a dramatic context allows the participant to 'partially and temporarily give up ones' separateness of identity', to achieve an empathetic state of being with the group involved in the play through the creation of shared objectives. This is much the same process whereby the needs of the collective become the emphasis in team sports, or in group dance. The notion of the collective, and the commonality of shared experiences of diagnostically grouped participants, can be defined as the 'intermediate area of expression' (Winnicott 1971: 9). This refers to the area of commonality shared by the collective within a drama or dance setting and which directly reflects the immersive play of a child. The process of shared play allows the participant to make sense of the world around them through an unchallenged, safe, experience within a culturally acceptable form of adult play, providing relief from the 'strain of relating inner and outer reality' (Winnicott 1971: 9).

Nevertheless, as for play within a sporting context, play within a drama or dance context differs from traditional notions of play in so much as the form of play is often not self-chosen or self-directed. Play in a drama context must be governed by mutually agreed rules in order for the play element to function. It is vital to have agreed modus operandi as to the nature and methods of play to be undertaken in the course of the therapeutic process, in order to reduce the adults' innate cynicism and suspicion and in order to create a mood of 'innocent playfulness' (Dunne 2007: 267). Thus, in order for play within a drama context to work, the drama facilitator has to assist 'the intellectualized adult to overcome his resistance against play' (Bach 1950: 226).

In the case of drama, play happens for one intrinsic purpose: to create and shape performance. Whether this performance is with the intention of sharing with an external audience, or for 'non-exhibitional' (Taylor and Warner, 2006) purposes (for social and cognitive development), it requires someone with the mantle of 'expert' to lead the play and to apply the rules and codes through which to shape the evolving art. Therein lies the most fundamental difference between the traditional notion of play (where the play activity is self-chosen and self-directed) and the notion of play within art forms, and specifically within drama or dance therapy. In order for drama or dance to take place, and for the therapeutic process to occur, play must be directed and shaped, whether through the facilitation of the drama or dance therapist, the director, the choreographer or dramaturg.

The therapeutic role of dance and drama

The benefit of dramatic play within this safe, creative environment is made explicit in the use of play within the phalanx of strategies deployed by the drama or dance therapist. Jones (2007: 175) suggests that drama therapy embodies the notion of play, both practically and conceptually, as a means of 'therapeutic intervention'. This may be through actual, active participation in drama games and warm-up activities or through the individual's playful relationship with themselves, their reality and the world around them, which allows for a 'heightened aesthetic distance … [which] loosens clients' habitual investment in over familiar reactions associated with their real life identities' (Weiner 2015: 13). Within drama therapy, unstructured play is not in itself a means to an end, but rather a starting point on the road to more developed drama-based activities, such as role play or structured improvisation, one of two key strategies utilized within the therapeutic context.

Although there are differing schools of thought as to what construes drama as therapy, a relevant definition is 'creative theatre as a medium for self-expression and playful group interaction and which base[s] their techniques on improvisation and theatre exercises' (Johnson 1984: 105). Drama and dance within a therapeutic context are tools by which the participant can make sense of the world around them, much in the same way the child does in play. This link between the play of the child and the creative therapies is most explicit in the developmental 'EPR' model suggested by Jennings (in Langley 2006: 26). This focuses on the three key elements of 'embodiment', 'projection' (often using ritual, puppets and objects as symbols), and 'role play', which form a triumvirate of strategies through which the adult in therapy can explore their world. Dramatic role play and storytelling often form a pivotal part of the therapy session as role play is seen to be 'a particularly favourable method for unlearning and relearning adaptive social behavior because it permits a symbolic trial and error social learning process which does not evoke realistic anxieties' (Bach 1950: 244).

Within the projection stage of therapy, the use of puppets (reflecting Klein's (1932) psychotherapeutic use of doll play with young children) allows the adult participant to identify with, project and voice their own thoughts and feelings. This is what Bach (1950: 226) terms the 'incognito protection of fiction', the safe space within which the participant can externalize thoughts and feelings through the comparative safety of 'other', allowing them to recognize, over time, their projected feelings as their own and thus performing a therapeutic function. The puppet as prop thus represents the externalisation of the *alter ego* for the participant, allowing them to express opinions and ideas within a protective framework and allowing the play activity to exist outside of 'ego depreciating censorship … in the protected world of make believe' (Bach 1950: 225).

In the same way that the 'make believe' play of the child facilitates an understanding of the world around them and expression of the self within that world (Jennings 1999), so play within a therapeutic drama framework for adults performs the same function, especially for those in 'marginalized' groups.

The efficacy of this triumvirate of strategies (embodiment, projection and role play) can be seen in a number of recent studies, such as in the use of myth and fairytales as a dramatic medium for storytelling and role play to explore the repressed feelings of sexual abuse survivors (Silverman 2004), or substance abusers (Dunne 2007), or in Cassin and Von Ransen's (2005) work with individuals with eating disorders, a disease associated with an obsessive and compulsive quest for perfection, where 'repetition of thoughts, emotions and behaviors causes a loss of spontaneity and identity' (Wood and Schneider 2015: 56).

We may ask what it is about play that produces an impact on behavior in these instances.

Play is about spontaneity and living in the moment, allowing for instinctive and immediate responses without overthinking, which is the very antithesis of the behaviors of those with eating disorders and similar compulsions. Much as play facilitates social and cognitive development in young children, play continues to serve a developmental function in adult play, drama, and dance therapy. As Chasen (2011: 70) states:

> Theatre and drama reflect, enact and engage processes and operations that occur within related systems of cognitive, emotional and social development, purposefully integrating polarised states of information and being.

By facilitating the process of play, we seek to achieve mastery of undesired behaviors and processes – in essence 'winning' over that which we seek to master – whether this be an eating disorder, a relationship or a game. Rubin (2008) suggests that drama as therapy allows for the creation of a connection between the hemispheres of the brain in an attempt to 'gain cognitive and affective mastery'. In effect, this implies that the processes of drama and play have a link to neurobiology, facilitating the creation and integration of new neural pathways and thus affording the individual the ability to connect with, and recognize, their condition (Seigel 2010).

Play in the form of re-enactment can also be identified in the use of drama as a strategy for resolving familial conflict ('psychodrama') within a therapeutic context (Chasin et al. 1989). This is enacted through the dramatic reconstruction of past events, allowing couples to reach a state of realization of 'the protagonist's phenomenology, empathising and frequently identifying with the protagonist's experienced truth' (Wiener 1996: 8). The process of dramatic reconstruction allows the participant to develop the skills and processes required to resolve difficulties and differences. Thus, it could be argued that the act of play through drama allows for the development of these 'mastery' skills within a non-judgemental environment and consequently affirms the ability of drama to impact on social and cognitive functioning.

Dance therapy also involves the connection of neural pathways, and in this way earns recognition as a holistic approach to therapy. As in drama therapy, dance therapy uses the whole body, including connection to the breath, using set exercises

140 Leanne Grundy

(including relaxation and breathing exercises) and physical play to improve conditions that affect co-ordination, balance and speech (ataxia). Dance also influences what Capello (2010) describes as 'psychosocial interactions ... supporting and enabling mutual communication' (as evidenced in the diagnosis and subsequent therapeutic treatment, through dance, of patients with mild to severe traumatic brain injury (Gueye cited in Capello 2010: 25).

Previous studies (Snow *et al.* 2003) have suggested that the impact of any therapeutic event is dependent on the participants' ability to spontaneously engage with the activity on a creative level, their attention span, and the ability to communicate with others and to 'assert oneself in performance' (Goyal and Keightly 2003: 338). The process also requires the participant to freely exercise the imagination as 'the use of imagination helps people disclose private parts of themselves that they would not confront directly' (Kedem-Tahar and Kellermann 1996: 5).

Griffins (1983) asserts that, in the facilitation of adult play through drama, there are four key areas of preparation for effective activity. These areas are time, safe space, appropriate materials and preparatory materials. Whereas the notion of play in a traditional sense negates the idea of structure or external control, drama therapy requires a facilitator (in this case the therapist) within the play space. The therapist as facilitator must create a safe environment of trust for, as Plaut states, 'The capacity to form images and to use these constructively by recombination into new patterns is – unlike dreams of fantasies – dependent on the individuals' ability to trust' (cited in Winnicott cited in LaMothe 2013: 68). The need for trust within a creative setting is of paramount importance, and effective interactions can only be produced within a milieu of mutual trust. The emphasis on trust is evident in traditional drama settings (such as the classroom or rehearsal space) where, at the formation of a new drama or dance group, considerable emphasis will be placed on trust games to form appropriate interactions. Trust is also an integral and essential starting point for the use of drama or dance as therapy, since it is only through the creation of mutual trust that a 'safe space' for creative exploration might also be created.

It could reasonably be suggested that the 'safe space' of a drama therapy workshop is a place where the individual can explore their perceived reality with impunity; examining their own behaviors and those of others through the form of play, which despite retaining many of the rules and structures of the 'real' world (as often seen in children's play) allows for the 'reordering, exaggerating, fragmenting' (Schechner 1988: 103) of those behaviors.

Conclusion

The benefits of play in the development of the cognitive, social, and emotional skills of the child are products of an organic process. However, within drama and dance therapy, the intrinsic benefits of play are planned-for and managed by the practitioner, who remains present throughout. Play, through dance and drama, is utilized implicitly for the purpose of facilitating change, whether emotional, behavioral or psychological. In order for the creative event to have therapeutic impact, an intrinsic understanding of the 'rules' of the art form is necessary for effective participation, much in the same way as play has its own implicit set of 'rules'. It is through play, and the rules of play, that the trained drama or dance therapist can apply and blur the boundaries between drama, dance and therapy. Winnicott summarizes this, stating that:

> It is in playing and only in playing that the individual child or adult is able to be creative and to use the whole personality, and it is only in being creative that the individual discovers the self

(Winnicott 1971: 54)

References

Bach, G.R. (1950) Dramatic play therapy with adult groups, *The Journal of Psychology*, 29: 225–246.

Brooks, S.L. (ed.) (2007) *The Use of the Creative Therapies with Sexual Abuse Survivors*, Springfield IL: Charles C. Thomas Publisher Ltd.

Capello, P.P. (2010) Innovative projects and special project in dance/movement therapy: 'The 2009 ADTA International panel', *American Journal of Dance Therapy*, 32 (1): 24 –32. Online. Available at http://thirdworld.nl/innovative-projects-and-special-populations-in-dance-movement-therapy-the-2009-adta-international-panel (accessed 22 February 2016).

Cassin, S. and von Ransen, K.M. (2005) Personality and eating disorders: a decade in review, *Clinical Psychology Review*, 25: 895–916.

Chasen, L.R. (2011) *Social Skills, Emotional Growth and Drama Therapy Inspiring Connection on the Autism Spectrum*, London: Jessica Kingsley Publishers.

Chasin, R., Roth, S. and Bograd, M. (1989) Action methods in systemic therapy: dramatising ideal futures and reformed pasts with couples, *Family Process*, 28 (2): 121–136.

Dunne, L. (2007) Drama therapy with sexual abuse survivors with substance abuse issues. In: Brooke, S. A. (ed.) *The use of creative arts therapies with sexual abuse victims*, Springfield: Charles C. Thomas: 261–279.

Goyal, A. and Keightley, M.L. (2008) Expressive art for the social and community integration of adolescenets with acquired brain injuries: a systematic review, *Research in Drama Education: The Journal of Applied Theatre and Performance*, 13 (3): 337–352.

Huizinga, J. (1950) *Homo Ludens: A Study of the Play-Element in Culture*, Eastford: Martino Fine Books (Reprint version 2014).

Jennings, S. (1999) *Introduction to Developmental Play Therapy*, London: Jessica Kingsley Publishers.

Jones, P. (2007) *Drama as Therapy Volume 1: Theory, Practice and Research*, 2nd ed., Abingdon: Routledge.

Kedem-Tahar, E. and Kellermann, P.F. (1996) Psychodrama and drama therapy: a comparison, *The Arts in Psychotherapy*, 23 (1): 27–36.

LaMothe, R. (2013) *Missing Us: Re-Visioning Psychoanalysis from the Perspective of Community*, Plymouth: Jason Aronson.

Langley, D. (2006) *An introduction to Dramatherapy,* London: Sage.

Praglin, L. (2006) The nature of the "in-between" in D.W. Winnicott's *Concept of Transitional Space* and in Martin Buber's *das Zwischenmenschliche,* Online. Available at www.uni.edu/universitas/archive/fall06/pdf/art_praglin.pdf (accessed 12 December 2015).

Rubin, S. (2008) Women, food, and feeling: drama therapy with women who have eating disorders, in Brook, S.L. (ed.), *The Creative Therapies and Eating Disorders*, Springfield, IL: Charles C. Thomas Publishing Ltd: 173–193.

Salen, K. and Zimmerman, E. (2006) *The Game Design Reader: A Rules of Play Anthology*, Cambridge, MA: MIT Press.

Schechner, R. (1988) *Performance Theory*, London: Routledge.

Seigel, D.J. (2010), *Mindsight: The New Science of Personal Transformation*, New York: Random House LLC.

Sheets-Johnstone, M. (2010) 'Why is movement therapeutic' – keynote address, 44th American Dance Therapy Association Conference, *American Journal of Dance Therapy* 32: 2–15.

Silverman, Y. (2004) The story within – myth and fairytale in therapy, *The Arts in Psychotherapy*, 31 (3): 27–135.

Snow, S., D'Amico, M. and Tanguay, D. (2003) Therapeutic theatre and well-being, *The Arts in Psychotherapy,* 30 (2): 73–82.

Stern, S. (1980). Drama in second language learning from a psycholinguistic perspective, *Language Learning*, 30 (1): 77–100.

Taylor, P. and Warner, C. D. (eds) (2006) *Structure and Spontaneity: The Process Drama of Cecily O'Neill*. Stoke on Trent: Trentham.

Wiener, D. J. (2015) Staging dramatic enactments to resolve conflicts in couples, *Drama Therapy Review*, 1 (1): 7–20.

Winnicott, D.W. (1971) *Playing and Reality*, London: Tavistock Publications.

12
ART FOR HEALTH

Julia Whitaker

This chapter will present a selection of current arts projects in Scotland's capital city, which are designed and delivered with the health and wellbeing of their participants in mind. They have been selected for their inherent qualities of 'playfulness' (Glyn and Webster 1992) which mark them out as having particular relevance to the theme of this volume.

Introduction

In 1947 the city of Edinburgh hosted its first 'festival of the arts', an initiative conceived to celebrate and enrich European cultural life after the Second World War. Like all the best-remembered parties, it was gate-crashed by uninvited performers who boldly staged their shows 'on the fringe' of the festival and today the Edinburgh International Festival and its famous 'Fringe' are renowned for being the largest arts festival in the world, with almost 300,000 additional visitors descending on the city for the month-long duration of the festival in 2015 (Convention Edinburgh 2015).

The festival's original remit to 'provide a platform for the flowering of the human spirit' (Fifield 2005: 263) lives on long after the visitors leave Edinburgh at the end of the season. The city's creative mission continues throughout the year under the guise of a range of local arts initiatives – many of which are designed to refocus attention on the wellbeing of the city's own inhabitants. In the words of Jimmy Reid (1972, cited in Danson and Trebeck 2013):

> The flowering of each individual's personality and talents is the pre-condition for everyone's development … The creative use of leisure, in communion with, and in service to, our fellow human beings can and must become an important element in self-fulfilment.

144 Julia Whitaker

Unity is health

The Arts and Health Diamond (McNaughton *et al.* 2005) has been applied in the selection of the following examples, recognizing the overlap between the intended and unintended consequences of any social intervention for individual and community wellbeing. This model categorizes art-for-health projects along two dimensions. The first dimension represents the *purpose* of any one initiative: whether this refers to engagement with the arts (with an assumed consequent benefit to health) or with health improvement *per se*. The second dimension represents the *focus* of the initiative – whether it is on the wellbeing of individuals or the health of communities. This is supported by the Department of Health (2007) who state that:

> The arts are, and should be clearly recognised as, integral to health and health services.

The concept of a relationship between the arts and healthcare delivery is not a new phenomenon and its history long pre-dates the foundation of the public health systems known today. The grandiose infirmaries *(asklepieia)* of Ancient Greece were majestic, temple-like halls designed to enhance the patients' sensory and spiritual experience of the healing environment (Cork 2012). The conviction that beauty and health are inextricably linked re-emerged in the fourteenth century in the form of the imposing religious frescoes of Catholic southern Europe, which were designed to inspire confidence in patients that they were being treated in institutions devoted exclusively to their wellbeing. By the sixteenth century, some hospitals in Europe were recognizing the possibility that painting and sculpture might represent more than merely inspiration or reassurance but might indeed be integral to the treatment itself, wielding a powerful psychological influence on the sick and their capacity for recovery (Cork 2012). The anatomical drawings of Leonardo da Vinci and Michelangelo in fifteenth- and sixteenth-century Italy, represent an entirely different purpose to art in healthcare: art as a means of communicating an understanding of the human body. This purpose has been reimagined for the twenty-first century in the digital artistry of Alexander Tsiaras (The Visual MD 2015).

The Victorians recognized that 'the lives of patients in hospitals and institutions should be made fuller and happier by pictures, plants and decorations' (Baron 1999: 9) and during the late nineteenth century various ambitious attempts were made to renovate the otherwise squalid hospitals of nineteenth-century Britain, most notably in Scotland. In Glasgow, the Kyrle Society originated in 1883 and aimed 'to bring the influences of natural and artistic beauty home to the people' (cited HeraldScotland 2015) and in Edinburgh, similarly lofty aspirations inspired the transformative endeavours of the Edinburgh Social Union (1885) at the city's Royal Infirmary and the Royal Hospital for Sick Children.

In more recent times there have been repeated attempts to organize and evaluate this now well-established connection between the arts and health

(Angus 2002; Dose 2006). Recent clinical studies have concluded that placing original artworks within the healthcare environment can, specifically, reduce levels of stress, anxiety and depression; reduce the length of hospital stays and the need for medication; and improve communication between patients and healthcare professionals (Staricoff *et al.* 2003). A study by Cuypers *et al.* (2012) is one of many (e.g. Castillo-Pérez *et al.* 2010; Gordon-Nesbitt 2015) to demonstrate that active participation in cultural activities is significantly associated with positive health and self-perceptions of wellbeing as well as with reductions in anxiety and depression.

Impact Arts (Training Provider of the Year, in the Creative and Cultural Skills Awards 2015) is a Scottish social enterprise that taps into the creative potential with the aim of enhancing social relationships on the understanding that good relationships are a key determinant of good health (Handley *et al.* 2015). The Craft Café project is a creative solution to reducing isolation and loneliness among the over sixties. In a safe, social and creative environment, participants learn new skills, re-connect with the community and re-define their social identity (Impact Arts 2015).

Research shows that 16 per cent of older people in the UK describe themselves as lonely. Loneliness and depression find their parallels in poor physical health in terms of blood pressure levels, immune system function, sleep quality and cognitive profile (O'Luanaigh and Lawlor 2008). The International Creativity and Aging Study found that those who had access to participatory arts programs had better health than those who did not. They made fewer visits to the doctor, required less medication and achieved lower scores on measures of depression and loneliness (Cohen *et al.* 2006).

The Craft Café aims to exploit the potential joyfulness that can be derived from creativity and self-expression when experienced in the company of others. Play has been described as an activity that produces both *immediate pleasure* and *involvement* (Sandelands and Buckner 1989). The playful pleasure of involvement in creative activity derives from the creative pursuit itself, rather than from the expectation of positive consequences, although these are many. Research evidence also suggests that the benefits of play in adulthood are likely to be immediate (Pellis *et al.* 2010). The Craft Café provides the dual benefits of mental and social stimulation: active participation in the creative arts fosters a sense of self-worth and personal fulfilment, whilst the opportunity to make new friends reduces feelings of loneliness and promotes a more positive outlook on life. Regular attendance is a key motivating factor, offering participants something to look forward to and representing a re-connection with community. An indirect consequence of the Craft Café has been an increase in exercise levels and a reduction in harmful behaviors (smoking, drinking, poor nutrition) among its users. Participants describe therapeutic effects of Craft Café attendance, whereby the discipline of creating artwork generates a sense of calm, reduces tension and contributes to a raised self esteem, with a brighter outlook on life. A number of participants reported significant positive effects on their mental wellbeing and on clinically diagnosed anxiety and depression; for some this led to a reduction in the level of medication required. As one Craft Café participant states:

> I'm eating less because I'm not as bored and feeling better about myself … it's therapy without it feeling like therapy.
>
> *(Impact Arts 2011: 21)*

The benefits of participation have also been shown to extend to the family members of participants; their new interests and engagement with life encourage more meaningful social interactions and a greater appreciation of art among the wider family. Family members of participants have indicated that since attending the Craft Café their parent or grandparent appeared more purposeful, more independent, safer, and less isolated; this provided a great source of comfort for relatives (Impact Arts 2011).

Another art-for-health project with cross-generational impact is Gallery Social, an initiative of the National Galleries of Scotland (2015) which offers regular tours at all four of its city-centre venues for people with dementia and their carers. Once a month, two artists host a three-cornered event which combines a multi-sensory experience with participation and an opportunity for socialization. The sessions are led by the same artists each time which gives a reassuring sense of continuity and allows relationships to develop (Saultz 2003). The 90-minute 'tour' purposely starts gently with an opportunity for participants to re-familiarize themselves with the environment, the tour facilitators and fellow participants. Resources, in the form of art publications, images or objects of artistic interest, provide cues for what is to follow and the sharing of 'tea and cake' brings participants together and re-defines the identity of the group. Group processes are always situation dependent and determined by systemic rules which may be either organized or chaotic, but which influence group behavior in a variety of unpredictable ways. Gallery Social practices an open acceptance that whatever happens in the group encounter is significant and has a bearing on how things unfold. Before the group enter the gallery space there is a demonstration of a practical art activity designed and tailored to the exhibition or artists to be viewed. Participants are invited to playfully explore and experiment with the artistic media and, freed from the pressure of defined expectations, can engage with the creative process without having to worry about making mistakes or 'getting it wrong'. Gallery Social culminates with a guided tour of a maximum of three works of art in the gallery proper, minimising the need for physical relocation and the associated potential for stressful disorientation.

The delicate balance of thinking, feeling and doing on the Gallery Social tour re-distributes the focus of attention away from the cognitive impairment which is the defining feature of dementia. An open-ended, playful attitude of curiosity and enthusiasm, which does not revolve around intellectual activity, allows participants to re-connect with their sense of self, untethered by their dementia diagnosis.

Research evidence from the Museum of Modern Art (MOMA) in New York, which operates a similar project for people with dementia, has identified several key factors that seem to contribute to the impact of these programs (Mittelman and Epstein n.d.). The role of the program leader, in particular their attitude and interaction with participants, is highlighted as being of overriding importance to the success of the program. The level of involvement of the program leader and the expression of genuine interest and appreciation for participants' contributions, rekindle feelings of self-worth. This observation reflects findings from the Health Development Agency (2000) report *Art for Health* which emphasized the quality of uniqueness belonging to specific initiatives – both in terms of content and mode of delivery – as a determinant of effectiveness. A sense of 'the personal' is inherent in all forms of artistic expression and this report acknowledges the key role of personality in building successful projects.

Gallery Social, like the 'Meet me at MOMA' project, combines opportunities for sensory and intellectual stimulation with opportunities for social interaction, both with accompanying family members and with others who share an interest in the arts. Regular attendance at the gallery tours, which are thoughtfully choreographed to follow a predictable sequence and rhythm, allows for the creation of a 'safe space' within which participants feel welcome and valued, in contrast to the loss of status often experienced by people with dementia in the wider community.

Anecdotal evidence from Gallery Social supports the finding that the positive emotions generated by the museum visits persist beyond the visits themselves. As with the Craft Café initiative described above, family members also benefit from the program in that they are able to share a pleasurable experience with their relative with dementia, to revive or discover a common interest, and to witness their relative perceived with respect and dignity.

Meg Faragher (2015), Families and Communities Learning Co-ordinator at the National Galleries of Scotland, says:

> I think the strength of our Gallery Social program is its emphasis on enjoying art and good company. These are the same reasons that many people have for visiting an art gallery and why should this particular audience be any different? We don't focus on medical or therapeutic outcomes; we simply want people to share a positive experience with friends or loved ones, meet others who may be going through something similar in their lives and to be stimulated by seeing something beautiful or thought-provoking. The practical element is always very 'light-touch' and something people can decide to do or not. We hope it invites people to connect with their own creativity in a playful way. We try to communicate information in a simple way, but certainly without 'dumbing down'. The wonderful thing about art is that there are often no right answers and no correct ways to feel or respond to a painting or a sculpture, diverse opinions and responses are valid and so conversations can be quite open and non-prescribed.

The two aforementioned projects have highlighted the benefits of active participation in appreciating and practising the visual arts, but the field of performance

148 Julia Whitaker

art is also uncovering its own unique potential for producing positive health benefits (as discussed in Chapters 9, 10 and 11).

A collaboration between creative teams at Oxford Brookes University and the University of Edinburgh resulted in the première of a new family opera, *Watching*, at the Royal Botanic Gardens Edinburgh in the Spring of 2015 (Watching Opera 2015) with the aim of improving public awareness of the importance of a good night's sleep through the playful intertwining of theatre, music and horticulture. Research in the field of sleep science has recently confirmed that healthy sleep is closely connected to both good physical health and improved cognitive function (Park 2014). However, changes to work and leisure patterns and pursuits and the infiltration of electronic media into every corner of contemporary life means that notions of what constitutes healthy sleep have become distorted. *Watching* relates the story of a sleepless night, taking as its inspiration the connections between the sleep cycles of plants and people and serves to widen accessibility to both music and a fundamental health message.

Watching uses music to tell its story and at the Scottish Storytelling Centre music and stories are being used as a way of reaching-out to a wide range of different people. The 'Arts of Memory in Later Life' project celebrates and nurtures the potential for creativity at all stages of life. Inspired by the premise that the greatest music is 'the music of what happens', this project draws on storytelling, poetry, song, visual memory and music to create and build healthful connections between individuals and communities.

'A Calendar of Memories' (Scottish Storytelling Centre 2014) represents the unfolding of a storytelling project, whereby professional storytellers make contact with groups of older people in care homes and day centers, meeting them once a month over the course of a year. The intention is to establish a sense of continuity and to build relationships with the monthly repetition of the group beating a rhythm in time with the changing seasons – different themes unfolding and developing over time. Stories are a way of making sense of our lives, of awakening the imagination and of reviving emotional memory. Shared within a group they build connections between people, offering inspiration and inviting response:

> Older people love hearing stories and telling theirs as they are given the chance to reminisce … The client benefits by gaining recognition. It is so important that we are seen. These things are important to all, especially to those whose short-term memory is faltering. Indeed, by stimulating the long-term memory with story interaction they are able, very able, to get a sense of worth and joy. You take them back to a time when life was sweet.
>
> *(Millie Gray, cited in Scottish Story Telling Centre 2014:10)*

Donald Smith (2015) writes that 'stories are the heartbeat of humanity, because they convey the music of what happens'. The sharing of stories 'eye to eye, mind to mind and heart to heart' (Scottish proverb) has transformative potential in the healthcare context. Across diverse communities and age-groups the value of storytelling is well recognized as a means of conveying positive health messages (Wilkin and Ball-Rokeach 2006), of helping to make sense of the patient journey (McWilliam *et al.* 1997), and of empowering service-users as agents of their own recovery (Høybye *et al.* 2005). It is the mutuality inherent in a storytelling interaction, the shared experience of respect, trust and empathy that creates a safe space within which new meanings can emerge, as connections between people and across place and time are established and reinforced.

Conclusion

Three common themes to emerge from a review of the inspirational projects discussed above, which place them in the realm of 'the playful', are continuity, communication and connection. The importance of continuity, of rhythm and repetition, lies in the value of having something to look forward to and knowing that it will follow a predictable pattern or set of rules. At the same time, there is an openness to the unknown and the unexpected – the security of a known rhythm allows for the creative emergence of the surprising and the unexpected. Engagement with the arts, whether it be through the expression or the appreciation of artistic talent, is a form of communication, a way of knowing oneself and of sharing oneself with others. Thus relationships or connections are formed and developed. The starting-point for the endeavour (whether intentionally health-driven or not) seems to be of less relevance to its health outcomes: it is the perceived value of 'art for art's sake' that has the greatest influence on the experience of wellbeing/self-esteem derived from engagement (Health Development Agency 2000). Art for health projects may be set within a particular social/health context but, allowed to grow organically from a dynamic impetus, they can transform themselves from 'health initiative' into 'play for health'.

References

Angus, J. (2002) *A Review of Evaluation in Community-based Art for Health Activity in the UK*, London: Health Development Agency.

Baron, J. H. (1999) A history of art in British hospitals, in Haldane, D. and Loppert, S. (eds), *The Arts in Health Care: Learning from Experience*. London: King's Fund Publishing: 4–23.

Castillo-Pérez, S., Gómez-Pérez, V., Calvillo Velasco, M., Pérez-Campos, E. and Mayoral, M. (2010) Effects of music therapy on depression compared with psychotherapy, *The Arts in Psychotherapy*, 37: 387–390.

Clift, S., Camic, P.M., Chapman, B., Clayton, G., Daykin, N., Eades, G., Parkinson, G., Parkinson, C., Secker, J., Stickley, T. and White, M. (2009). The state of arts and health in England, *Arts and Health,* 1 (1): 6–35.

Cohen, G.D., Perlstein, S., Chapline, J., Kelly J., Firth, K.M., and Simmens, S. (2006) The Impact of Professionally Conducted Cultural Programs on the Physical Health, Mental Health, and Social Functioning of Older Adults, *The Gerontologist,* 46 (6): 726–734.

Convention Edinburgh (2015) *Creative Capital*, Online. Available at www.convention edinburgh.com/why-edinburgh/facts-and-figures/creative-capital/ (accessed 13 December 2015).

150 Julia Whitaker

Cork, R. (2012) *The Healing Presence of Art*, New Haven, CT: Yale University Press.

Cuypers, K., Krokstad, S., Holman, T.L., Knudsten, M.S., Bygren, L.O. and Holmen, J. (2012) Patterns of receptive and creative cultural activities and their association with perceived health, anxiety, depression and satisfaction with life among adults: the HUNT study, Norway, *Journal of Epidemiology and Community Health*, 66 (8): 8 698–703.

Danson, M. and Trebeck, K. (2013) *No More Excuses. How a Common Weal Approach Can End Poverty in Scotland*, Biggar: The Reid Foundation.

Department of Health with Arts Council England (2007) *A Prospectus for Art and Health*, London: Department of Health.

Dose, L. (2006). National Network for the Arts in Health: lessons learned from six years of work, *Journal of the Royal Society for the Promotion of Health*, 126 (3): 110–112.

Faragher, M. (2015) Personal conversation with Julia Whitaker [unpublished].

Fifield, C. (2005) *Ibbs and Tillett: The Rise and Fall of a Musical Empire*, Farnham: Ashgate.

Glynn, M., and Webster, J. (1992) The adult playfulness scale: an initial assessment, *Psychological Reports*, 71(1), 83–103.

Gordon-Nesbitt, R. (2015) *Exploring the Longitudinal Relationship Between Arts Engagement and Health*, Manchester: Arts for Health.

Handley, S., Joy, I, Hestbaek, C. and Marjoribanks, D. (2015) *The Best Medicine? The Importance of Relationships for Health and Wellbeing*. Doncaster, UK: Relate.

Health Development Agency (2000) *Art for Health. A Review of Good Practice in Community-based Arts Projects and Initiatives which Impact on Health and Wellbeing*, London: Health Development Agency.

HeraldScotland (2015) Putting art in the hands of the people, *Herald Scotland*, 7 July 2007 Online. Available at www.heraldscotland.com/ (accessed 13 December 2015).

Høybye, M.T., Johansen, C., Tjørnhøj-Thomsen, T. (2005) Online interaction. Effects of storytelling in an internet breast cancer support group, *Psycho-Oncology*, 14 (3): 211–220.

Impact Arts (2011) *Craft Café. Social Return on Investment Evaluation*, Glasgow: Social Value Lab.

Impact Arts (2015) *Older People: Craft Café*, Online. Available at www.impactarts.co.uk/content/our-work-older-people/ (accessed 13 December 2015).

McNaughton, J., White, M. and Stacey, R. (2005) Researching the benefits of arts in health, *Health Education*, 105 (5): 332–339.

McWilliam, C.L., Stewart, M., Brown, J.B., McNair, S., Desai, K., Patterson, M.L., del Maestro, N., and Pittman, B.J., (1997) Creating empowering meaning: an interactive process of promoting health with chronically ill older Canadians. *Health Promotion International*, 12 (2): 111–124.

Mittelman, M. and Epstein, C. (n.d.) *Research: Meet me at MOMA Project*, Online. Available at www.moma.org/momaorg/shared/pdfs/docs/meetme/Resources_NYU_Evaluation.pdf (accessed 13 December 2015).

National Galleries of Scotland (2015) *Gallery Social Programme*, Online. Available at www.nationalgalleries.org/education/gallery-social-programme/ (accessed 13 December 2015).

O'Luanaigh, C. and Lawlor, B.A. (2008) Loneliness and the health of older people, *International Journal of Geriatric Psychiatry*, 23: 1213–1221.

Park, A. (2014) The power of sleep, *Time Magazine*, 11 September 2014 Online. Available at www.time.com (accessed June 2015).

Pellis, S., Pellis, V. and Bell, B. (2010) The function of play in the development of the human brain, *American Journal of Play*, Winter: 278–296.

Sandelands, L.E., and Buckner, G.C. (1989) Of art and work: aesthetic experience and the psychology of work feelings, in Cummings L.L. and Staw B.M. (eds), *Research in Organizational Behavior, Vol. 11*. Greenwich, CT: JAI Press: 105–131.

Saultz, J.W. (2003) Defining and measuring interpersonal continuity of care. *Annals of Family Medicine,* 1 (3): 134–143.

Scottish Storytelling Centre (2014) *A Calendar of Memories*, Edinburgh: Scottish Storytelling Centre.

Smith, D. (2015) Essay of the week: the power of storytelling. *HeraldScotland*, 18 October 2015 Online. Available at www.heraldscotland.com/arts_ents/books_and_poetry/13876854.Essay_of_the_week__The_power_of_storytelling/ (accessed 13 December 2015).

Staricoff, R.L., Duncan, J.P. and Wright, M. (2003) *A Study of the Effects of the Visual and Performing Arts in Healthcare*, Online. Available at www.publicartonline.org.uk/resources/research/documents/ChelseaAndWestminsterResearchproject.pdf (accessed 7 September 2015)

The Visual MD (2015) Image Library, Online. Available at www.thevisualmd.com/images/ (accessed 13 December 2015).

Watching Opera (2015) *Watching*, Online. Available at www.watching.eca.ed.ac.uk (accessed 13 December 2015).

Wilkin, H.A. and Ball-Rokeach, S.J. (2006) Reaching at risk groups. The importance of health storytelling in Los Angeles Latino media, *Journalism,* 7 (3): 299–320.

13
PLAY AND SOCIAL THERAPY

Eric Fleming

Garvald Edinburgh is a Scottish charity offering creative opportunities and support for people with learning disabilities. Inspired by the ideas of the educator and philosopher Rudolf Steiner (1861–1925), it is an example of a social therapy approach which recognizes the importance of the social environment to the development of personal potential. Steiner is popularly quoted as saying:

> A healthy social life arises when the whole community finds its reflection in the mirror of each person's soul, and when the virtue of each person lives in the whole community.
>
> *(Rudolf Steiner) (unsourced)*

Garvald aims to help its individual members to experience personal fulfilment through making a meaningful contribution to their community and so to society as a whole. Since its establishment in 1969, Garvald Edinburgh has extended the range and reach of the creative opportunities offered to people with learning disabilities in Edinburgh and the surrounding area, to include arts and craftwork, drama and horticulture. Working in community with others – whether through preparing a meal, giving a performance, working on a joint arts project or celebrating a festival – creates connections that gently allow people to reveal parts of themselves to others in a process of personal and interpersonal growth.

Craft-based learning opportunities and festival celebrations are seen as core activities by organizations influenced by the principles of social therapy. The underlying rationale stems from cultural influences popular in the late 1800s and early 1900s when Steiner was developing his theories. Art movements such as Arts and Crafts, Symbolism and Art Nouveau had spread throughout Europe and promoted alternative forms of expression and ways of being which were in contrast to the recent domination of Classicism and the rational thinking associated with that style of art and architecture. In social therapy, craft-based activities, seasonal and Christian festival celebrations are seen to augment skills – practical, artistic and social – in addition to fostering a sense of community. These impulses are motivated by a desire to seek a more balanced view of human development; especially a concern for feelings and our connection to nature. For this chapter on the arts and health, I will describe possible encounters with play in both these domains and discuss how play and playfulness can contribute to individual and group engagement. Positive engagement signifies that individuals and groups are involved to the extent that they are 'realizing potential', the potential to develop and achieve, with an affirmative impact on health and wellbeing.

Many health and social care professionals who engage in training as part of their continuing professional development will note the occasional reference made to 'having a sense of humor'. This is typically offered as a means of survival or, more positively, as a useful 'tool' and is discussed in more detail in Chapter 21. However, humor and playfulness are commonly reduced to the level of being a mere 'hooking-in' device, designed to motivate, distract or capture the attention of an individual or an audience; to lighten the mood and 'bond' with service-users. Whilst this may be useful, it is often where its usefulness is thought to end. However, there is the potential for playfulness to be seen as a motif which echoes throughout a process of learning and development and which facilitates the engagement of service-users in the less cited concept of 'serious play' (Brown 2008).

The notion of serious play signifies play on a deep level, akin to a profound immersion in a condition of experiment and discovery. When an activity is craft-based, then the aspiration to facilitate individuals and groups into this state of being is a worthwhile goal, as this indicates a heightened mode of creativity and exploration. However, as mentioned above, exploration of serious play is rarely evoked in regard to the aim of realizing potential or the promotion of health and wellbeing. It is with this in mind, that this exposition of the concept of play in the context of the Glass Studio at Garvald Edinburgh may be used to illustrate how embracing playfulness and serious play can contribute to effective craft-based therapeutic education.

Running a glass studio according to the principles of social therapy is an exciting, rewarding and challenging experience. In a craft-based studio of this nature, the chief concern is how to engage adults with learning disabilities in meaningful activity, 'meaningful' being suggestive of creative, educational and therapeutic purpose. Depending on the personality of the studio leader and the particular methodology they adopt, play may be utilized to facilitate involvement and inclusion in this endeavour. Humor can be an effective and fruitful way of forging bonds between the leader and individual members of the group and with the group as a whole.

In the past creativity, or 'being creative', was often used in an unspecified way to suggest artistic ability, or an artistic 'type'. However, the merits of promoting lateral or creative thinking in relation to problem-solving and decision-making have increasingly found their place in such fields as business and design (McGuinness 2015). Whilst we all have unique tendencies towards different strengths and weaknesses, and great artists have been lucky enough to unlock their creativity successfully, most people have the ability to imagine and day-dream – abilities related to innovation. Most of us would recognize the inherent creativity of our dream world, when we can remember parts of dreams. Tapping into imaginative thoughts and images, and to the fluid associations that creative thinking offers, is used in the Glass Studio as a gateway into the development of ideas and themes. Encouraging free-play of the imagination and 'flights of fancy' in a safe environment, where people trust that this will be appreciated and responded to in a positive and encouraging way, promotes the emergence of new ideas and possibly unusual associations.

To support this happening, what is needed is a fluid arena of possibility, an atmosphere where there is no such thing as a wrong idea, a wrong perspective, a wrong line or wrong texture. In making a sketch, every type of line or form of mark-making has its possibilities for experimentation and inclusion. Technical and structural necessities with regards to glass-forming can be addressed later-on in the process, but even the boundaries of these requirements can be 'played around with' and reinvented. It is through embracing the possible, taking risks and accommodating a level of uncertainty, that lucky accidents may lead to innovation. Throughout the design process in the Glass Studio, an integral aspect of teaching and making methodology, facilitating engagement through serious play, becomes most apparent. There are several steps to the process: research to generate ideas on the theme; development of ideas through sketching and/or collage; model-making/prototyping in card, plastic or wood; and then making the piece in glass. Serious play marks an attitude of experiment and invention throughout the sketching and model-making stages. Drawings, collages or models are often broken up and re-joined in different ways, to push and pull the range of forms available and 'discover' previously unknown possibilities.

Play and the experience of one member of the Glass Studio

The use of playfulness as dialogue is made manifest in the case study of one member of the Glass Studio. Peter is a 57 year old male with a moderate learning disability. He attended a special school and then moved-on to council run adult training centers for 19 years. Peter describes this time as 'boring': that they watched a lot of television or did 'boring' repetitive activities and that 'nothing ever changed'.

Peter is a shy, self-conscious individual and, although he can be vocal and articulate, he lacks self-confidence and does not readily initiate conversation or seek help or support from others. When Peter arrives at the Glass Studio in the mornings he appears unsure and hesitant; he sits very still and does not attract attention. Since he does not move around or get involved without encouragement, there are associated risks to both his physical health and general

Play and social therapy **155**

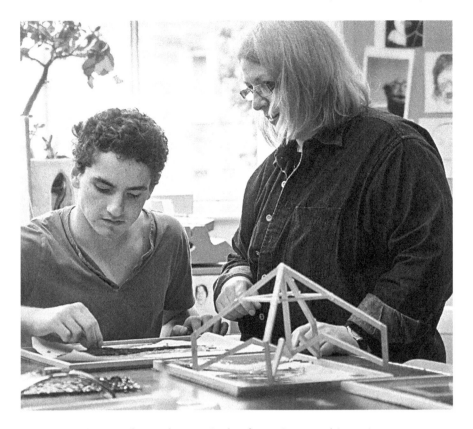

FIGURE 13.1 Serious play marks an attitude of experiment and invention

wellbeing. To the onlooker, Peter would appear to be depressed, disengaged and isolated within the group.

However, within the spirit of acceptance and appreciation that we strive to create at Garvald, Peter has revealed an animated eagerness to share his point-of-view, especially in regard to items in the news. He might listen quietly to a discussion before intervening with mock outrage, laughing at the ridiculousness of a situation. This aspect of his personality – being always ready to laugh at 'the powers that be' – is infectious and, if facilitated, can stimulate other participants into taking-up the same playful tone. The consequential atmosphere of playful interaction then opens-up an effective route into a further and more serious interchange of burgeoning ideas. Elements of active listening, acceptance, participation and imagining heats the air with creative energy, nurturing a heightened sense of motivation and purpose. At this point, more serious ideas can be introduced and developed in this atmosphere of creative possibility.

At both levels of the interaction – in playfulness and in serious play – Peter thrives in his own quiet way, observant yet absorbed in whatever he is involved

156 Eric Fleming

with. Since joining the glass workshop, Peter has proved capable of learning several glass techniques that he is able to perform independently with some support. He involves himself at all stages of the design process, offering and responding to suggestions, and is justly proud of his achievements. Peter's playfulness is integral to the process of generating a creative energy in the Glass Studio which can be transformational not only for Peter as an individual but for the group as a whole.

Social therapy, play and the celebration of festivals

As referred to earlier, during the mid- to late 1800s and early 1900s there was a rediscovery in Britain and Europe of craft-based work and its inherent value. This came about as a reaction to what was seen as the unhealthy development of factory-based employment and a general disengagement with nature and former rural ways of life. The use of crafts and the values associated with them are well documented by such thinkers as John Ruskin and William Morris in the nineteenth century and, more recently, by Richard Sennett (2009) in his book *The Craftsman*.

Craft-based work involves working more closely with materials, often natural materials, and learning a range of skills which result in tacit or 'embodied knowledge' (Sennett 2009: 44). Intellectual concerns or 'thinking skills' are less important when hands, body and the senses work in integration. Decisions are made in response to what 'feels' right, rather than to any externally imposed concept of 'rightness' and, when completely absorbed, the maker is less aware of the self, less aware of the spinning wheels of the mind. Problems are temporarily forgotten, hunger goes unnoticed. The power of craftwork rests on this re-balancing of body, feelings and mind. Traditionally, craftwork is often experienced in the context of a workshop and embodies an experience of collaboration and mutual support along the lines of an apprenticeship model. Engagement in a shared endeavour means that individual interests become subdued and less distinct and competition is sacrificed for mutual achievement.

The philosophy of Rudolf Steiner, which underlies the work of Garvald Edinburgh and other similar organizations sharing a common ethos, offers an additional layer of understanding in this regard. Steiner had taken a professional interest in Johan Wolfgang von Goethe's (1749–1832) perspective on nature which had in turn been influenced by Goethe's correspondence and dialogue with Friedrich Schiller (1759–1805), one of the first thinkers who attempted to define the role of play in human development. According to Schiller (1793) the integration, through an instinct for play, between a person's 'sensuous impulse' (related to our physical being) and the 'form impulse' (related to our moral being) results in harmony between these two forces and 'living form', the equivalent in modern terms of the realization of a universal latent potential for self-actualization. Goethe found great merit in Schiller's mission but thought it too conceptual and proposed a more intuitive interaction between the self and nature which involved 'active

Play and social therapy **157**

imagination' and a 'delicate empiricism' – themselves key components of play itself. This approach saw the human being as the most sensitive and reliable 'instrument' for gaining insights into the world of nature and was in direct contrast to Newtonian methodology which sought an objective approach, repressing the possible 'contamination' of the human element.

Goethe felt that Schiller's project could have a greater impact if delivered in the form of symbolic, narrative imagery and so wrote the fairy-tale, 'The Green Snake and the Beautiful Lily' (cited in Allen 1979). Steiner famously claimed that the whole of his own philosophy, Anthroposophy, could be found in this fairy-tale. The strength of fairy-tales is that they activate the imagination; we have to abandon the logic of a linear narrative to allow the story to communicate metaphorically in a dreamlike, symbolic way. The images and the feelings that we generate through correspondence with the symbolic narrative and metaphor integral to fairy-tales, enable us to process aspects of human experience that are enigmatic or that may be a cause of anxiety; for example, coming to terms with difficult circumstances such as illness or death. Serious play has a role in this process through our ability to recreate the related stories during active image- and form-building within us. This is a capacity that adults can retain from childhood, if they are given the opportunity and encouragement to do so. Through developing our innate capacity to gain insights by engaging aesthetically with our environment, via the arts or nature, we can reach a state of mental and emotional equilibrium.

The writing of Gadamer (cited in Grondin 2001), in more recent times, sought to show that Schiller's ideas on play, as related to individual subjective experience, have the potential to extend beyond the individual and to become active in a more communal capacity through group gatherings such as festivals or conferences. This is eloquently expressed in the following observation by Grondin (2001):

> In a festival it is clear that those who participate in it are embedded in a play that goes beyond their subjective choice, activity, and intending. Who would ever want to 'objectify' a festive mood? It is simply there and we 'share' it. A festival – as every work of art, yes, as every understanding – has its being in its accomplishment and the community'
>
> *(Grondin 2001: 46)*

At Garvald, a sense of play goes beyond the individual craft workshops to re-emerge in the collective planning and celebration of festivals. Whilst in the workshop, projects are developed on a more individual basis, the coming together at particular points during the year to celebrate embodies a feeling of belonging, signifying community. Members of the Glass Studio have been involved in creating dramas on the theme of Michaelmas and other seasonal festivals and, whilst such dramas are typified by playfulness, humor and joy, there are underlying motifs which appear within the core themes (for example, light and dark, life and decay and endurance in the face of challenges). Serious play is at the root of this gravity, in that entertainment and joy, become the vehicle for underlying messages

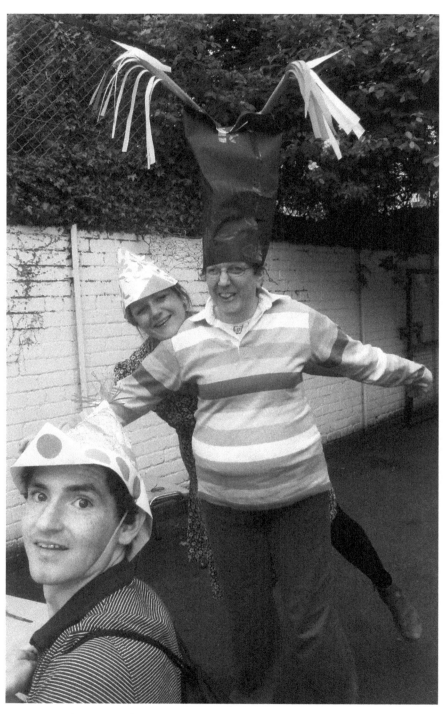

FIGURE 13.2 A sense of play re-emerges in the celebration of festivals

Play and social therapy **159**

and awareness of our connection to processes of life and death. This kind of symbolism is aimed at generating resolve through acting on our aesthetic sensibilities. Gadamer describes what we experience at these times in terms of the occasion 'taking us up': rather than us using the event for our individual benefit we momentarily surrender our sense of self into *being* 'taken up' in play as a collective happening. A merging of the self with the greater group is transformative to the extent that the self is subdued and identity is momentarily a community identity. This community identity endorses a common ethos or culture within which every member is bonded in a powerful way. The sense of belonging to something warm and embracing, something socially nourishing and enduring, serves to transform our vulnerability to isolation and disengagement into a wellspring of resilience and meaningful purpose.

References

Allen, P. M. (1979) *Goethe: The Fairy Tale of the Green Snake and the Beautiful Lily.* Edinburgh: Floris Books.

Brown, T. (2008) *Tales of Creativity and Play. TED Serious Play Conference,* Online. Available at www.ted.com/talks/tim_brown_on_creativity_and_play (accessed 13 December 2015).

Grondin, J. (2001) *Play, festival and ritual in Gadamer on the theme of the immemorial in his later works.* A paper delivered for a symposium at University 'Mozarteum' in Salzburg, Germany, Online. Available at www.mapageweb.umontreal.ca/grondinJ/pdf/play_festival_ritual_gadam.pdf (accessed 5 August 2015).

McGuinness M. (2015) *Lateralaction,* Online. Available at http://lateralaction.com/articles/lateral-thinking/ (accessed 9 August 2015).

Schiller, F. (1793) *Letter XIV, Letter's on the Aesthetic Education of Man,* Online. Available at www.gutenberg.org/files/6798/6798-h/6798-h.htm (accessed 9 August 2015).

Sennett, R. (2009) *The Craftsman,* London: Penguin.

14

PLAYING WITH WORDS

Sandie Dinnen and Alison Tonkin

This chapter aims to give a theoretical understanding of what health literacy means and explores how this can be used to benefit those working in and using healthcare services. Deconstructing examples of health literacy strategies and applying these to practice can lead to new and different approaches to healthcare which better engage service-users and which can help them during what are often difficult and emotional times in their lives. The chapter looks at how we can use some very simple and effective ways to understand how each of us feels about ourselves and about those we interact with, and offers ideas for how we can be helped to feel more in control of our lives both as practitioners and as service-users, through the use of humor, storytelling and play.

Introduction

Health literacy is a concept that has been in existence since the 1970s. The original research focuses on the definitions of health literacy and its impact on healthcare practice. This in turn has led to our greater understanding of health promotion and the huge value that peoples' understanding of health issues has in maintaining positive health and wellbeing, as well as preventing and treating disease. Kaksawadia (2013) suggests that 'one of the most subtle, but most powerful ways we can either empower or belittle others is in the language we use' and that includes the language we use to convey health-related messages.

Health Literacy is now seen as a fundamental component of the pursuit of health and wellbeing, both at an individual and at a societal level, particularly as rates of chronic health conditions rise (Day 2009). As society and healthcare systems become increasingly complex, enabling people to become 'health literate' presents new challenges (World Health Organization (WHO) Regional Office for Europe 2013). Health Literacy is increasingly being recognized as a 'significant public health concern' on a global scale (NHS Scotland 2014). Health literacy goes beyond an ability to read the literature available and encompasses activities such as understanding instructions on prescription medicines, attending appointments, completing consent forms, way-finding in a healthcare setting and reading healthcare brochures and information leaflets (Day 2009). This recognizes the complex level of cognitive functioning necessary to engage with health-related information, with skills such as reading, listening, analysing and decision making all being part of the process. As a result, health literacy has become an important facet of public health policy around the world as 'poor Health Literacy adversely affects people's health. Literacy has been shown to be one of the strongest predictors of health status along with age, income, employment, status, education level and race or ethnic group' (WHO Regional Office for Europe 2013: iv). Health Literacy is a social determinant of health (Health Literacy 2015) and addressing the issues surrounding health literacy could facilitate a reduction in health inequalities (NHS Scotland 2014). Simply put:

> Those of us with poor Health Literacy have the highest burden of health. Those of us with the lowest Health Literacy generally have double the rates of poor health outcomes, complications and death, compared to those who have the highest abilities.
>
> *(NHS Scotland 2014: 9)*

Defining health literacy

Thirty years after the Ottawa Charter was first published in 1986, one of the biggest innovations in health promotion has been the recognition that health-related messages need to be shared within the context of *how* and *where* people operate on a daily basis (Ewles and Simnett 2003). As an international milestone in the movement towards the twenty-first-century public health agenda, the Ottawa Charter had five overarching themes, two of which specifically link to health literacy. These were:

- Creating supportive environments
- Developing personal skills through information and education in health and life skills

> *(Ewles and Simnett 2003: 14).*

The drive to promote 'Health Literacy friendliness' (WHO Regional Office for Europe 2013: iv) within the context of people's daily lives has resulted in a proliferation of definitions and conceptual models, leading to much debate in terms of what is deemed effective practice and good advice.

Sørensen *et al.* (2012) undertook a systemic review of health literacy definitions and conceptual models and the content analysis of 17 definitions yielded a new and comprehensive definition:

Health Literacy is linked to literacy and entails people's knowledge, motivation and competence to access, understand, appraise and apply health information in order to make judgements and take decisions in everyday life concerning healthcare, disease prevention and health promotion to maintain or improve the quality of life during the life course.

(Sørensen et al. 2012)

As an outcome of the review, Sørensen et al. (2012) also produced an integrated model of health literacy which conceptualizes the core competencies and dimensions which impact on health literacy.

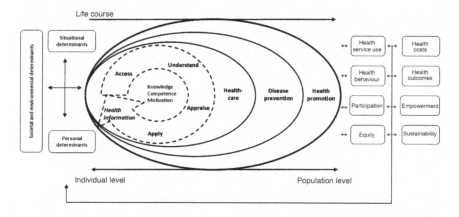

FIGURE 14.1 Integrated model of Health Literacy (Sørensen et al., 2012, kindly reproduced under Creative Commons Attribution License)

As noted in Chapter 2, conceptual frameworks linked to health often fall within the realms of biopsychosocial models, and developing effective and appropriate health literacy at both individual and community levels demands that the aspects that determine health (such as social, political and environmental factors) are addressed.

More recently, the WHO has provided a simpler statement that reflects elements of the definition offered by Sørensen et al. (2012).

Health Literacy is defined as the cognitive and social skills which determine the motivation and ability of individuals to gain access to, understand and use information in ways which promote and maintain good health.

(WHO 2015)

The WHO (2015) goes on to describe how health literacy should move beyond the obvious measures of having written pamphlets and materials available, through the extension of this information to the point where people are confident to engage fully with the service they are using. This concept identifies traditional ideas of health education as being the starting point, rather than the end point, on a person's journey through the healthcare system. Health Literacy in its fullest sense should allow those using the service to understand the wider context of what is happening to them, including political and social factors which influence health. This greater understanding empowers people to make decisions which are better informed and, in doing so, gives them the confidence to address many of the difficulties they are facing. The WHO (2015) provide a good example of this, citing a campaign to eradicate malaria in Mexico and Central America without the use of the highly toxic chemical DDT. The first aspect was educating people to understand the causes of malaria though poster campaigns, and various other methods. By understanding the need to keep their homes and surrounding areas free of standing water, to manage their drainage systems, to cover water containers and by working in local groups to clean their neighbourhoods, there was a 63 per cent reduction in malaria in those regions.

Exploring health literacy in practice

As shown in the previous example, the necessity for people to engage in the self-management of their own and their family's health, requires information to be sought, rights and responsibilities to be understood, and ultimately, decisions to be made. In order for this to be successful, skills and knowledge that enable people's participation in the healthcare process are required. Historically, these skills and knowledge have been assumed (Hoffman-Goetz *et al.* 2014; Nielsen-Bohlman *et al.* 2004), resulting in ineffective campaigns and costly interventions that often exclude the very people who need to engage with the health message being conveyed. The scale of this problem was explored in 2011 when the European Health Literacy Survey was undertaken in eight countries. When the report was released in 2012, a key finding was that, on average, 47 per cent of respondents were at risk of limited health literacy, with levels varying across the eight countries (The HLS-EU Consortium 2012). These findings are mirrored in England where 43 per cent of working age adults will struggle to calculate the dose of paracetamol for a child, and in the US where the cost to the economy of inadequate health literacy is estimated to be in the region of $106–$236 billion per year (NHS Scotland 2014). So how can health literacy be improved and what role can play and playfulness offer in its development?

Here in the UK, governments are proactive in educating the population through health promotion and usually adopt a typically British approach: humor is often used to send us effective messages. The recent campaigns to raise awareness among young men of the dangers of testicular cancer are an excellent example of how to reach a group of people who are likely to be less engaged with the health system (Whiteford and Wordley 2003; Peate 1997).

In order to inform men aged 18–35 years of how to identify if they were at risk from testicular cancer, J. Walter Thompson Advertising (2015) produced a

164 Sandie Dinnen and Alison Tonkin

campaign using a glamour model to engage and educate this group. Its aim was to reduce stigma, to make this something young men could talk about and ultimately to lead them to a website where they could find all the information they needed if they had concerns for their own health. This approach may be criticized for its political incorrectness but it does show an insightful understanding of the target audience.

The Male Cancer Awareness Campaign (2015) has also produced a raft of humorous ideas and characters that raise awareness of the disease and how to spot any early signs of it. These have included a 'Going Commando' day which raises awareness of male cancer in general; the 'Skyballs' and 'Mr Testicles' campaigns linked to testicular cancer; 'James Bum 002' linked to bowel cancer; 'Near Naked Man' linked to prostate cancer; and a campaign to raise awareness of male breast cancer. All of these are designed to appeal to young men and all use humor and language that most young men can identify with. It is still too early to measure the impact of these campaigns in terms of earlier presentation for investigation and potential treatment, but from the media responses it can be assumed that the campaign is getting the messages out to the target audience.

An alternative approach has been developed by GIANTmicrobes®, a toy company based in America who manufacture plush soft toys resembling microbes. GIANTmicrobes® (2011a) describe the toys as 'stuffed animals that look like tiny microbes – only a million times actual size! They're humorous, educational, and fun'. Originally designed as a simple educational tool for teaching young children about the importance of washing their hands, the company has grown considerably since it started in 2002 and now manufactures over 100 designs that can be used for a diverse range of purposes. Each microbe is scientifically based on an image of the real microbe, and can be used by health professionals, educators or by friends and families as a means of safe engagement in potentially embarrassing or tricky conversations. One cited testimony on the website stated 'My boyfriend needed a hint', linked to Porphyromonas gingivalis – bad breath (GIANTmicrobes 2011c).

As an example of an effective health promotion strategy, gift boxes have been produced around festivals or celebratory themes, such as the Heart Warming™ Mini Microbe Box which was released for Valentine's Day containing a sperm cell, egg cell, Kissing Disease, Penicillin and pink Amoeba. Alternatively, you could also purchase the Heart Burned™ Mini Microbe box (Figure 14.1) which contains Herpes, Pox, HPV, chlamydia and penicillin microbes (GIANTmicrobes 2011b).

A similar approach has been taken by the *Iheartguts* Company from the United States. The company was founded in 2005 by illustrator Wendy Bryan Lazar, and makes plush cartoon internal organs, lapel pins, T-shirts and posters (Iheartguts 2015a). There are now over 50 different lapel pins featuring different organs and glands of the body and 29 plush toys which can be used by practitioners undertaking the delivery of health education:

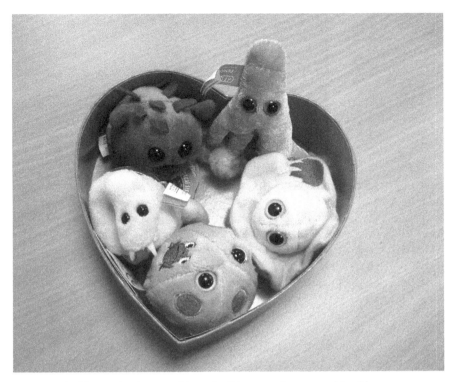

FIGURE 14.2 Giant microbes provide a playful approach to sexual health

> I'm a nurse and a diabetes educator and I've turned the giant sticker set into magnets and I use them in my group diabetes education classes when we talk about pathophysiology/complications of diabetes. My students are all adults, but who doesn't like smiley cartoon organs helping you learn about your chronic condition? I use brain, heart, liver, kidney, stomach, intestines, and pancreas is the star of the show… I [also] wear a pancreas lapel pin on my badge as my own little 'diabetes educator' marker.
>
> *(Diana D. (cited in Iheartguts 2015b)*

They can also be used by people who have a chronic health condition:

> I have been living with Crohn's Disease for 12 years now. Just last month I had my second surgery to remove more of my intestines. My best friend came to the hospital with a new set of intestines for me. Not only was it incredibly hilarious but it was also helpful too. The intestine pillow works amazing as a post-operative cough pillow to hold tight to your abdomen. During my month long stay in the hospital I showed off my pillow to all of the staff and they loved it.
>
> *(Krystal B. cited Iheartguts 2015b)*

166 Sandie Dinnen and Alison Tonkin

Kystal B. (Iheartguts 2015b) shows the very personal way in which people deal with illness and this clearly demonstrates, that a major factor in ensuring people receive, understand and engage with messages sent as part of a health literacy strategy, is how the message is communicated. This is covered in more detail in Chapter 22. Knowledge of how to communicate messages, in a world which can often be complex and difficult to understand, can encourage practitioners to think carefully about not just what they are saying but, just as importantly, how it is being said.

Professor Albert Mehrabian pioneered his work in the field of communications in the 1960s (Chapman 2012). His research has been widely quoted and misquoted in the intervening years but much of what he found is still relevant for health practitioners today. Mehrabian established that our body language can say as much as, if not more than, our verbal language but he also researched how our communications are received, understood and remembered. He identified that only 7 per cent of received meaning comes from the words spoken, that 38 per cent comes from the way in which words are said and that 55 per cent derives from facial expression. For people who are highly anxious, who have dementia or learning disabilities the rates of understanding are likely to be even lower than those given above (Chapman 2012). When working at face-to-face level, the language used needs to be clear and pitched at an appropriate level for the person listening. Visual aids can be used to support a conversation, as shown in Figure 14.1. The body language of the practitioner conveys strong messages to the listener and in turn much of the listeners' reaction to that conversation will be evident in their own body language. The more relaxed people are in the communication cycle the more effective it will be.

Promoting health literacy is about more than giving people the opportunity to understand their situation and giving them the knowledge to make choices at a difficult time. It is also about how people are supported through their journey and how to make their lives as stimulating and enjoyable as possible in difficult circumstances. Often this is about practitioners being able to listen and provide opportunities for activities that will distract people from their problems and help them to enjoy a better quality of life.

In 2008 the Alzheimer's Society Magazine *Living with Dementia* reviewed research on the communications skills of people with dementia (Bradley 2008). The findings of a small American study at that time noted that, although people with this syndrome often found it difficult to communicate and had difficulty remembering words, it did not mean that they had forgotten the meaning of the words themselves (Harley *et al.*, cited Bradley 2008). When translated into practice these findings are significant.

People with dementia need to be given the time to try and work out alternative ways of communicating their messages and often this will be through a description of the object or event, rather than direct reference to the main topic under discussion. In *A Life Like Other People's*, Alan Bennett (2009: 210) tells of a conversation he had with his mother who had dementia:

Except now her language is beginning to go, and planted in front of a vast view over Somerset she laughs and says, 'Oh, what a lovely … lot of it about.

It is clear to Bennett's mother that she is discussing the scenery and he also knows exactly what she is trying to say. People with dementia need more time to be able to express what they want to say and, for those working with this patient group, Bennett's account of his mother's struggles provides a helpful insight into the challenges they face.

The Alzheimer's Society (2015b) provides an extensive range of fact-sheets with the most popular being available in written or audio versions. The fact-sheet relating to communication explains how frustrating and upsetting trying to communicate can be for the person with dementia, and it provides plenty of suggestions to enhance the communication process, one of which is the use of humor:- 'humor can help to bring you closer together, and may relieve the pressure. Try to laugh together about misunderstandings and mistakes – it can help' (Alzheimer's Society 2015a). This type of advice and guidance enables people with dementia and the loved ones who care for them, to devise shared strategies to make living with a degenerative condition such as dementia more manageable for all concerned, especially when language skills may vary from day to day and time to time (Alzheimer's Society 2015a). Having adequate information and support helps to empower people to 'live well with dementia' enabling them to enjoy a good quality of life and to remain active within their communities (Alzheimer's Society 2015b). Written in positive and enabling language, the guidance provides helpful examples of how health literacy should reflect the needs of the user group, giving hope and practical advice. This is demonstrated through the comments of one person who uses a local Alzheimer's Society branch:

> My time is well spent here. We talk and encourage one another while laughing at ourselves on occasion. There is a good feeling of camaraderie. We understand both our feelings and our needs.
>
> *(Alzheimer's Society 2010)*

A major supermarket chain has taken this message on board and is trialling a checkout designed specifically for people with dementia. The staff have been trained in working with people with dementia by an NHS specialist nurse and the checkout is set-up with clear visual aids linked to coinage and written information about memory loss and sources of help on display. This approach is to be applauded as it acknowledges the needs of their customers and removes some of the stigma attached to dementia (ITV News 2015).

The effects of laughter have been well proven, yet this is something that is often not considered in the everyday world of healthcare. Giving people something to laugh at goes some way towards providing the stimulation necessary for maintaining physical and mental wellbeing and perhaps also gives them something to talk about afterwards. Humor certainly enhances the quality of life and recent research identifies the value of humor in health transactions (Cann and Kuiper 2014). Humor helps people to relax and to take their thoughts away from those things which are worrying them. For a space of time, humor can help to relieve pressure and stress and to create a more pleasurable world for patients and staff alike. McGhee (2007) identifies that, as the body relaxes with humor, certain physiological changes take place; the cellular immune system can be enhanced, pain can be reduced and laughter provides cardiac exercise. In India there are groups of people who meet regularly for laughter classes. The participants talk about the positivity of their experiences and about how laughing for a short time every day enhances the quality of their lives, improving their wellbeing and providing a social event (Agarwal 2014). This is something that can easily be replicated in everyday practice and some American hospitals now offer laughter clinics to support patients with cancer (Mcreaddle and Payne 2011). Laughter yoga and laughter therapy have become worldwide phenomena, with the growing recognition that laughter is another route to positive health.

It is interesting to note that adults may use self-deprecating humor to deal with difficult situations. Therefore, it is important for the practitioner to recognize this and to also be able to understand and empathize with the feelings that lie beneath the humor. These self-deprecating jokes can provide an opportunity to open up a conversation with a patient to find out what is really worrying them and to perhaps allay some of their fears. This also demonstrates how humor can enable us to see things from differing perspectives and for patients can allow a sense of balance to be regained (Gesell 2014).

Humor is one valuable source of communication and storytelling is another. All of us have a story to tell, but not all of us have someone to listen to our stories. Patients who have the opportunity to tell their own stories provide practitioners with an insight into their lives. With greater knowledge of their patient, the practitioner can devise strategies to help retain memory and keep their history alive, through the creation of memory books or life stories or to gain a greater understanding of what makes them happy, including their likes and dislikes (deVries 2013). This is the rationale behind the *This is me* tool which has been developed by the Alzheimer's Society (2015c) and supported by the Royal College of Nursing for people with dementia. Originally designed for when people go into hospital, its use has been extended to include communication with professionals in any setting, providing information about the person's needs and preferences.

It is not just the patient who can benefit from storytelling. TimeSlips is a research project that examines the attitudes of practitioners towards people with dementia (George *et al*. 2011). The project aimed to improve understanding between older people and the medical practitioners who were treating them. TimeSlips is a creative storytelling program that measured the attitudes of fifth-year medical students to people with dementia before and after they have engaged in group storytelling sessions over a period of time. The research concluded that the group-based storytelling did indeed improve the attitudes of the medical students, many of whom went on to include this in their own practice, and in turn can only

Playing with words **169**

be of benefit to the patients with dementia and to the patient-professional relationship (George *et al.* 2011).

The use of picture stories is particularly effective for people with limited language skills. This includes newcomers to a country, or for people with low level literacy skills, for whom the social determinants of health mean that the community are more likely to face disease (Wahowiak 2014). Picture stories keep wording to a minimum, giving just enough information to convey the required message. Cartoons and comics provide a valuable platform for sharing health-related information in this way. For example, in 2012 in Fall River, Massachusetts where 50 per cent of people speak Portuguese, the rate of diabetes among this community was 11.3 per cent, which was 2 per cent higher than the national average for the United States. Dobbins and McLane (cited Wahowiak 2014) created a one-panel comic strip called 'Dica de Diabetes' that explained different aspects of diabetes directly to the Portuguese community. This was released through the local, weekly Portuguese language journal, resulting in new patients attending local clinics in the following weeks as a direct result of having read the comic. Fotonovelas (photo-driven comics) are also an important source of 'edutainment' and these often use a soap-opera style, with the bulk of the message being presented through images. In Southern California, fotonovelas are particularly popular with the Hispanic and Latino communities and 'because they're easy to read and understand, people learn new things about chronic conditions they may have had for years' (Wahowiak 2014).

This strategy can also be used as part of language enhancement programs such as ESOL (English for Speakers of Other Languages) courses, whereby health literacy can be tailored to the specific needs of a particular community (Singleton 2004). Stories tend to feature cartoon characters, avoiding the need to disclose personal experiences. This is an effective strategy which was instigated in 2007 by NHS Tower Hamlets in a project entitled ESOL Health and Humor (n.d.). Designed to allow ESOL tutors to embed health-related topics into ESOL classes, NHS Tower Hamlets have developed ten health packs and a website with resources that acts as a repository for practitioners all around the world.

The concept of narrative graphics has been extended by Graphic Medicine, a website that was started in 2007 by Ian Williams, a physician and artist from North Wales. The website 'explores the interaction between the medium of comics and the discourse of healthcare. We are a community of academics, health carers, authors, artists, and fans of comics and medicine' and is supported by the Wellcome Trust (Graphic Medicine 2015a). The site works on a number of levels, providing a vehicle for sharing experiences for the whole medical community, including practitioners, patients, caregivers and families, all of whom have stories to share, allowing creative reflection on what can be complicated and difficult experiences (Graphic Medicine 2015b).

By listening to and telling stories together practitioners can gain a much greater understanding of what their patients value and what matters to them, impacting positively on the way they are treated throughout their health journey. Humor and storytelling are both creative forms of therapy that require communication skills, imagination and provide proven physical and mental benefits to those involved in the process. Play is an equally creative therapeutic medium of promoting and supporting health literacy.

Traditionally we tend to think of play as something for children. In reality adults do play; they play card games, computer games, puzzles and word games, all of which stimulate and engage our thinking processes, distract us from our day-to-day routine and concerns, as well as providing a sense of achievement. As with all activities, it is important that game-playing should be a positive experience and that it does not cause frustration, so games may need to be adapted to a person's level of ability. It is also important to remember that these players are adults and although the game, or the language around the game, may need to be simplified, the person playing the game is still an adult and needs to be treated as such. All of these activities provide physical and mental benefits for the people involved, with the proviso that they are engaged with as a matter of choice. As with anyone in a difficult, painful or complex situation, it is vital that people have a voice in the activities undertaken and that they are given choices about what they do and do not wish to take part in (Alzheimer's Society 2010).

Conclusion

Health Literacy has moved on considerably from the original definition. It is the role of practitioners to provide people with the information they need to make informed choices about their healthcare choices, in a manner most suited to their particular needs and context. However, more than that, it is also the duty of healthcare providers to ensure that people who are using health services have their rights to knowledge respected and are given the time to ask questions. Practitioners have available a raft of knowledge and skills to allow this to happen. As professionals, it is important to continue to build on existing skills to enable those using the healthcare system to have as good an experience as is possible according to their own particular circumstances. A greater understanding of health literacy and of the benefits to patients and health professionals alike will improve the healthcare experience for all involved. The skills to make people laugh, to forget about their troubles, even for a short space of time, to be involved and active and to remain a valued member of their community should never be underestimated.

References

Agarwal, S. (2014) *Spreading a Smile*, Online. Available at http://timesofindia.indiatimes.com/life-style/health-fitness/health-news/Spreading-a-smile/articleshow/45020491.cms (accessed 21 October 2015).

Alzheimer's Society (2010) *Living with Dementia Booklets: Keeping Involved and Active,* Online. Available at www.alzheimers.org.uk/site/scripts/download_info.php?fileID=731 (accessed 19 October 2015)

Alzheimer's Society (2015a) *Communicating,* Online. Available at www.alzheimers.org.uk/site/scripts/documents_info.php?documentID=130 (accessed 19 October 2015).

Alzheimer's Society (2015b) *Living with Dementia*, Online. Available at www.alzheimers. org.uk/site/scripts/documents.php?categoryID=200342 (accessed 19 October 2015).

Alzheimer's Society (2015c) *This Is Me Tool*, Online. Available at www.alzheimers.org.uk/ thisisme (accessed 19 October 2015).

Bennett, A. (2009), *A Life Like Other People's*, London: Faber & Faber Ltd and Profile Books.

Bradley, C. (2008) *Living with Dementia November 2008: Communication skills*, Online. Available at www.alzheimers.org.uk/site/scripts/documents_info.php?documentID= 783&pageNumber=3 (accessed 21 October 2015).

Cann, A. and Kuiper, N. (2014) Research on the role of humor in wellbeing and health, *Europe's Journal of Psychology*, North America, 10, August 2014. Online. Available at http://ejop.psychopen.eu/article/view/818 (accessed 18 October 2015).

Chapman, A. (2012) *Mehrabian's Communication Research: Professor Albert Mehrabian's Communications Model*, Online. Available at www.businessballs.com/mehrabiancommun ications.htm (accessed 18 October 2015).

Day, V. (2009) Promoting health literacy through storytelling, *The Online Journal of Issues in Nursing*, 14 (3) Manuscript 6.

deVries, K. (2013) Communicating with older people with dementia, *Nursing Older People*, 25 (4): 30–37.

ESOL Health and Humor (n.d.) *What is ESOL Health and Humor?* Online. Available at www.esolhealthandhumor.org/index.html (accessed 19 October 2015).

Ewles, L. and Simnett, I. (2003) *Promoting Health: A Practical Guide*, 5th ed., The Netherlands: Baillière Tindall.

George, D., Stuckey, H., Dillon, C. and Whitehead, M. (2011) Impact of participation in TimeSlips, a creative group-based storytelling program, on medical student attitudes toward persons with dementia: a qualitative study, *The Gerontologist*, 51 (5): 699–703.

Gesell, I. (2014) *The Healing Power of Humor and Play*, Online. Available at www.health literacyoutloud.com/2010/04/27/hlol-36-the-healing-power-of-humor-play/ (accessed 19 October 2015).

GIANTmicrobes (2011a) *Learn about GIANTmicrobes®*, Online. Available at www.giantmi crobes.com/uk/content/learnaboutgiantmicrobes.html (accessed 5 December 2015).

GIANTmicrobes (2011b) *Heart Boxes*, Online. Available at www.giantmicrobes.com/ uk/products/heart-burned.html (accessed 5 December 2015).

GIANTmicorobes (2011c) *Why do People like GIANTmicrobes®?* Online. Available at www.giantmicrobes.com/uk/ (accessed 5 December 2015).

Graphic Medicine (2015a) *About Graphic Medicine*, Online. Available at www.graphic medicine.org/about/ (accessed 21 October 2015).

Graphic Medicine (2015b) *Book Series*, Online. Available at www.graphicmedicine. org/book-series/ (accessed 21 October 2015).

Health Literacy (2015) *Why is Health Literacy Important?* Online. Available at www.health-literacy.org.uk/ (accessed 18 October 2015).

Hoffman-Goetz, L., Donelle, L. and Ahmed, R. (2014) *Health Literacy in Canada: A Primer for Students*, Toronto: Canadian Scholars Press.

Iheartguts (2015a) *About us*, Online. Available at http://iheartguts.com/pages/about-us (accessed 21 October 2015).

Iheartguts (2015b) *Testimonials + Compliments*, Online. Available at http://iheartguts.com/ pages/testimonials/ (accessed 21 October 2015).

ITV News (2015) *UK's First Dementia Friendly Checkout Opens in Chester*, Online. Available at www.itv.com/news/granada/2015-10-20/uks-first-dementia-friendly-checkout-opens-in-chester/ (accessed 21 October 2015).

Kaksawadia, A. (2013) *The Power of Words,* PLOS. Blogs. 10 January 2013 Online. Available at http://blogs.plos.org/publichealth/2013/01/10/the-power-of-words/ (accessed: 17 October 2015).

Male Cancer Awareness Campaign (2015) *Home,* Online. Available at www.malecancer.org/ (accessed 18 October 2015).

Mcreaddle, M. and Payne, S. (2011) Humour in health-care interactions: a risk worth taking, *Health Expectations,* 17: 332–344.

McGhee, P. (2007) *Humor and Health,* Online. Available at www.holisticonline.com/ Humor_Therapy/humor_mcghee_article.htm (accessed 18 October 2015).

Nielsen-Bohlman, L., Panzer, A. and Kindig, D. (eds) (2004) *Health Literacy: A Prescription to End Confusion,* Washington, DC: The National Academies Press.

NHS Scotland (2014) *Making it easy: A Health Literacy Action Plan for Scotland,* The Scottish Government.

Peate, I. (1997) Testicular cancer: the importance of effective health education, *British Journal of Nursing,* 6 (6): 311–316.

Singleton, K. (2004) *Picture Stories for Adult ESL Health Literacy,* Online. Available at www.cal.org/caela/esl_resources/Health/ (accessed 19 October 2015).

Sørensen, K., Van den Broucke, S., Fullam, J., Doyle, G., Pelikan, J. Slonska, Z., Brand, H. and (HLS-EU) Consortium Health Literacy Project European (2012) Health literacy and public health: a systematic review and integration of definitions and models, *BMC Public Health,* 12: 80.

The HLS-EU Consortium (2012) *Final Report: Executive Summary (D17) The European Health Literacy Project (HLS-EU),* The HLS-EU Consortium.

Thompson Advertising, J. Walter (2015) *Male Cancer Awareness Campaign,* Online. Available at www.jwt.com/en/london/work/rhiantouchesherself/ (accessed 18 October 2015).

Wahowiak, L. (2014) *Comic Books and Cartoons for Better Health,* Online. Available at www.diabetesforecast.org/2014/10-oct/comic-books-and-cartoons-for.html?referrer= https://uk.search.yahoo.com/ (accessed 21 October 2015).

Whiteford, A. and Wordley, J. (2003) Raising awareness and detection of testicular cancer in young men, *Nursing Times,* 99 (1): 34–36.

World Health Organization Regional Office for Europe (2013) *The Solid Facts: Health Literacy,* Copenhagen: Geneva: World Health Organization Regional Office for Europe.

World Health Organization (2015) *Track 2: Health Literacy and Health Behaviour,* Online. Available at www.who.int/healthpromotion/conferences/7gchp/track2/en/ (accessed 18 October 2015).

15
PLAYING WITH TECHNOLOGY

Debbie Tonkin and Alison Tonkin

This chapter will explore how technological advances have changed the face of both play and healthcare provision. The utilization of play-based technology to develop games designed to encourage physical activity, and the application of technical know-how for tracking health and fitness, means that technology has also found its place in health education, enhancing patient engagement and enabling the sharing of play-based experiences. As noted by Goldstein (2013): 'Where people play and with whom is increasingly virtual and remote, and this trend is likely to continue. At the same time, new technologies free us from chairs and computer screens to allow mobile and active play, virtual and otherwise'.

Introduction

Technology has advanced to such an extent that we all carry portable gadgets and devices that have become integral to our work and social lives (Topol 2013). Smartphones and tablets are used daily to work on-the-go, to catch-up with friends and family wherever we may be, and to keep up to date with the latest news and trends (Ofcom 2015a). Smart technology is also used to monitor various aspects of our lives, including those related to our health and wellbeing.

In the UK, internet usage has increased by 27 per cent over the past ten years with nine out of every ten adults now going online for between ten and 20 hours each week (Ofcom 2015a). Although the number of people searching for health-related information on the internet has remained relatively stable over the past ten years, at around 16 per cent (Ofcom 2015a), the advancement of technology has enabled the creation of apps and games designed to improve and maintain our health and wellbeing through play. Innovative means have been used to recommend forms of exercise, to monitor and record exercise levels and food intake, and to provide the motivation to undertake exercise that, in an ever-increasingly busy world, we wouldn't otherwise do (Lyons *et al.* 2014). The widespread use of social media websites such as Facebook and Twitter creates opportunities for individuals to interact with others sharing common medical conditions whilst also providing the means for sharing resources and research into specific conditions for a wide variety of different target audiences (BBC WebWise 2014).

What is technology and how has it changed in recent years?

The Oxford English Dictionary (2015), defines technology as 'The branch of knowledge dealing with the mechanical arts and applied sciences', and goes on to explain that the term can be used to describe the study, application, and products of this knowledge. According to Buchanan (2015a), 'technology is the systematic study of techniques for making and doing things' and has a history dating from 3000 BC to the present day. The period of transition from the nineteenth into the twentieth century is of most significance to the developing role of technology in healthcare, as it saw major advances leading to the discovery of new drugs such as aspirin, x-rays, vaccines and anaesthetics (Buchanan 2015b). In recent years, healthcare settings have had to adapt in order to keep up with both technological advances and the changing lifestyles of service users. One of the biggest contributing factors to this change is the creation of the World Wide Web in 1992 (Encyclopaedia Britannica 2015). The internet has become increasingly influential on the way western healthcare has been organized and delivered over the last 14 years and we now expect to have our hospital notes recorded electronically, to receive confirmation of medical appointments via text message or email, and use apps on our smartphones to monitor recommended changes in diet and exercise.

School students have access to iPads, smartboards and computer games designed specifically for teaching purposes, alongside other interactive learning aids that would have been unimaginable even as recently as a decade ago. Today's children are learning in completely different ways from those of previous generations. Prensky (2001) proposes the concept of d*igital natives* and *digital immigrants* to describe generational differences in present-day interactions with technology. Digital natives are those who have been brought up alongside the advancement of technology and therefore feel more at ease using it than digital immigrants, who have had to learn to adapt to using technology as a means of social communication. This includes things such as using the internet rather than books for research into a topic, using text messages and emails rather than letters to communicate, and using digital diaries rather than paper organizers (Prensky 2001). The use of social media is also related to age, with the 25- to 34-year age group showing the most prolific usage in the UK. Across the globe, the use of social media is significantly reduced in those above 55 years of age – Prensky's so-called 'digital immigrants' (Ofcom 2013).

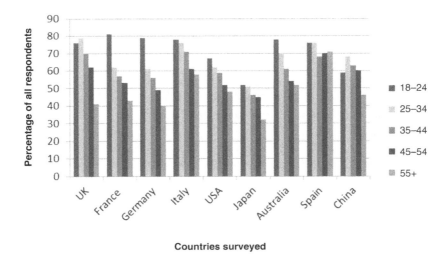

FIGURE 15.1 Weekly use of home internet connections to visit social networking sites (Ofcom 2013)

The use of technology in healthcare has undergone parallel changes over the course of the last 20 years. The modern NHS has a number of webpages and resources that derive from advancements in technology, including the NHS Choices (2015) website, which helps users to locate service information relevant to a specific geographical area or specific medical conditions. In hospitals and GP surgeries, iPads are used to distract children and vulnerable adults during treatment procedures and general health information is disseminated on screens in waiting rooms. Doctors' appointments can be made online, whilst tablets and patient portals are making patient engagement a more meaningful experience (Fluckinger 2015). There is even an iPad app which provides 'augmented reality to overlay complex vascular systems during operations', such as complex liver surgery, thus reducing possible complications and shortening the length of the surgery (Apple 2015).

Play-based technology for health and wellbeing

Technology is being used both to improve healthcare services and in the promotion of health and wellbeing through the creation of games and apps which use play as a means of looking after oneself both physically and mentally.

Videogames and exergames

Videogames have been held responsible for increased inactivity and reduced physical fitness among the young and for replacing the healthy outdoor play of

176 Debbie Tonkin and Alison Tonkin

previous generations (Campbell 2011). However, in response to these criticisms, and with the advancement of technology, videogames have been created which can track the movement of the player and simulate physical exercise whilst the game is being played (Lyons *et al.* 2014).

Exergames are games that demand movement from the player, this movement being detected by sensors and through the use of remote controls which determine the game process (Brox *et al.* n.d.). One of the first exergames to acquire widespread popular usage, was the Dance Mat for PlayStation One. This involved the user responding to audio and visual prompts to step on buttons incorporated in the 'dance mat' in a prescribed sequence. Further advancements in the field led to the 'Wii fit' which was released in 2007 and which became the first high profile game to record fitness statistics such as height, weight and BMI (Nintendo 2015). Interaction with the game via an interactive board enabled weight and movement to be picked-up, and users exercised whilst playing the game, having their progress monitored and recorded at each subsequent play session. The success of Wii fit led to other gaming platforms creating similar games, such and the Xbox Kinect (Microsoft 2015). Although these so-called exergames are designed to increase physical activity and reduce the effects (such as obesity) of sedentary gaming, the findings have been disappointing. When tested under laboratory conditions, adults and children recorded moderate to vigorous physical activity levels during the game-play, but when similar exergames were played within the home environment, subjects were found to be no more active than children who played inactive games (Stross 2012). This phenomenon is well known and suggests that, although there may be an increase in energy expenditure during the exergame, subjects compensate by doing less physical activity throughout the rest of the day (Stross 2012). These findings pose the challenge of how exergames can be used to motivate adult users to become more active.

Lyons *et al.* (2014) undertook research with 50 young female adults aged 18 to 35 years examining levels of engagement, enjoyment and energy expended whilst playing the active 'Dance Dance Revolution' game. Enjoyment of the game was identified as the key mediator, linking directly to engagement with the game and the amount of energy expended. Enjoyment is a psychosocial factor which has also been linked to player movement in non-traditional exergames, such as Guitar Hero, which can induce significant movement activity extraneous to the completion of the gaming task (Lyons *et al.* 2014). It has also been found that the enjoyment derived from listening to music during exercise acts as a distraction from the performance of the exercise itself and is known to be associated with decreased pain perception (Lyons *et al.* 2014).

Competency and the ability to actively engage with a game are also considered to be crucial factors for perceived enjoyment (Lyons *et al.* 2014). This is significant when considering the use of exergames by people who are 'functionally compromised', such as stroke-patients and the elderly. Wüest *et al.* (2014) have shown that gaming strategies can be used for rehabilitation and can be particularly effective for the management of motor movements in people who have suffered a stroke (Wüest *et al.* 2014). However, changes in information-processing and movement skills among this patient group mean that alternative approaches to exergaming need to be found (Brox *et al.* n.d.). In a study looking at the balance skills required for standing and walking, Wüest *et al.* (2014) produced an exergames rehabilitation program, which could be tailored to the individual's progression. Conventional, 'off the shelf', video games were found to be over-complex, highlighting the need for physical and cognitive limitations to be factored into the design and implementation of exergames used for rehabilitative purposes. The research team used Gentile's motor-skill taxonomy as the theoretical framework for the exergame, developing a total of six basic games, each of which demonstrates the importance of providing treatment that is simultaneously engaging and challenging in order to inspire commitment to the rehabilitation process (Wüest *et al.* 2014). This is exemplified in reference to the exergames *Scarecrow* and *Fruit Basket*.

In the game *Scarecrow*, a scarecrow avatar is used to practice standing quietly. The game *Fruit catcher* features an avatar who tries to catch fruit falling from a tree in a basket balanced on its head, requiring controlled weight-shifts by the player to enable optimal positioning of the avatar (Wüest *et al.* 2014).

A modified-game approach can also be used to enhance balance in the elderly for whom falls represent the leading cause of disability and injury (Garcia *et al.* 2012). Traditional fall-prevention interventions are often perceived as 'boring', leading to high dropout rates. In contrast, the use of a Kinect-based gaming experience not only improves engagement but also allows for player performance to be quantified in terms of motor function demonstrated during the game (Garcia *et al.* 2012). Van Diest *et al.* (2013) also noted that adherence to traditional programs aimed at fall prevention was low. They analysed 13 papers linked to exergaming and postural control, including two involving healthy subjects and nine concerning elderly people with age-related impairment of postural control. All the studies reported high levels of enjoyment and motivation to play the exergames, and several of the studies also demonstrated an increase in balance ability (van Diest *et al.* 2013). An additional benefit identified by some of these studies, was the social aspect of exergaming for elderly people living in the community.

Brox *et al.* (n.d.) note that regular physical activity is important for both physical health and psychological wellbeing and that exergames enable the elderly to combat social isolation and loneliness through the social interaction that online exergames provide. Fun is identified as the fundamental motivation for engagement with the exergame, demanding that games designed for this purpose must first be acceptable to the target group. These games typically rely on biofeedback mechanisms but the Wii has been found to be too fast for the elderly and consistently provides negative feedback when used with this age-group (Brox *et al.* n.d.). Games specifically designed for the elderly, such as dance mats and Eyetoy games which use cameras to track movement, have been found to be more suitable than conventional alternatives. Players have also been shown to be more involved in exergames when others are spectating or participating alongside (Brox *et al.* n.d.). Multiplayer games require players to work together collectively through a social platform and this can be an effective means of promoting intergenerational gaming (Cantwell *et al.* 2014).

Another example of the use of modern technology has been the development of a biofeedback game that uses meditation to improve heart rhythm and mindfulness, through the tracking of 'heart rate variability and skin conductance' (Healthy Heart Meditation 2015). Guided relaxation and meditation games enable players to 'build stairways with your breath, open doors with meditation, juggle balls with your laughter' through a game that is played on a computer using an ear lobe sensor and which involves travelling around virtual worlds through the *Wild Divine Journey* (Healthy Heart Meditation 2015).

The digitization of doodling provides another example of the playful application of technology to promote emotional wellbeing. With numerous apps now devoted to screen-based doodling (Morais 2015), Kate (cited Graham 2015) notes that doodles 'offer time and space for over-loaded brains to empty out, and allow the deeper, more imaginative processing, which is essential for wellbeing, to take place'.

The health benefits are plentiful, as described by Sue Doodles (2010):

> My name is Sue and I love to doodle. I love the zen of black and white, and I love to play in riotous color… I have a doodle ritual. Every night before I go to bed, I [doodle] for an hour or so. I unwind. I don't eat after 8 pm. I sleep like a baby. I have great dreams.

The gamification of healthcare

Gamification is defined as 'applying game design techniques, game mechanics, and/ or game style to non-game applications to solve problems, engage audiences and to make otherwise mundane tasks more fun and engaging' and, in the context of healthcare, this is turning 'users into players' (Nuvuin 2015a). Trent (2015) suggests that gamification makes life more like a game by reducing the seriousness that is often associated with the adoption of healthy habits and with trying to achieve personal health goals. The use of gratification and reward is the cornerstone of gamification, through its appeal to the limbic structures of the brain (Trent 2015).

Gamification is mainly represented in health and wellness apps linked to self-regulation and management, disease prevention and medical education-related simulations (Nuvuin 2015a). Play-based strategies utilized within these apps fall into three categories:

1 Progress bars are used to measure success
2 Players can share their progress and results with other users or friends, inducing a competitive spirit to encourage better use of the service

Playing with technology **179**

3 Positive reinforcement through the award of stars, medals, virtual gifts and badges, all of which provide a sense of achievement and motivation to do more (Nuvuin 2015a).

Monitoring technology is not only used for recording data on exercise, but also on food and calorie intake. There are many apps which can be used to assist in weight loss and weight management and not all of these utilize positive reinforcement to encourage the user. 'CARROT fit' aims to 'transform your flabby carcass into a Grade A specimen of the human race' through a variety of motivational means, including 'inspiring, threatening, bullying, bribing, ridiculing and insulting, to push "chubby humans" into losing their extra pounds' (Nuvuin 2015b). Users of the app manually input their personal data and earn rewards if they lose weight which include 'workout tips, cat facts and watching your friend eat a bag of potato chips'. Failure to lose weight garners the wrath of the Carrot Overlord in the form of a sinister voiceover and various humorous animations which insult and shame the user into trying harder. It should be obvious that this approach to weight-loss tracking is not suited to everyone but, for those with a sense of humor, it represents another, novel approach to user engagement (Nuvuin 2015b).

There are also apps that reward some players based on the failure of others. The Pact mobile app by GymPact uses actual monetary rewards and losses as motivational incentives to the achievement of weight and fitness goals. If personal goals are achieved each week, players can earn money from the losses incurred by others who do not manage to keep 'their pact' (Kim 2015).

Apps are also being designed which help people affected by chronic, long-term conditions, such as diabetes. The addition of a gaming element has been found to help with disease self-management (Kim 2015). An example of one such app is 'mySugr', which helps users to understand how they need to modify their diet. Fun and laughter are espoused to help people manage diabetes through the use of 'externalized representation – the diabetes monster' (Johnson 2015). 'MySugr' advocates the view that living with diabetes is not as bad as it is often portrayed to be, suggesting that 'it's the people we know with diabetes who inspire us to bring the coolness into diabetes, and the beauty into diabetes, and the elegance and witty humor and pleasurable experience into diabetes' (Johnson 2015). The diabetes monster needs to be 'tamed' each day through the inputting of data via the 'mySugr' Logbook app, action which is then rewarded by feedback from an animated monster – 'it entertains, praises or teases. Now even more' (mySugr 2015). The app description says it all:

> Sometimes tame, sometimes cheeky mySugr Logbook is a charming diabetes logbook app that's full of attitude. It makes your diabetes data useful in everyday life with elements of fun, gamification, and immediate feedback through your diabetes monster! Stay motivated and involved in your diabetes therapy, today!
>
> *(mySugr 2015)*

The unique contribution made by the diabetes service company responsible for the mySugr range of apps and training materials, is that many of the mySugr team actually live with diabetes themselves and have used their personal knowledge and experience in the development of these innovative products. Fredrik Debong co-founded mySugr in 2010 and has discussed his experience of having Type 1 diabetes since early childhood in a TED talk. Debong stresses how play and play-based strategies have helped him to cope with living with diabetes (Debong 2014), especially when fear became the driving force for managing his condition, likening this state to living with 'a diabetes monster'. Following several years of non-compliance with treatment which resulted in serious health consequences, Debong began to treat his diabetes as if it were a game, and 'subconsciously began rewarding myself for doing things that I should'. The notion of rewarding positive disease-management subsequently became intrinsic to Debong's way of coping with his diagnosis as he found a way to re-enter the 'game' of managing his diabetes. 'Using games and modern technology, mobile phones and web browsers – can it be that simple, can it work?' (Debong 2014). The diabetes monster that Debong lived with for so long, is now represented through the Logbook app, which helps people to remain engaged with their diabetes therapy. Debong concludes his TED talk by referring to his team as digital natives who have 'attacked' the field of medicine, suggesting that healthcare has become part of a new digital revolution (Debong 2014).

In addition to gaming platforms which encourage players to exercise and apps that can encourage healthy behavior change, hundreds of apps and devices exist which can also be used alongside each other to monitor fitness levels during physical activity. An example of this is Fitbit (2015), which is a mobile app based on the concept 'that fitness is not just about gym time. It's all the time'. Fitbit can be used to monitor heartbeat and sleep behavior and as a pedometer, suggesting that small steps towards fitness can have as big an impact as dedicated physical activity. Fitbit also promotes the role of socialization, suggesting that 'Fitness is more fun with friends and family' and allows for the sharing of achievement badges as well as providing a platform to encourage friends and families, through the use of group challenges, a leader board, cheers and taunts (Fitbit 2015). A recognition of the need to achieve interconnectivity between personal devices has resulted in the Internet of Things (IoT) which allows 'previously unconnected devices to communicate and share data with one another' (Ofcom 2015b). The potential for this new connectivity to enable the monitoring of fitness and activity levels across multiple devices could encourage a more personalized commitment to individual health and encourage a healthier lifestyle (Ofcom 2015b). However, there have been reports that the use of fitness bands may actually result in some users gaining weight, suggesting weight loss is more of an art than a science (Urist 2014). Lofton (cited Urist 2014) suggests 'calorie counting on a wristband doesn't give you a full picture of your lifestyle – even when you're tracking your number of steps or hours slept. Are you spreading calories throughout the day or eating a lot before bedtime? Are you much more active some days of the week but not others? Urist (2014) provides a concluding comment, suggesting the 'weight loss is still too complex for even the niftiest tracking device'.

Social media

Social media websites such as Facebook and Twitter have grown in popularity since their creation in 2004 and 2006 respectively. These sites have a fundamental role in promoting groups that meet to discuss and advise on health and wellbeing. There are a multitude of localized groups which meet to encourage weight-loss or the sharing of personal experience of certain health conditions. Whilst these groups do not fit neatly into the category of 'play', they encourage socialization among like-minded people and can be seen to represent a kind of virtual 'recreation ground' for the present age. Facebook has recently incorporated the facility to add 'how you're feeling' to your status update, using emoticons to show other people your current state of wellbeing. Facebook also provides users with the opportunity to play games with their friends, some of which are related to health and wellbeing. An example of this is Fitness City, created in 2011, which invites users to open their own 'fitness center' with the wellness of its members its ultimate goal. Suggestions as to how to meet members' needs include:

> Spinning classes, yoga, massages, swimming, weight lifting, beauty treatments, wine therapy sessions, paddle tennis, contrast baths, Pilates, self-defence training, Tai Chi… There's all you need to equip your fitness center and to expand it. Do pay attention to your members' requests: each of them has different lifestyles and needs.
>
> *(facebook 2015)*

Promoting fitness centers as the 'perfect place to take care of your body and mind and feel better', this game uses a social messaging platform to promote a health education message which reflects a generous interpretation of what constitutes healthy behavior.

Social media platforms such as Facebook and text messaging have been employed to promote physical activity among African American women who reported a physically inactive lifestyle (Joseph *et al*. 2015). Information material promoting physical activity, health topics for discussion, and engagement opportunities were posted weekly on the group Facebook wall, and backed-up by motivational text messaging and self-monitoring through a goal-setting program. Facebook users of this program showed positive results, including a decrease in sedentary behavior and an increase in light physical activity, suggesting that culturally-sensitive programs using social media platforms can contribute to behavior change programs (Joseph *et al*. 2015).

Twitter is a microblogging platform that allows short snippets of information to be posted using 140 characters or less. Srinivas (2015) has identified ten 'super-smart Twitter feeds to follow', stating that each 'approaches health in a novel way'.

For example, ZDoggMD has 11.8K followers and uses humor and medical satire to promote health-related messages. However, it has also been found that people who use tweets to express negative emotions and anger have a high rate of heart disease mortality, whilst positive tweets describing positive experiences and optimism have been shown to be protective factors against heart disease (Curtis 2015).

Kath Evans, the NHS England lead on patient experience for children and young children, is a prolific tweeter, and strongly advocates the use of social media for connecting people anywhere, at any time and on any topic. Using Twitter as a playful tool, the role of social media has an enormous potential for doing good by,

> bringing attention to issues that previously may have been ignored as well as supporting the development of networks and shared knowledge, bringing new ideas and fresh voices to complex issues. Since experience is a key marker of quality, it has a big role to play in the healthcare process.
>
> *(Evans 2015)*

Conclusion

The advancement of technology during the last decade has seen the rise of a multitude of innovative ideas which have been harnessed by gaming companies to support attempts to promote health and fitness in an era of sedentary activity. Play and playfulness have facilitated the realization of many of these ideas as a means of engaging the users of new products and apps, demonstrating that living a healthily lifestyle can also be fun. Play can also facilitate the personal acceptance of a medical diagnosis, transforming the mundane routine of daily monitoring into a game or challenge, as well as providing education and information. Exergames, apps and social media have all been created and used in an attempt to promote healthier lifestyles, which for a generation becoming increasingly busy and decreasingly active, may revolutionize the move towards more personalized and patient-centred healthcare services. Modern healthcare services face an ongoing challenge to keep pace with a growing cohort of techno-savvy service users and to take advantage of all that modern technology has to offer in the way of engagement, communication and the provision of patient-centered services.

References

Apple (2015) *Life on iPad: New eyes for hands-on surgery*, Online. Available at www.apple.com/ipad/life-on-ipad/new-eyes-for-hands-on-surgery/ (accessed 22 February 2016).

BBC WebWise (2014) *What Are Social Networking Sites?* Online. Available at www.bbc.co.uk/webwise/guides/about-social-networking (accessed 29 November 2015).

Buchanan, R. (2015a) *Perceptions of Technology: Science and Technology,* Online. Available at www.britannica.com/technology/history-of-technology/Perceptions-of-technology (accessed 29 November 2015).

Buchanan, R. (2015b) *History of Technology,* Online. Available at www.britannica.com/technology/history-of-technology (accessed 29 November 2015).

Brox, E., Luque, L., Eversten, G. and González Hernández, J. (n.d.) *Exergames For Elderly: Social Exergames to Persuade Seniors to Increase Physical activity,* Online. Available at www.helmholtz-muenchen.de/fileadmin/JOIN/PDF/PID1790829-Exergames.pdf (accessed 29 November 2015).

Campbell, D. (2011) Children growing weaker as computers replace outdoor activity, *The Observer,* 21 May 2011. Online. Available at www.theguardian.com/ (accessed 29 November 2015).

Cantwell, D., Broin, D., Palmer, R. and Doyle, G. (2014) *Motivating Elderly People to Exercise Using a Social Collaborative Exergame with Adaptive Difficulty.* Online. Available at www.helmholtz-muenchen.de/fileadmin/JOIN/PDF/Motivating_Elderly_People_To_Exercise_Using_a_Social_Collaborative_Exergame_with_Adaptive_Difficulty_Poster.pdf (accessed 29 November 2015).

Curtis, S. (2015) Angry tweeting 'could increase your risk of heart disease'. *Daily Telegraph,* 22 January 2015 Online. Available at www.telegraph.co.uk (accessed 29 November 2015).

Debong, F. (2014) *Diabetes — Time for a Change | Fredrik Debong | TEDxVienna,* Online. Available at www.youtube.com/watch?v=W61QWmvmzwQ (accessed 29 November 2015).

Encyclopaedia Britannica (2015) *World Wide Web WWW,* Online. Available at www.britannica.com/topic/World-Wide-Web (accessed 29 November 2015).

Evans, K. (2015) Connect – the power of social media, *Experience of Care Lead for NHS England, Kath Evans, Shares 10 Ways to Build Quality Care Experiences for and with Children, Young People and Their Families,* 30 November 2015 Online. Available at www.pickereurope.org (accessed 1 December 2015).

facebook (2015) *Fitness City App Page,* Online. Available at www.facebook.com/fitnesscityfan/info?tab=page_info (accessed 29 November 2015).

Fitbit (2015) *Fitbit: Find your Fit,* Online. Available at www.fitbit.com/uk/whyfitbit (accessed 29 November 2015).

Fluckinger, D. (2015) *How Health IT Drives Patient Engagement, Improvise Healthcare Workflow,* Online. Available at http://searchhealthit.techtarget.com/feature/How-health-IT-drives-patient-engagement-improves-healthcare-workflow (accessed 29 November 2015).

Garcia, J.A., Felix Navarro, K., Schoene, D., Smith S.T. and Pisan, Y. (2012) Exergames for the elderly: towards an embedded Kinect-based clinical test of falls risk, *Studies in Health Technologies and Informatics,* 178: 51–7.

Goldstein, J. (2013) *Technology and Play,* Online. Available at www.scholarpedia.org/article/Technology_and_Play (accessed 29 November 2015).

Graham, S. (2015) *National Doodle Day: Could Doodling be Good for Your Mental Health?* Online. Available at www.rscpp.co.uk/content/features/doodle-day-mental-health.html (accessed 1 December 2015).

Healthy Heart Meditation (2015) *Wild Divine Meditation Biofeedback Game,* Online. Available at www.healthy-heart-meditation.com/biofeedback-game.html (accessed 29 November 2015).

Johnson, S. (2015) mySugr and Colgate Total®. *mySugr blog,* 12 November 2015 Online. Available at www.mysugr.com (accessed 29 November 2015).

Joseph, R., Keller, C., Adams, M. and Ainsworth, B. (2015) Print versus a culturally-relevant Facebook and text message delivered intervention to promote physical activity in African American women: a randomized pilot trial, *BMC Women's Health*, 15: 30.

Kim, J. (2015) *Gamification in Healthcare Isn't Just about Playing Games,* Online. Available at http://searchhealthit.techtarget.com/opinion/Gamification-in-healthcare-isnt-just-about-playing-games (accessed 29 November 2015).

Lyons, E., Tate, D., Ward, D., Ribisl, K., Bowling, M. and Kalyanaraman, S. (2014) Engagement, enjoyment, and energy expenditure during active video game play, *Health Psychology*, 33 (2): 174–181.

#MatExp (2015) *About #MatExp,* Online. Available at http://matexp.org.uk/about-matexp/ (accessed 18 December 2015).

Microsoft (2015) *Xbox: The Future of Fitness,* Online. Available at www.xbox.com/en-GB/xbox-360/fitness (accessed 29 November 2015).

mySugr (2015) *Diabetes Logbook.* Online. Available at https://mysugr.com/logbook/ (accessed 29 November 2015).

Morais, B. (2015) The future of doodling, *The New Yorker*, 19 October 2015, Online. Available at www.newyorker.com (accessed 3 November 2015).

NHS Choices (2015) *Home Page,* Online. Available at www.nhs.uk/pages/home.aspx (accessed 29 November 2015).

Nintendo (2015) *Wii Fit,* Online. Available at www.nintendo.com/games/detail/hoiNtus4JvIcPtP8LQPyud4Kyy393oep (accessed 29 November 2015).

Nuvuin (2015a) *Gamification*, Online. Available at http://nuviun.com/digital-health/gamification (accessed 29 November 2015).

Nuvuin (2015b) *Lose Weight or Get Shamed by This Sadistic Talking App,* Online. Available at http://nuviun.com/content/lose-weight-or-get-shamed-by-this-sadistic-talking-app (accessed 29 November 2015).

Ofcom (2013) *Social Networking in the UK is Most Popular among Respondents Aged 25 to 34,* Online. Available at http://stakeholders.ofcom.org.uk/market-data-research/market-data/communications-market-reports/cmr13/international/icmr-5.27 (accessed 27 November 2015).

Ofcom (2015a) *Adults' Media Use and Attitudes: Report 2015,* Ofcom.

Ofcom (2015b) *Promoting Investment and Innovation in the Internet of Things Summary of Responses and Next Steps,* Ofcom.

Oxford English Dictionary (2015) *Technology*, Online. Available at www.oed.com (accessed 29 November 2015).

Prensky, M. (2001) Digital natives, digital immigrants part 1, *On the Horizon*, 9 (5): 1–6.

Srinivas, S. (2015) Ten super-smart health Twitter feeds to follow now, *The Guardian*, 19 February 2015, Online. Available at www.theguardian.com/ (accessed 29 November 2015).

Stross, R. (2012) 'Exergames' don't cure young couch potatoes, *The New York Times*, 23 June 2012 Online. Available at www.nytimes.com/ (accessed 29 November 2015).

Topol, E. (2013) How technology is transforming health care, *U.S. World and News Report*, 12 July 2013, Online. Available at http://health.usnews.com/ (accessed 29 November 2015).

Trent, J. (2015) 7 Best gamification fitness apps for 2015, *Nuvuin*, 1 January 2015, Online. Available at www.nuviun.com (accessed 29 November 2015).

Urist, J. (2014) My fitness band is making me fat: users complain of weight gain with trackers, *Today: Health and Wellness,* 16 July 2014, Online. Available at www.today.com (accessed 7 December 2015).

van Diest, M., Lamoth, C., Stegenga, J., Verkerke, G. and Postema, K. (2013) Exergaming for balance training of elderly: state of the art and future developments, *Journal of NeuroEngineering and Rehabilitation*, 10: 101.

Wüest, S., van de Langenberg, R. and de Bruin, E. (2014) Design considerations for a theory-driven exergame-based rehabilitation program to improve walking of persons with stroke, *European Review of Aging and Physical Activity*, 11 (2): 119–129.

16
ASPIRE LEISURE CENTRE

Inspiration through integration

Claire Weldon

This chapter explores the Aspire National Training Centre (ANTC) which was originally set up to offer rehabilitation facilities for people who had suffered spinal cord injuries. The ANTC is the first fully-accessible training center in Europe for disabled and non-disabled people and play-based activities and techniques are an integral part of the program offered to all members of the center. The chapter will also explore how innovative practice in this area is being shared from an international perspective.

Introduction

According to Unicef (2014) 'Play in all its forms is the right of every child' and the 'right to play' is protected by the United Nations Convention on the Rights of the Child article 31 (Unicef 2012). Play and sport allow children to develop social skills, express emotions, gain confidence, improve physical and mental skills and develop important life-skills. These skills continue developing throughout the individual's lifetime and the value of play and recreation does not diminish with increasing age. In fact, because adults continue to develop new neural networks that allow them to continue to learn throughout their lifespan, they also benefit from continuing to play (Goldstein 2012).

Play has always been an integral part of communal living and social cohesion since earliest times. In his *Definitive Guide to Play*, Sissons (cited in Mark's Daily Apple 2015) writes that, at the end of a day's 'work', our hunter-gatherer ancestors might 'wrestle, race, have throwing contests, or even just hang out and groom each other. This was pure, unadulterated leisure time, and plenty of it'. Play was about more than just having fun and also served to establish and maintain social ties, strengthening 'the collective power and safety of the tribe'. From ancient times to the present day, adults have engaged in structured group play – or sport – as a demonstration or test of physical strength and skill; as a route to social status and belonging; and as a source of shared fun and entertainment. Sport is 'well recognized internationally as a low-cost and high impact tool for development and a powerful agent for social change. It is a culturally accepted activity that brings people together and unites families, communities and nations' (Sport Matters 2015). Participation levels appear to be good among the general public as noted in a report by the Department for Culture, Media and Sport (2011) which found that 53 per cent of the adult population played some form of sport whilst 68 per cent walked and 10 per cent cycled, for health and recreation. The main reasons for participating in sporting activity were identified as health benefits, socializing and fun (Department for Culture, Media and Sport 2011).

The history of disability sport

Disability sport has evolved over time with the first organized event being held in 1911 (Disability Sport 2014), culminating in the biggest celebration of disability sporting excellence at the 2012 London Paralympic Games which further revolutionized disability sport in the United Kingdom (UK). The London Games led to disability sport events being broadcast alongside mainstream events, giving disabled athletes the recognition that they have long deserved. Winning the rights to broadcast the Games was fiercely contested, eventually being won by Channel 4, who provided extensive coverage that 'took over Channel 4 for the duration' of the Games (British Library n.d.).

The first organized disability sporting event was the International Silent Games, now known as the Deaflympics, held in Paris in 1924 (International Committee of Sports for the Deaf 2015). It has been held every year since its inception (with the exception of wartime) and is thus the longest running disability sporting event. The *Cripples Olympiad* was organized in the United States in 1911 but it was not until the end of the Second World War that organized disability sport really became established, when Ludwig Guttmann used sport as a method of rehabilitation for injured and wounded war veterans at Stoke Mandeville Hospital. Silver (cited Mandeville Legacy 2014) described how

> [Guttmann] … knew that sport can make an amazing difference to the life of a person with a spinal cord injury. It aids rehabilitation. It decreases the need for long-term healthcare and medical treatment because of the healthy lifestyle. It restores independence enabling people to undertake everyday tasks more easily including dressing, transferring in and out of their wheelchairs to the car, bath and bed. Finally, it motivates disabled people by giving them new goals and increases confidence and self-belief.

In 1948 Guttmann organized the Stoke Mandeville Games for the veterans at the hospital and the success of these games meant that they soon developed into an international competition, evolving into what we now know as the Paralympic

Games. In the United States in the early 1960s, Eunice Kennedy Shriver held a day camp for children and adults with special needs. This camp aimed to provide an opportunity for individuals with learning and developmental disabilities to participate in play and recreation (Special Olympics 2012). The Special Olympics movement grew out of this first camp and in 1968 the first Special Olympics World Games was held.

The Paralympic Summer Games were first held in Rome in 1960, with the first Winter Games taking place in Sweden in 1976. These have been held every four years since, usually starting shortly after the Olympic or Winter Olympic Games. The first Paralympic Summer Games had 400 competitors from 23 countries; the number of competitors has increased over the years to more than 4,000 in 2012, with an increased number of sports and disabilities now represented. Disabled athletes have also competed in the mainstream Olympic Games, the first in 1904. Whilst this is not a common occurrence, it highlights the potential for greater inclusiveness in the Games.

In 2014, the first Invictus Games were held in London. Their aim was to 'use the power of sport to inspire recovery, support rehabilitation and generate a wider understanding and respect for those who serve, or have served, their country' (Help for Heroes n.d.). Four hundred competitors from 13 nations took part in events such as swimming, wheelchair rugby and basketball, as well as rowing, cycling and athletics.

Where are we today?

Approximately 19 per cent of the UK population are disabled. Seventeen per cent of these were born with a disability but most disabled people become disabled during their lifetime. The Papworth Trust (2013) state that 'the prevalence of disability rises with age. In 2011/12, 6 per cent of children were disabled (0.8 million), compared to around 16 per cent of adults of working age (5.8 million) and 45 per cent of adults over the state pension age (5.3 million) are also disabled'. With an aging population, and in the light of what we know about the link between aging and disability, it is likely that the majority of the population will experience some form of disability during their lifetime. Healthcare providers, and society at large, need to consider the personal, social and economic impact that this increase in numbers may have and the adjustments needed, in relation to both attitudes and services, to accommodate this changing picture.

Attitudes about integration

Attitudes towards disability have changed over time, as demonstrated by the evolution of accepted models for understanding disability. The most commonly referred to models of disability are the 'medical model' and the 'social model'. The medical model is the oldest model of disability and focuses on the individual's medical condition, using this to determine what they can and cannot do at any point in time; whether this is likely to change; and what help is needed. Under the medical model, the responsibility rests with the individual to adapt-to and to fit-in with society. In contrast, the social model emphasizes the responsibility of society to remove the barriers that prevent a disabled person's access to facilities and services. The shift towards a social model of disability is reflected in a parallel shift in the language used to refer to disabled members of society. In the UK, the term 'disabled people' is generally used in preference to 'people with disabilities'. It is argued under the social model that, whilst an individual's impairment is an individual problem, the concept of 'disability' is created by societal factors, such as a lack of wheelchair access to public transport or to public and private facilities (Glasgow Centre for Inclusive Living n.d.). The social model of disability was evident during the 2012 Paralympic Games with the widespread recognition and celebration of what disabled individuals are capable of. However, it is not only the physical barriers to participation that need to be challenged; unless there is a parallel change in attitudes towards disabled people, there will remain social barriers to full acceptance and integration of disabled athletes in the sporting world and elsewhere.

Aspire Leisure Centre is one of the few fully-accessible leisure centers world-wide. Aspire shares its knowledge and expertise internationally to help other centers increase access to their facilities and to show that there are sound business opportunities for doing this. However, there is a dearth of fully-accessible sports and leisure centers worldwide which means that many disabled individuals do not have full access to exercise facilities. This inhibits participation in sport and recreation and denies disabled users the holistic benefits that physical activity has to offer. There are two exceptions, Inspire and the Steadward Centre:

Inspire is a Maltese charity that believes 'everyone has a right to equality and inclusion' and their mission is 'to try to help everyone with a disability achieve this' (Inspire 2013b). The Inspire Leisure Centre is 'the only fully-accessible fitness facility in Malta' and part of the organization is dedicated to the provision of a wide variety of therapeutic and educational services to the Maltese community (Inspire 2013a).

Similarly, the Steadward Centre for Personal and Physical Achievement in Alberta, Canada aims to 'create, disseminate and apply knowledge of physical activity, athletic development and motor skill development specific to persons experiencing disability' (University of Alberta 2015).

Aspire and the Aspire Leisure Centre

Aspire Leisure Centre is 'the first leisure centre in Europe for disabled and non-disabled people' (Association for Spinal Injury Research, Rehabilitation and Reintegration 2015), providing fully-accessible sport and leisure facilities for people of all ages and abilities. The center includes a swimming pool, dance studio, fitness studio, sports hall and café and also runs a range of exercise classes. It is attached to the London Spinal Cord Injury Centre at the Royal National

Orthopaedic Hospital (RNOH) but is operated independently of it. Aspire and the Aspire Leisure Centre show how, with positive attitudes, full access to sporting and recreational pursuits is achievable and, furthermore, that integrated facilities can benefit both disabled and non-disabled members of the community.

The concept underlying this initiative followed discussion which identified a lack of adequate rehabilitation facilities available to patients at the London Spinal Unit. This lack was seen to compromise the care provided to this specific patient group and Aspire was established in 1982, since when it has developed as a fully integrated facility.

Architect Andrew Walker was appointed to design the building. As a result of having a spinal injury himself, Walker had a unique insight into the requirements of disabled people and his design has enabled a broad range of people to use the facilities. The concept of integration lay at the heart of what Walker and Aspire wanted to achieve: Aspire was to be a place where disabled and non-disabled people could come together to exercise, to work or to socialize. Integration was to be the *norm* and the focus rested firmly on a *can do* attitude. At the time of its inception, legislation requiring buildings to be fully accessible had yet to be implemented, making the inclusive design of the Aspire building even more innovative. Due to the nature of the organization, Aspire attracted disabled workers who helped to develop the organization further, changing both attitudes and service delivery. Aspire employs fitness instructors, reception staff and maintenance staff who are themselves disabled, further extending the original concept of an integrated sports facility.

Aspire operates as a registered charity providing support for people who have been paralysed by spinal cord injury. It offers a broad range of services including: Aspire Grants, Aspire Housing, Aspire Independent Living Advisors, Aspire Assistive Technology, a Welfare Benefits Advice Service and Aspire Campaigns. These services enable those with spinal cord injury to improve their quality of life and provide the support to enable them to do this.

In order to fund these valuable services, Aspire organizes a range of fund-raising events, many of which have a sporting theme. These events include: swimming, in the comfort of the local swimming pool as well as in open water (the Aspire Channel Swim), multi-sport events, cycling and running. These events are open to all who are able to take part, regardless of ability.

The Aspire Leisure Centre is an inclusive environment designed to enable individuals both to access the center and to participate in physical activity. The removal of barriers, both physical and attitudinal, enables users to actively engage in the activities of their choice. All those using the center know that they will be able to achieve full access to the facilities on offer: the integration of non-disabled and disabled users is considered so commonplace that an individual's ability or disability does not stand-out as their defining feature. The ethos of Aspire is one of support and encouragement, with service-users supporting each other on personal, social, emotional and physical levels. Social relationships are developed and support networks established, leading to an increase in the use of the facilities and a consequent increase in participation in physical activity.

How does Aspire promote health and wellbeing?

The sport and play-based techniques used at the Aspire Leisure Centre contribute to the six aspects of health (Tonkin and Etchells 2014). The six aspects of health (physical, social, mental, emotional, spiritual and societal) show how different areas of health and wellbeing develop and evolve throughout the course of the lifespan.

Physical health is developed through participation in physical exercise whereby the individual develops muscle tone, endurance or improved core stability. Social relationships are also created at the Aspire Leisure Centre: the center is unique in that the friendly and inclusive atmosphere fosters an environment where new friendships are formed and developed. There is a freedom to interact with other disabled and non-disabled people, which is often absent in wider society. This inclusive environment contributes to a greater willingness to exercise and to engage with others, with consequent positive effects for both physical and social health.

The atmosphere of acceptance and inclusivity at the Aspire Leisure Centre also helps users to nurture their emotional health and mental wellness. Spending time with others who have a similar disability, or who face similar difficulties and challenges, can help an individual to learn new ways of managing their own thoughts and feelings and, in turn, to maintain a positive state. Practices such as yoga and 'water walking' (based on the principles of Tai Chi) address the individual's spiritual health needs and can serve to sustain the quest for emotional and spiritual equilibrium.

Societal perceptions of disabled people are widely variable, as are the experiences of disabled members of society. Disabled individuals frequently have to deal with negative attitudes and to overcome social barriers to inclusion and acceptance. The inclusive nature of the Aspire Leisure Centre allows service-users to spend time in a non-judgmental environment where commonly encountered barriers have been removed or reduced and where they can aspire to reaching their full potential. One member of the Aspire Leisure Centre, who sustained a spinal cord injury, said: 'Being at Aspire helps to bring back normality. You can wheel in and feel normal. It is a place where it is more normal to be disabled than able bodied'.

The majority of environmental factors that affect health are linked to the location in which the individual spends most of their time. The Aspire Leisure Centre provides a positive environment for people on a regular basis. Some center users visit once a week, or less frequently, whilst others visit on a daily basis. For those who visit the center regularly, the environment has wide-reaching health benefits.

The swimming pool

Aspire's swimming pool is 25 m in length with ramped access. The center has several water-based wheelchairs so that wheelchair users can transfer themselves and push straight into the pool; this benefits many other center users, including those with limited mobility. The temperature of the swimming pool is maintained at 31°C to help reduce muscle spasms and to allow non-swimmers to exercise without getting too cold. A range of aqua classes are available. These include aqua-aerobics as well as aqua-therapy and 'dip' sessions for those who are nervous about swimming in a general session. Swimmers can also use the pool to do rehabilitation exercises. One-to-one swimming lessons are available to all adults, and physiotherapists at the RNOH use the pool with in-patients as part of their rehabilitation programs.

The fitness studio

The fitness studio has a range of equipment suitable for both disabled and non-disabled users. Much of the equipment is suitable for wheelchair users and the fitness instructors devise individualized programs according to specific need. A range of specialized services are offered including: a GP referral program; cardiac rehabilitation; a 'senior fitness' session; and 'assisted exercise' whereby a qualified instructor will assist disabled users during their training session. All fitness instructors are trained to help disabled users maximize their fitness potential and many of them also have training in working with older adults.

The dance studio

The dance studio at Aspire Leisure Centre is used for a variety of exercise classes, such as Pilates, yoga and aerobics, as well as by the CandoCo dance company. CandoCo was founded in 1991 and is a company of disabled and non-disabled dancers who tour in the UK and internationally. CandoCo was developed after a series of workshops for those with spinal injuries held at Aspire Leisure Centre.

The sports hall

A range of activities take place in the sports hall and these include activities for individuals who are disabled as well as for older adults. 'Over fifties' badminton sessions are run twice a week and the London Titans wheelchair basketball team and the London Wheelchair Rugby Club both train at Aspire Leisure Centre and are open to new members.

Exercise classes

Group exercise classes take place daily. All classes are accessible but some classes are aimed at specific levels or at those who are disabled. Accessible classes, such as Krank cycling, have adapted bikes for wheelchair users. Classes such as aerobics and yoga are all accessible and specialist classes for disabled users are also offered, including chair-based exercise and water walking.

InstructAbility

The aim of InstructAbility is to 'support disabled people into a fitness career where they can encourage other disabled people to access leisure facilities and enjoy an active lifestyle'. (Association for Spinal Injury Research, Rehabilitation and Reintegration 2015). InstructAbility is run in conjunction with the YMCA and offers a recognized qualification which can lead to employment or further training. Admission criteria for a place on the InstructAbility course include: having a disability; experience of using a gym; and being able to work to a level 2 academic standard.

Parasport

The Aspire Leisure Centre has the facilities to offer a range of parasports at all levels, including to elite athletes. Wheelchair rugby and wheelchair basketball are currently played at the center which has also hosted wheelchair football. Tennis, table tennis and bowls can all be played and the center has the facilities to offer archery and canoeing. The gym facilities allow para-athletes to train for events such as marathons and rowing.

Rehabilitation and sport

The RNOH use the facilities at the Aspire Leisure Centre for some of their rehabilitation programs. The RNOH has a Spinal Cord Injury Centre and also runs pain management and rehabilitation programs including the 'Active Back' and the 'Complex Regional Pain Syndrome' programs. Patients can participate in a range of sporting activities as part of their rehabilitation, including swimming, bowls, tennis, archery and table tennis, as well as using the gym. The National Institute of Clinical Excellence (NICE) state that professionals should 'advise people with low back pain that staying physically active is likely to be beneficial' and that 'exercise programs may include the following elements: aerobic activity, movement instruction, muscle strengthening, postural control, stretching' (NICE 2009). Participation in a range of sporting activities during a rehabilitation program enables patients to try activities under supervision and thus discover what is achievable. This may encourage them to continue exercising after their rehabilitation has finished, with the hope of also improving their pain levels.

The remainder of the chapter focuses on two case studies – Joe and Graham.

Joe

Joe sustained a spinal cord injury at the age of 19. He was working on a roof when he slipped and fell 45 feet, injuring his spinal cord. He was taken to his local hospital for emergency treatment and later transferred to a Spinal Injury Centre 100 miles from his own home. Joe sustained his injury in the 1970s when treatment for spinal cord injuries was very different from today and he spent 13 weeks just lying in bed. After this period, he did receive some physical rehabilitation but this was ward-based, rather than personalized, with all patients on the ward doing similar exercises. Six months after his injury, Joe was discharged from hospital and returned to live in the family home, which was only partially accessible, and he strove to become as independent as possible. A further six months after discharge from hospital, Joe secured a job at Remploy, an organization providing jobs for disabled people. During his time at Remploy, Joe developed friendships and started attending a Physically Handicapped and Able Bodied (PHAB) club.

Prior to his injury, Joe had been a 'sporty person', playing football at weekends and training during the week; following his injury, Joe looked for opportunities to become active once again. Joe started to play table tennis in a league with able-bodied people and each year he attended the Stoke Mandeville Games where he could participate in snooker, table tennis and basketball. Joe's interest in disability sport developed further when, in 1973, he watched an international basketball game at Stoke Mandeville Hospital. Joe found basketball to be an exciting sport and so joined a local club – 'local' in this case meaning 50 miles from his home. Club involvement provided the opportunity to play the sport at a higher level, in a league with other disabled people. During the summer months, teams met fortnightly to play against each other, although training between these events was not possible as most sports centers remained inaccessible. Despite the lack of local facilities, Joe succeeded in playing basketball for Great Britain between 1984 and 1988.

Joe continues to develop his sporting ability. He regularly goes out for long 'pushes' in his local area and coaches wheelchair basketball.

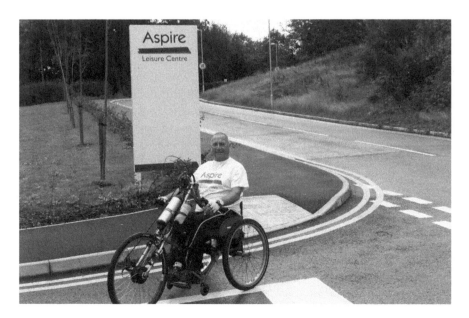

FIGURE 16.1 Joe setting out on a 'long push'

Joe's sporting achievements were ultimately recognized with his nomination to carry the Olympic torch during the torch relay in 2012.

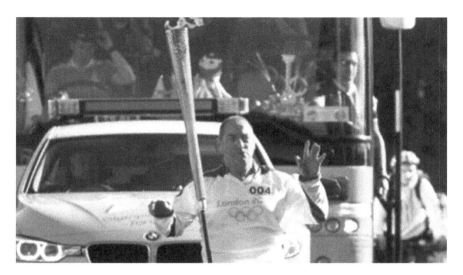

FIGURE 16.2 Joe carrying the Olympic torch during the Torch Relay prior to the London Olympics

Joe's interest in sport following his injury, both motivated and supported his drive for independence with consequent benefits for all aspects of his health and wellbeing.

Sport enabled Joe to improve and maintain his physical fitness. When he left hospital he was underweight but was able to develop muscle tone and strength through exercise. Sport has allowed Joe to meet new people and to develop long-term friendships, some of which endure to this day. People with spinal cord injuries, from around the country, meet together at sporting events where sport is only one of many opportunities for socializing. Joe has learnt a range of new skills through sport. After deciding to pursue basketball at a competitive level, he taught himself the necessary skills by reading books and then going to the local sports centre to practice them. Depression and anxiety were common amongst Joe's fellow patients on the wards of the spinal unit, although these conditions were not fully diagnosed. Sport offered Joe a break from the daily routine of hospital life. The routine of bladder and bowel management and the effort involved in getting dressed and making meals can be difficult to manage; sport provides an escape from the monotony of routine with a positive impact on emotional health. Through sport, Joe was able to develop new interests and friendships. He was able to grow into a new 'Joe' and to create a life for himself after spinal injury. He is now able to talk about the events that happened to him and about his experience in hospital in a manner that is suggestive of robust spiritual health. A big change in Joe's life

196 Claire Weldon

came with meeting and marrying his wife post-injury. When Joe sustained his injury, it was unusual for the public at large to encounter a disabled person in the course of day-to-day life. Once Joe became more involved in sport he found that people accepted his disability and helped him when he needed it. The staff at Joe's local sports center helped him to participate in activities, even though there were no accessible facilities. This demonstrates that, over the past few years, society has become more accepting of disabled people and this has also meant that Joe has been able to engage with a greater range of opportunities.

Graham

Graham was born with a disability and has used a wheelchair since three years of age. He attended a primary school for children with special needs where he participated in wheelchair skills lessons and this led to a developing interest in sport. At 8 years of age, Graham first tried wheelchair racing. He started attending his local wheelchair racing club, the closest being over an hour's journey from his home, where he raced for seven years between the ages of 8 and 15 years old.

Graham started attending a mainstream secondary school at 12 years of age. He was not allowed to participate in physical education lessons in case he injured another pupil but, when he reached 14, the school arranged for him to attend the local gym during physical education lessons. This further developed his interest in sport and started him on his chosen career path. In 1995 Graham started a National Vocational Qualification (NVQ) in sport and recreation, spending one day a week at college and four days a week at the Aspire Leisure Centre. Once qualified, he was employed by Aspire Leisure Centre as a fitness instructor. Graham has tried a variety of sports including table tennis, archery, basketball, badminton, swimming and circuit training and has completed the London Marathon twice. In 2000 he completed the Marathon in a racing chair in just under 3 hours and in 2012, using his day chair, he completed the course in 5 hours and 7 minutes.

Being a fitness instructor means that Graham is in the gym daily and this helps to keep him fit and motivated which, in turn, helps him to motivate others. Graham believes that being a disabled fitness instructor has helped other disabled people to see what is possible. Working at the Aspire Leisure Centre has led to Graham developing many social relationships. Its close proximity to the London Spinal Cord Injury Centre allows him to talk to the patients in the wards when they are at their most vulnerable and to show them what can be achieved post-injury. Graham's friendly and caring nature also facilitates a valuable rapport with his clients during one-to-one sessions. Training as a fitness instructor has helped Graham to develop his intellectual skills and he has gained several professional qualifications. He is required to undertake annual continuing professional development through which he can acquire new skills and complete further educational qualifications. Evidence suggests that being active helps to maintain positive mental health and to protect against the likelihood of depression and anxiety. Graham has found his ideal job and says that he is where he wants to be in life. Working at

Inspiration through integration 197

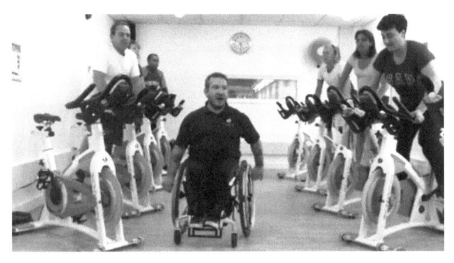

FIGURE 16.3 Graham instructing a Spin class

Aspire Leisure Centre has been a positive experience for Graham but he does not think he would do the same job in a 'regular' gym due to previous negative experiences. For the most part, Graham has found his experience of working in the fitness industry to be a positive one and he feels totally accepted by the Aspire Leisure Centre community.

Conclusion

Integrated sport is a healthy way for all adults to play together. The Aspire Leisure Centre provides inspirational proof that disability need not be socially divisive nor be a barrier to participation in playful pursuits. When disabled and non-disabled people play together then it can be mutually beneficial for the development of all aspects of health.

Acknowledgments

Many thanks to Laura, Brian, Hannah, David, Joe, Graham and Alex for all their help in the compilation of information for this chapter. All your help and support has been very much appreciated.

References

Association for Spinal Injury Research, Rehabilitation and Reintegration (2015) *What We Do*, Online. Available at www.instructability.org.uk/what-we-do? (accessed 25 July 2015).
British Library (n.d.) *The Media and the Paralympics*, Online. Available at www.bl.uk/sportandsociety/exploresocsci/sportsoc/media/articles/paramedia.html (accessed 16 December).

Department for Culture, Media and Sport (2011) *Adult Participation in Sport*, Online. Available at www.gov.uk/government/uploads/system/uploads/attachment_data/file/137986/tp-adult-participation-sport-analysis.pdf (accessed 3 December 2015).

Disability Sport (2014) *A Brief History of Disability Sports*, Online. Available at www.disabilitysport.org.uk/a-brief-history-of-disability-sports.html (accessed 16 December 2015).

Glasgow Centre for Inclusive Living (n.d.) *GCIL Support*, Online. Available at www.gcil.org.uk/ (accessed 28 November 2015).

Goldstein, J. (2012) *Play in Children's Development, Health and Well-being*, Brussels: Toy Industries of Europe.

Help for Heroes (n.d.) *The Invictus Games*, Online. Available at www.helpforheroes.org.uk/sports-recovery/major-events-archive/invictus-games/ (accessed 25 July 2015).

International Committee of Sports for the Deaf (2015) *History*, Online. Available at http://deaflympics.com/icsd.asp?history (accessed 16 December 2015).

Inspire (2013a) *Inspire Fitness Centre*, Online. Available at http://inspire.org.mt/fun-facilities/fitness-centre/ (accessed 16 December 2015).

Inspire (2013b) *What We Do*, Online. Available at http://inspire.org.mt/what-we-do/ (accessed 24 July 2015).

Mandeville Legacy (2014) *Sport as Rehabilitation: New Approaches to Physiotherapy*, Online. Available at www.mandevillelegacy.org.uk/page_id__22_path__0p4p13p.aspx (accessed 16 December 2015).

Mark's Daily Apple (2015) *The Definitive Guide to Play*, Online. Available at www.marksdailyapple.com/the-definitive-guide-to-play/ (accessed 3 December 2015).

The National Institute for Clinical Excellence (NICE) (2009) *Low Back Pain: Early Management of Persistent Non-specific Low Back Pain*, Online. Available at www.nice.org.uk/guidance/cg88/chapter/1-Guidance (accessed 14 October 2015).

Papworth Trust (2013) *Disability in the United Kingdom 2013 Facts and Figures*, Papworth Trust.

Special Olympics (2012) *Eunice Kennedy Shriver: One Woman's Vision*, Online. Available at www.eunicekennedyshriver.org/ (accessed 16 December 2015).

Sport Matters (2015) *Why sport?* Online. Available at www.sportmatters.org.au/why_sport.php (accessed 24 July 2015).

Tonkin, A. and Etchells, J. (2014) Promoting health and wellbeing, In: Tonkin, A. (ed.) *Play in Healthcare: Using Play to Promote Child Development and Wellbeing*, Abingdon: Routledge: 110–125.

Unicef (2014) *Why Sport?* Online. Available at www.unicef.org/sports/index_23624.html (accessed 24 July 2015).

Unicef (2012) A summary of the UN Convention on the Rights of the Child, Online. Available at www.unicef.org.uk/Documents/Publication-dfs/betterlifeleaflet2012_press.pdf (accessed 16 December 2015).

University of Alberta (2015) *The Steadward Centre* for Personal & Physical Achievement, Online. Available at www.steadwardcentre.ualberta.ca/en/AboutUs.aspx (accessed 16 December 2015).

17

THE FACILITATION OF PLAY AND PLAYFULNESS THROUGH ALTERNATIVE HEALTHCARE PROVISION

Julie Dakin and Alison Tonkin

This chapter looks at the role of complementary and alternative healthcare and their contribution to a holistic approach to health and wellbeing that lies beyond the realms of a westernized approach to mainstream healthcare. The therapeutic use of acupuncture provides the main focus for the chapter, which brings together ancient and modern approaches to medicine.

Introduction

Play makes us feel better and acts as an energizing life force. Complementary and alternative medicines are concerned with healing the body, mind, soul and spirit and acknowledge that the life force (known as Qi in the East) is vital to all of us. If we suffer from pain, be it mental or physical, it tends to erase the 'joie de vivre' from life. When we are in pain we are neither able, nor want, to engage with others and are disinclined to undertake pleasurable pursuits such as spending time outside in nature or playing with children or grandchildren and, as a result of this diminished engagement, our health can deteriorate still further.

Complementary and alternative medicines (CAM) have evolved over thousands of years (Barnett and Shale 2012) emanating from a range of differing cultures and traditions to provide an alternative means of addressing illness, either in isolation or alongside conventional medicine (Royal College of Psychiatrists 2015). In contrast to the medicalized approach to healthcare adopted by Western societies, wherein disease is treated as a separate entity to health (Tseui 1978), CAM are thought to be more 'humanistic' in nature, focusing on holistic or 'integrative care' that is linked to addressing individualized wellbeing needs (Franzel *et al.* 2013). Playfulness is considered to be an essential component of wellbeing (Proyer and Ruch 2011) and it may be that a complementary approach to healthcare provision can enhance the patient experience so as to facilitate playfulness and all its associated benefits.

Both Eastern and Western approaches to medicine originated as holistic means of promoting healing through the use of natural remedies, such as plants and herbs (Mantri 2008). The divergence of medical traditions is associated with Vesalius' dissection of the human body in 1539, enabling human anatomy to be revealed, and consequently studied in detail, for the first time. From this point forward, the traditional unity of mind and body rapidly dissipated and the scientific, empirical foundations of modern medicine emerged (Mantri 2008). These differences are summarized in Table 17.1.

TABLE 17.1 Simplistic overview of differences between traditional medical and CAM approaches to treatment and the promotion of health and wellbeing

TCM approach	Western approach
Mind and body are seen as one	Mind and body are seen as separate entities
Holism and individualized	Focus on the disease or illness
Subjective – rely on patient narrative and observation	Objective – rely on test results
The human body is seen as a miniature version of the universe	The body is seen as a 'machine' that needs to be finely tuned for optimum performance
Health is supported by a harmonious relationship between *yin* and *yang* and diseases result from an imbalance between the two opposing forces	Biomedical view of health has led to value judgements that mean the treatment for physical illness is unchallenged whereas emotional consequences often go unnoticed
Functioning of the body is explained by five elements – fire, earth, wood, metal, and water	Functioning of the body is linked to mechanized physiology whereby medicine is grounded in scientific explanation
Qi is a vital energy flowing through the body and is crucial for the maintenance of health	Energy fields are not considered significant and do not contributed to clinical diagnosis or treatment

With the dissociation of the mind from the physical body, acknowledgement of how emotions contributed to overall wellbeing was marginalized in Western medicine and this affected how patients were (and still are) perceived and treated (Finston 2015). 'Real illnesses' such as those that result from physical injury or disease are tangible and regarded as suitable for treatment, whereas issues related to mental illness which cannot be observed are often considered to be 'less real and more the result of character flaws' (Finston 2015). Nature does not recognize such a 'split' and in Eastern medicine individuals are perceived as being responsible for managing their emotions as much as for the health of their physical body. This is of particular significance when considering stress-related illness, which may not initially manifest itself in physical changes but may result in the body ceasing to function as efficiently and effectively as it might (Finston 2015).

Play can be considered as an alternative or complement to traditional therapies and can help to counter the effects of modern lifestyle trends. For example, Sultanoff (2002) promotes the use of *breath play* as a means of countering excessive workloads and 'over-stressing', which can lead to dysfunction which is reflected in our patterns of behavior. Sultanoff (2002: 213) suggests that the term *breath play* 'invites safe participation [which] conveys welcome and acceptance, for both adult and (inner) child, making room for whatever comes forth, through playful, open exploration'. Breath play 'combines elements of imagination and visualization, sensing and feeling, focusing, affirmation and physical alignment' in order to capture the natural rhythm of the breath, which can then be utilized as a natural healer (Sultanoff 2002: 215). Singing and chanting are also considered to be spontaneous forms of breath play, offering an inclusive practice that is the 'sacred fabric of community'. Sultanoff (2002: 223) summarizes his work on breath play by suggesting we should: 'Sing for your health and wellbeing, for your upliftment, for the joy of creation … most importantly, sing for no reason at all'.

Traditional Chinese Medicine (TCM) acknowledges the role of play in healing, with playfulness being one of the characteristics of the Fire Element, which is associated with joy and laughter (Schiesser 2015). In Traditional Chinese Medicine, the heart is said to belong to the Fire Element and it is also associated with joy and considered to be the 'ruler of all other organs' (Suttie n.d.). Living a joyful and fulfilling life, that has meaningful relationships at its core, is seen to contribute to a healthy heart, and play is a contributory factor in this process. The notion of realignment, of refocusing of the body's own capacity to heal naturally, is of particular relevance to a non-westernized approach to health and wellbeing and is a common theme which runs throughout the differing approaches featured in this chapter.

Underlining concepts of complementary and alternative medicines

The Chinese believe that everything in the universe, including the body and mind, is a delicate balance of Yin and Yang. Yin is described as nourishing, dark, cool, night, substance, interior, whereas Yang is the polar opposite – energy, light, heat, day, function and exterior. Everything is on the spectrum between the two poles and everything is perceived as mutually creating and transforming: for example, day moves gradually into night and back again. The concept of Yin and Yang helps to explain how the polar opposite moods of depression and playfulness transform from one to the other as health is restored.

The concept of Qi is absent from Western medicine. Qi is defined as the body's life force and flows through everything that is alive; when Qi stops flowing, life ends (Tse 2014). The Chinese believe that we are born with a certain amount of Qi, which we must nurture and replenish for a long, happy and healthy life. The amount of Qi within each person depends on the health (mental and physical) of the parents and on the condition of the universe at the time of conception –

whether there were storms or other natural catastrophes occurring or whether it had been a beautiful day with the birds singing. The quality of food and drink consumed, the work/life balance achieved, and the state of the emotions all have a direct effect on Qi and can generate good health or illness, happiness and playfulness or withdrawal and depression.

Chronic pain is one of the most debilitating, long-term health conditions and has a detrimental effect on both physical health and emotional wellbeing. In an article by van Hecke *et al.* (2013) it was noted that chronic pain occurs in 20 per cent of the population of Europe, affects more women than men, and is more common in older people. The incidence of chronic pain is also detrimental to society as a whole, and it is estimated that, in financial terms, it costs the economy more than €200 billion per year in Europe and $150 billion in the USA. Van Hecke *et al.* (2013) further note that 'management [of chronic pain] in the community remains generally unsatisfactory, partly because of a lack of evidence for effective interventions'. Patients who suffer from chronic pain have been shown to have altered brain activation although it is suggested that, in the early stages of chronic pain, these brain changes may be reversible after effective treatment (van Hecke *et al.* 2013). This suggestion alone should galvanize the medical profession to seek evidence of effective remedial options, including from the field of complementary and alternative therapies, whose efficacy is often undervalued due to a lack of 'clinical evidence'.

The effective management of chronic pain is particularly important when the pain is associated with advanced cancer of which it can be the major symptom in up to 70 per cent of cases and which seriously affects quality of life (Ling 2013). Integrating TCM with treatment modalities such as chemotherapy and radiotherapy has been shown to alleviate some of the symptoms generated by these treatment regimes. For example, acupuncture can alleviate symptoms of nausea and TCM is effective in relieving cancer-related fatigue (Ling 2013). Emotional care is an essential treatment consideration for patients with advanced cancer and 'transference of attention' is advocated as a means of diverting concentration away from the disease, in an effort to achieve a more tranquil mental state. In the consideration of emotional care, the 'seven emotions of TCM', which include 'joy, anger, worry, anxiety, sadness, fear and fright' can be applied through activities such as reading, playing chess or a musical instrument, as well as fishing and painting – all of which have playful elements that can achieve transference of attention, leading to improved therapeutic outcomes (Ling 2013).

In most instances, complementary therapies aim to return the patient to health and to allow for re-engagement with normal activities, be it work, rest or play. This can be exemplified in the following reference to acupuncture:

> maintaining and promoting mobility and comfort are the key to a happy life. Acupuncture and physical rehabilitation therapy can be instrumental in this regard and benefit a [patient] in ways that are not always achievable with traditional … medicine alone.
>
> *(Frank, cited Cornell University Veterinary Specialists 2015)*

Following completion of the treatment interventions, the patient sample were shown to be more energetic, became more playful and appeared to be happier following the use of acupuncture (Cornell University Veterinary Specialists 2015). This was also noted by Alnorthumbria Veterinary Group (2015) whose patients 'can respond with a noticeably improved sense of well-being after treatment – they are brighter, more playful and alert'.

Although these examples relate to animals, and the initial sessions may require the use of 'treats, warm laps and comfort-inducing acupuncture points', the animals appear to have fun and show signs of relaxation, recognizing acupuncture as a positive experience that they eagerly return to (Cornell University Veterinary Specialists 2015). The fact that animals show these benefits seems to challenge the idea of a placebo effect for acupuncture. Animals and people are known to respond to, and benefit from, acupuncture in a similar manner (Alnorthumbria Veterinary Group 2015). Therefore, it is suggested that humans also benefit from the facilitating role of acupuncture, particularly in the management of chronic pain (Cornell University Veterinary Specialists 2015), enabling them to return to a playful disposition which is so often compromised when living with such pain.

Everything needs to be in balance for health to blossom and TCM holds that we need to eat healthily, with the occasional treat, and to have enough free time to do the things that make us happy in order to balance the stresses of twenty-first century living. Play and playfulness are essential activities for re-balancing health and the following exploration of different therapeutic approaches provides an overview of how CAM can provide alternative means of restoration, enabling an 'abundance of Qi' to flow smoothly through the body and to optimize health and wellbeing (Tse 2014).

The essential role of relationships

Relationships between CAM practitioners and their patients are considered a first priority and complementary therapists typically spend more time in consultations (Franzel *et al.* 2013) than their often overstretched medical counterparts. CAM practitioners are interested in finding the root of a referred problem, for example whether a patient suffering from insomnia has a long-buried worry about a past life-event or experience. Palmer (2015) suggests that a consultation with a TCM doctor in China finds its parallel in a visit to a CAM practitioner in the West whereby:

> You spend half an hour or longer talking with a nice, kind, probably quite wise person about your health, your lifestyle, the stresses you're under, and they give you some sensible advice about diet, looking after yourself, and perhaps a dose of spiritual guidance on top.

The efficacy of TCM is strongly associated with the *jingyan* (the experience of the practitioner) which is seen as 'individualized and localized … passed down from

204 Julie Dakin and Alison Tonkin

master to favoured apprentice' (Palmer 2015) and the ability to pick up on the cues essential for the selection of the most appropriate therapeutic elements. Playfulness has much to offer to the therapeutic relationship.

Play can be used to offer alternative routes of engagement or exploration, often through the use of humor which can help to 'shift' people into a different state of self. According to Coulter and Rushbrook (2010: 26) 'through play we are better able to develop trust and intimacy; or rather it appears to accelerate the process'. This can be important when gaining a holistic overview of the patient, and teasing out cues and minor details that may change the focus of the issues being addressed. Some of the questions that need to be asked concern personal and potentially embarrassing matters, both for the patient and the practitioner (Tse 2014). Playfulness provides a shared language, allowing practitioners to understand the true nature of their patient, although it is noted that humor is aversive to some people and that in some cases it can actually be detrimental to the therapeutic relationship (Coulter and Rushbrook (2010).

The range and breadth of complementary therapies

Acupuncture is one example of a range of therapies that come under the collective term, Traditional Chinese Medicine (TCM). TCM has been incorporated into mainstream healthcare systems and is a $60 billion industry in mainland China and Hong Kong, with roughly 12 per cent of healthcare provided within TCM facilities (Palmer 2015). This includes the conventional medicine provided within these institutions, demonstrating the possible integration of Western medicine and TCM. The contrasting conceptualization of illness is a defining factor when comparing these two approaches to treating people. TCM emphasizes an individualized and personalized approach to caring for the patient (Franzel *et al.* 2013), incorporating elements such as personal growth, holism, self-activation, wellbeing, integrative care and alliance, all of which are taken to contribute to the individual's medical treatment (Franzel *et al.* 2013). This is in stark contrast to the scientific and empirical approach to illness practiced in Western medicine (Mantri 2008).

CAM includes many different practices, designed both to treat disease and to promote health. These practices derive from a wide range of cultures and traditions with some, such as TCM, dating back more than 2,500 years (National Centre for Complementary and Alternative Medicine 2013). The most popular CAM methodologies are summarized in Table 17.2.

Although the link to play is not always obvious, returning the body to a state of balance whereby playful dispositions can be expressed is a common thread underlying all these methodologies. Play can be used or facilitated in a number of ways and a more detailed contextual background is provided, to demonstrate why play is seen as a supportive mechanism with much to offer these age-old traditions.

TABLE 17.2 Main benefits to health and wellbeing of a selection of CAM techniques

Therapy	Description	Main benefits to health and wellbeing
Acupuncture – Traditional Chinese	The use of slender needles placed in acupuncture points along channels over the body	Rectifies and harmonizes the body's energy and expels pathogens by strengthening the immune system, enhancing circulation, regulating hormones, increasing energy and reducing stress.
Alexander Technique	Teaches improved posture and correct movement, over-riding learned bad habits	'Feeling better' and moving in a more relaxed way, thus avoiding unnecessary tension and pain.
Aromatherapy	Massage using essential oils obtained from flowers, bark, stems, leaves or roots	Altering the mood by stimulating brain function and improving cognitive, psychological or physical wellbeing
Bach Flower Remedies	Solutions of brandy and water containing extreme dilutions of flower material	Altering the mood and improving emotional well-being
The Bowen Technique	Gentle rolling movements to release the fascia, leaving short spaces of time between each move to allow healing	Relaxation and improved flexibility
Chinese Herbal Medicine	Prescription of different herbs and plant material taken as tinctures, tablets, powders or boiled up in a 'tea'	Restores the balance and harmony between Yin and Yang by clearing blockages and depletions of Qi and vitality. Disease prevention
Homeopathy	Taking an extreme dilution of a substance, causing health reducing symptoms to encourage the body to heal	Triggers the body's natural system of healing for both physical and psychological symptoms
Reflexology	Massaging of (mainly) the hands and feet until sensitive areas are reduced or eliminated	Pain and anxiety relief leading to rejuvenation, relaxation and better sleep
Reiki	Spiritually guided life-force or energy-flow using the laying on of hands	Stress reduction and relaxation that promotes healing
Shiatsu	Massage with fingers, thumbs and palms including stretching, joint manipulation and mobilization	Supports and strengthens the body's natural ability to heal and balance itself. Addresses physical symptoms and psychological, emotional and spiritual needs

206 Julie Dakin and Alison Tonkin

Traditional Chinese Acupuncture

There is a growing body of evidence from Western scientific research that demonstrates the effectiveness of acupuncture for treating a wide variety of conditions. From a biomedical viewpoint, acupuncture is believed to stimulate the nervous system, influencing the production of the body's communication substances – hormones and neurotransmitters. The resulting biochemical changes activate the body's self-regulating homeostatic systems, stimulating its natural healing abilities and promoting physical and emotional wellbeing (British Acupuncture Council 2015). Like the Western concept of 'nerve-energy potential' and the *prana* (life force) of Indian philosophy and medicine, ch'i (Qi) is a dynamic force in constant flux (Manaka and Urquhart 1995: 23).

Traditional Chinese Acupuncture is an ancient therapy developed thousands of years ago to keep the body and mind in a healthy, balanced state and to prevent disease. Disease and injury are regarded as unavoidable hazards of life and acupuncture is therefore used to restore balance and health. The oldest known text describing acupuncture is the *Nei Ching Su Wen* (Classic of Internal Medicine), dating to approximately 2600 BC. Manaka and Urquhart (1995) suggest that it can be reasonably assumed that the Chinese people developed an awareness that specific points on the body became touch-sensitive following a particular illness or organ malfunction. By recording the locations of these points, and their link to the relevant vital bodily organ, connecting lines could be drawn to create a chart to represent the channels by which energy (Qi) flowed through the body. In this way, the physical body acquired a heart meridian, a liver meridian and so on, and these became the energy (Qi) pathways upon which acupuncture has an effect.

In Chinese medicine each organ of the body is associated with its various functions and its interactions with other organs. Each bodily organ is also associated with an emotion, an element, a season, a color, a taste, a type of body tissue and a developmental stage of life. For example, the kidney system can be affected by the emotion of fear and its element is water, whilst the liver is affected by anger and its element is wood. The heart is thought to be affected by joy and its element is fire; 'too much' joy (over-excitability) results in disharmony (see Table 17.3). The elements are generated and destroyed in a cyclical interaction, which is used to explain why and how some of the organs interact with each other. Sometimes the interpretations arising from Traditional Chinese Acupuncture are in accord with Western medicine: The *Nei Ching Su Wen* states 'the heart fills the pulse with blood... and the force of the pulse flows into the arteries and the force of the arteries ascends into the lungs' (Lewith 1998:19). At other times an organ unknown to conventional medicine is used to explain how part of the body works e.g. the *San Jiao* or 'triple burner' which is concerned with the flow of fluid through the body.

Study Stack (2015) have produced a range of online activities that allow people to generate 'flash-cards' to help them learn the TCM points used for acupuncture. The site suggests that flash-cards can be a way to have 'serious fun' whilst studying

TABLE 17.3 The five phases (Liang 2004)

	Wood	Fire	Earth	Metal	Water
Yin Organ	Liver	Heart	Spleen	Lung	Kidney
Yang Organ	Gall bladder	Small intestine	Stomach	Large intestine	Bladder
Season	Spring	Summer	Late summer	Autumn	Winter
Color	Green	Red	Yellow	White	Black
Taste	Sour	Bitter	Sweet	Acrid	Salty
Development	Birth	Growth	Transformation	Harvest	Storage
Tissues	Sinews	Vessels	Muscles	Skin	Bones
Affects	Anger	Joy	Thought	Sadness	Fear

and offers users the choice of generating their own cards or sharing those previously been made by other people. The site also offers other playful means of learning TCM points including Hangman, crosswords, matching activities, quizzes and a game called 'Chopped', whereby players need to re-assemble 'chopped-up' words to solve clues about different conditions and acupuncture points (Study Stack 2015). Playful activity as a means of learning and sharing strategies for effective learning can also be extended to coloring activities. Hutchinson (2015) has produced *The Acupuncture Point Functions Colouring Book* as a practical and fun way to learn about the functions of acupuncture points 'on the twelve primary points and the eight extra channels. Students are invited to color and doodle their way through the sequence of images on each channel' (Hutchinson 2015). In this instance, the main educational purpose of the activity has additional benefits as both coloring (discussed in Chapter 8) and doodling (discussed in Chapter 15) are recognized as therapeutic play techniques, as well as just being fun (Williams 2015).

The Alexander Technique

The Alexander Technique is a method for teaching people to 'unlearn' bad habits of posture and to get rid of harmful tension created in the body as a result of these habits (Arnold 2013). The Alexander Technique consists of a number of different techniques for carrying-out everyday tasks and movements in a balanced way that does not cause harm to the body. Many people who practice these techniques experience a general feeling of lightness throughout their bodies and describe the sensation as being like 'walking on air'. Since the physical state directly affects both mental and emotional wellbeing, people often say that they feel much calmer and happier, even after just a few Alexander lessons. This often results in less personal and interpersonal tension and a greater ability to cope with life in general (Brennan 2013) and so re-ignites a motivation for engagement in pleasurable activities, in play and in recreation. Clappison (n.d.) even challenges people to 'see if the

208 Julie Dakin and Alison Tonkin

Alexander Technique can restore some of that playful sense of freedom that you were born with? [and if not] discover when and how your habits might make that freedom less likely'.

The Bowen Technique

The Bowen Technique originated in Australia and is a method of gently bringing the body back into balance. The practitioner's hand performs single rolling movements over parts of the body to release the fascia and the practitioner then leaves the treatment room to allow the body to adjust itself. After an interval, the practitioner returns to perform another similar move, repeating this process several times. During application of the Bowen Technique, the autonomic nervous system slows down, leaving the patient relaxed and the body able to work in peace. In this peaceful state, the brain becomes aware of the areas that need to heal and allows energy and nerve impulses to flow for therapeutic effect (Zainzinger and Knoll 2007). The Bowen Technique is used to treat many conditions, including those caused by lack of flexibility. Many people enjoy sport as a way to exercise, relax and socialize, but conditions such as a hamstring strain can interfere with potential enjoyment of the sporting activity. A randomized controlled trial studied the effects of the Bowen Technique on hamstring flexibility and showed improvement that was maintained for the week following treatment with no further intervention (Marr *et al.* 2011).

Chinese Herbal Medicine

Chinese Herbal Medicine, like acupuncture, is based on the balance between Yin and Yang. When this harmony is damaged by disease or illness the practitioner diagnoses the pattern of imbalance from the patient's signs and symptoms and prescribes the appropriate herbal mix to correct it. Herbal remedies are available for skin diseases including eczema and psoriasis; gynaecological and gastro-intestinal disorders; blood disorders; respiratory, rheumatological and urinary conditions; and psychological problems. The Register of Chinese Herbal Medicine (RCHM) (2015) explains that Chinese Medicine 'places great emphasis on lifestyle management in order to prevent disease before it occurs'. It also 'recognizes that health is more than just the absence of disease and it has a unique capacity to maintain and enhance our capacity for wellbeing and happiness'.

The Rocky Mountain Herbal Institute (RMHI) (n.d.) recognizes the 'tedium of rote memorization' and advocates the use of a playful, problem-solving approach to learning. The Institute has developed 'Herbal Think-TCM', an interactive game module to help students learn clinical Chinese herbology (RMHI n.d.). Using 'realistic clinical puzzles', students are given permission to make mistakes, a sentiment expressed in the statement: 'as long as you eventually learn the material, your scores will reflect this, and your earlier mistakes will be forgiven and forgotten' (RMHI n.d.). Applying elements of gaming into training programs offers learners

Playfulness through alternative healthcare provision **209**

a more engaging experience (O'Brien 2015); the increasing use of gamification within healthcare is discussed in detail in Chapter 15.

Aside of the activities noted above, there is a distinct lack of games or play-based techniques to aid learning and practice within TCM. Whereas Western medicine has successfully utilized new technologies to produce games, simulations and apps to engage both users and practitioners, it would appear that the multi-faceted nature of TCM cannot be simulated in a meaningful or robust manner. TaiChiCentral (2011) discusses the expansion of the classic 'Rock, Paper, Scissors' game by one of the characters in the popular US television series, 'Big Bang Theory'. In the series, this playground game is extended by including 'Lizard' and 'Spock' as possible outcomes in order to 'increase the randomness of the outcome'. An unsuccessful attempt was subsequently made to apply this variation of the game to the 5-Element Theory (TaiChiCentral 2011). Gu (2013: 65) applied theoretical physics to try to simulate the possible actions and consequences relating to the five elements using the 'Rock, Paper, Scissors, Lizard and Spock' metaphor and concluded that 'the randomness in the Five Elements is very high that it exceed the scale for the game to be completely controlled'. TaiChiCentral (2011) suggests that 'adherence to a metaphor, which was initially meant to simplify difficult concepts, becomes what some modern technologists might call 'simplexity'. It makes the whole thing impossible to understand'. Perhaps the essence of TCM, and the fundamental reality of alternative healthcare approaches, is best explained by the fact that, whilst games may be useful in learning basic concepts, it is their practice and experience that set them apart from more linear, cause-and-effect approaches (Luger 2005).

Conclusion

Complementary and alternative healthcare approaches are linked to 'balance' and a focus on returning the body to a balanced state. Alternative approaches to healthcare can both facilitate and be facilitated by playfulness and playful activities. Play enhances the individual's capacity to 'be at one' in body and mind, generating an abundance of Qi that flows throughout the body for optimal health. This is neatly summarized by Prodoehl (2012) who states:

> What never ceases to amaze me about Chinese Medicine is its holistic nature. The playful balance between all of the organs and substances within the body, and the dynamic the body has with its environment … but it's when we put it all together that the magic takes place.

References

Alnorthumbria Veterinary Group (n.d.) *Acupuncture*, Online. Available at www.alnorthumbriavets.co.uk/index.php?page=acupuncture (accessed 19 July 2015).

210 Julie Dakin and Alison Tonkin

Alzheimer's Society (2015) *Complementary and Alternative Therapies,* Online. Available at www.alzheimers.org.uk/site/scripts/documents_info.php?documentID=134 (accessed 19 July 2015).

Arnold, J. (2013) *The Complete Guide to the Alexander Technique,* Online. Available at www.alexandertechnique.com/at.htm (accessed 4 May 2015).

Barnett, J.E. and Shale, A.J. (2012) The integration of complementary and alternative medicine (CAM) into the practice of psychology: a vision for the future, *Professional Psychology: Research and Practice* 2012, 43 (6): 576–585.

Brennan R. (2013) *What is the Alexander Technique?* Online. Available at www.alexander technique.com/at.htm (accessed 4 May 2015).

British Acupuncture Council (2015) *Research,* Online. Available at acupuncture.org (accessed 24 July 2015).

Clappison, J. (n.d.) *Alexander Technique,* Online. Available at www.thewellbeing centre.info/alexander-technique.html (accessed 5 December 2015).

Cornell University Veterinary Specialists (2015) *Acupuncture,* Online. Available at www.cuvs.org/services-acupuncture.php (accessed 18 July 2015).

Coulter, N. and Rushbrook, S. (2010) Playfulness in CAT, *Reformulation,* Winter: 24–27.

Finston, P. (2015) *Why are Eastern and Western Treatments so Different?* Online. Available at http://acu-psychiatry.com/what-is-world-medical-wisdom/basic-differences-between-eastern-and-western-medicine/ (accessed 27 November 2015).

Franzel, B., Schwiegershausen, M., Heusser, P. and Berger, B. (2013) Individualised medicine from the perspectives of patients using complementary therapies: a meta-ethnography approach, *BMC Complementary and Alternative Medicine,* 13: 124.

Gu, S. (2013) *From Rock Scissor Paper to Study and Modeling of Chinese Five Elements,* Online. Available at www.diva-portal.org/smash/get/diva2:686368/FULLTEXT01.pdf (accessed 5 December 2015).

Hutchinson, R. (2015) *The Acupuncture Point Functions Colouring Book,* Singing Dragon.

Lewith, G. (1998) *Acupuncture Its Place in Western Medical Science,* Suffolk: Green Print.

Ling, Y. (2013) Traditional Chinese Medicine in the treatment of symptoms in patients with advanced cancer, Annals *of Palliative Medicine,* 2 (3): 141–152.

Luger, T. (2005) *The Perpetual Problem,* Online. Available at www.chineseherb academy.org/articles/idt_tcm.shtml (accessed 5 December 2015).

Manaka, Y. and Urquhart, I. (1995) *The Layman's Guide to Acupuncture,* New York: Weatherhill Inc.

Mantri, S. (2008) Holistic medicine and the western medical tradition, *American Medical Association Journal of Ethics,* 10 (3): 177–180.

Marr, M., Baker, J., Lambon, N. and Perry, J. (2011) The effects of the Bowen Technique on hamstring flexibility over time: a randomized control trail, *Journal of Bodywork Movement Therapies,* 15 (3): 281–290.

National Center for Complementary and Alternative Medicine (2013) Traditional Chinese Medicine: An Introduction. National Center for Complementary and Alternative Medicine.

Palmer, J. (2015) *Do Some Harm,* Online. Available at http://aeon.co/magazine/health/james-palmer-traditional-chinese-medicine/ (accessed 15 August 2015).

Prodoehl, C. (2012) *Mechanisms of Menstruation: the Chinese Medicine Perspective,* Online. Available at http://cgicm.ca/2012/04/mechanisms-of-menstruation-the-chinese-medicine-perspective/ (accessed 9 May 2016).

Proyer, R. and Ruch, W. (2011) The virtuousness of adult playfulness: the relation of playfulness with strengths of character, *Psychology of Well-Being: Theory, Research and Practice,* 1: 4.

O'Brien, J. (2015) *Play to Win! The Gamification Benefits In Workplace Training*, Online. Available at http://elearningindustry.com/gamification-benefits-in-workplace-training (accessed 5 December 2015).

Register of Chinese Herbal Medicine (2015) *About Chinese Herbal Medicine*, Online. Available at rchm.co.uk (accessed 24 July 2015).

Rocky Mountain Herbal Institute (RMHI) (n.d.) *HerbalThink-TCM 4.0*, Online. Available at www.rmhiherbal.org/herbalthink/ (accessed 5 December 2015).

Royal College of Psychiatrists (2015) *Complementary and Alternative Medicines 1*, Online. Available at www.rcpsych.ac.uk/healthadvice/treatmentswellbeing/complementary-therapy.aspx (accessed 22 February 2016).

Schiesser, M. (2015) *The Five Elements*, Online. Available at www.innerjourney seminars.com/the-five-elements.html (accessed 19 July 2015).

Study Stack (2015) *Flash cards: TCM Points*, Online. Available at www.studystack.com/flashcard-784047 (accessed 5 December 2015).

Sultanoff, B. (2002) Breath work, in Shannon, S. (ed.), *Handbook of Complementary and Alternative Therapies in Mental Health*, San Diego, CA: Academic Press: 209–227.

Suttie, E. (n.d.) *Chinese Medicine Living: The Heart*, Online. Available at www.chinese medicineliving.com/blog/medicine/organs/the-heart/ (accessed 19 July 2015).

TaiChiCentral (2011) Five Element Theory vs Rock Paper Scissors Lizard Spock, *TaiChiCentral*, 15 April 2011 Onine. Available at http://community.taichicentral.com/five-element-theory-vs-rock-paper-scissors-lizard-spock/ (accessed 5 December 2015).

Tse, H. (2014) *The Nature of Qi: Part 1*, Online. Available at www.chinesefootreflexology.com/nature-of-qi/ (accessed 27 November 2015).

Tseui, J. (1978) Eastern and western approaches to medicine, *Western Journal of Medicine* 128 (6): 551–557.

van Hecke, O., Torrance, N. and Smith, B. (2013) Chronic pain epidemiology and its clinical relevance, *British Journal of Anaesthesia*, 111 (1): 13–18.

Williams, Z. (2015) Adult colouring-in books: the latest weapon against stress and anxiety, *The Guardian*, 26 June 2015 Online. Available at www.theguardian.com (accessed 5 October 2015).

Zainzinger, M. and Knoll, S. (2007) *Bowtech: The Original Bowen Technique*, Gloucester: BoD(Books on Demand).

18

PLAYFUL DESIGN

Alison Tonkin

Play and playfulness are often reflected within the design process, from the initial concept and planning phase through to the completed project. Healthcare is benefiting from playful design, in concepts such as outdoor gyms and adult playgrounds through to the promotion of healing environments, which use color, shape, form and light to promote relaxation and feelings of emotional wellbeing. The scope of playful design and its application in the healthcare context is vast, ranging from individual, personalized features, to work and living spaces in areas such as wards or communal homes. This includes the buildings that house healthcare facilities as well as those designed for whole communities who share a common need. With the recognition that design is considered to be a collaborative process involving a number of players, play-based strategies can be utilized to facilitate engagement across differing perspectives and levels of expertise, as well as featuring in the completed product.

Introduction

According to the Design Council, 'good design makes things simple so that you can get on with enjoying your life', a statement that is equally applicable to the provision of care (Hunter 2014). Owing to the complexity and scope of design, finding a single definition that encompasses all the differing elements is problematic. For the purposes of this chapter, Miller (2014) provides a simple definition suggesting that:

> Design is the thought process comprising the creation of an entity.

Play is known to trigger creativity (Robinson *et al.* 2015) and this is not just for people who are considered to be 'right-brain' dominant. Neuroscience shows that personality types such as the creative, free-spirited, 'right brainer' and the 'logical left brainer' have been falsely categorized (Novotney 2013). However, those who

Playful design **213**

are considered to be more logical in their thought processes may require help to 'access' their inner creativity, and this is where playful strategies can enhance the creative process. In most instances, the process of play focuses on the actual experience as opposed to any outcome (Robinson *et al.* 2015) but increasingly, the components of game play and their associated thought processes are being utilized as part of the design process. The concept of *Playful Design* has been described as 'the use of game thinking and playful elements in the design of user experiences in non-game contexts' (Tsekleves 2015). This is useful when considering how the design process needs to capture the knowledge perspectives of users, staff and stakeholders throughout the life of a design project, from the initial concept right through to the 'creation of an entity', and how that entity works in reality.

The process of healthcare design is neatly summarized in a publication by ArtCare (2014) entitled *Robust Healthcare Design*. ArtCare is the Arts in Health provider for Salisbury NHS Foundation Trust, which has patient and staff experience at the core its work and utilizes this experience to facilitate evaluation and planning of everything they do. With the emphasis on participatory engagement, this publication sums up how the process of participatory design can provide benefits to all engaged in the service.

The growing recognition of design as a means of transforming healthcare practice through innovation is an exciting area of healthcare service provision, particularly with its potential to enhance *person-centeredness* (Lab4Living 2015a). The fact that there is no simple method, no single solution, no fixed end-point in the design process, presents a 'wicked problem' in that it is working on the problem that 'might well bring forth a better solution' (Lexicon/ft.com 2015). Lab4Living (2015a) see this 'wicked problem' as an opportunity, stating:

> This is where we argue design's strength lies, where we can draw on a tradition of creative and divergent thinking to address these fundamental and yet practical challenges to our societies' health.

Gray (2009) suggests that the playful evolution of humans as a species has seen the elaboration of biological and cultural characteristics, enabling the creation of new functions of play. These are now being utilized within the design process, particularly in the promotion of cooperative and sharing strategies that enable the participation of a whole range of players, all of whom have perspectives to offer and knowledge to contribute. Play and playfulness feature in a number of the projects presented on the Lab4Living (2015b) website, such as a collaborative, multidisciplinary project involving artists, musicians, social scientists and surgeons, exploring surgical simulation as an artistic medium. Using spherical filming techniques, this allowed surgeons to reflect on the patient view during a surgical procedure, something that many surgeons would not ever have experienced or perhaps even considered (Lab4Living 2015b).

A more obvious link to play is the use of Lego Serious Play whereby the users' service experience can be imagined, or played-out, through the medium of this

214 Alison Tonkin

popular construction toy. The experience under consideration is enacted as a group activity, with different elements of the user story represented from different perspectives: the user, staff member and relevant environmental context are represented in the form of a Lego scenario, providing a safe arena within which open discussion can take place. Once set up,

> you literally walk through the service moments, taking pictures with a digital camera and ideally with another person, imagining what the various actors are doing, saying and feeling. It can be useful to enact the walk through using various different personas, and under different imagined situations.
>
> *(Better Services by Design 2015a)*

The use of *personas* is becoming increasingly popular, especially when considering generational aspects of service use. For example, during the early part of design planning for the Park Nicollet Women's Center in Minneapolis (US), AECOM worked with administrators and clinicians to develop four key patient types: 'young professional women, young mothers, middle-age menopausal women, and the elderly. The effort illustrated how each patient journey through its new facility was different' (Cahnman 2014). This led to the identification of opportunities to enhance the patient experience through the use of art, lighting placement and speciality furniture, all of which contributed to the promotion of a healing environment (Cahnman 2014). The act of creating personas can be achieved through playful interactions, collating various sources of information about similar people to create a character that is representative of that particular user-group (Better Services by Design 2015c). Involving service-users themselves is by far the most effective means of capturing the lived experience, especially as 'the individual patient is the one common denominator across all their care experiences, making them a natural source for information across healthcare boundaries, health professionals, services and care settings' (O'Hara and Isden 2013). However, this can be a time-consuming process and participation might be perceived as a negative experience; participants may not enjoy the experience or may feel that their concerns have not been taken on board (van Amstel and Hartmann 2011). This is particularly true for some service-users who feel that their involvement is tokenistic and undervalued, despite the fact that they bring insight from a different perspective, albeit with a different level of tacit knowledge and experience. Gray (2009) suggests that 'playfulness and the signals associated with it (such as laughter)… [can be used to] promote ways of cooperating and sharing with one another'. Perhaps more importantly, Gray (2009) sees play and humor as a means of creating equity and as a means by which the human drive towards dominance can be overcome.

Cultures of creativity

Holistic healthcare design is a highly complex process involving a large number of different participants and covering a range of physical and practical demands

Playful design **215**

(Garde 2013). Gauntlett and Thomsen (2013: 5) extol the virtue of 'cultures of creativity', suggesting that:

> creativity arises not exclusively in individuals, or in culture, but in the interaction between the two. Both sides are important: the imaginative individual, who originates new ideas, and the stimulating, supportive culture which both inspires those ideas and helps them to flourish.

Garde (2013) advocates the utilization of a participatory design process in order to facilitate this cross-fertilization of ideas. Participatory design uses a set of design principles and values that enables all practitioners who have a role in the project (user, worker, designer or researcher) to become active participants and fully engaged in the design process. However, this requires 'dedicated facilitation' as the development of new ideas needs to be supported by appropriate design tools that enable visualization and imagination of future design (Garde 2013). This highlights an issue in terms of abstraction skills, in that users and workers may lack the capacity to envisage the finished project before building has begun, meaning the optimum contribution comes once the building has been completed, at which point changes are difficult to make. However, the use of 'ludic explorations of future scenarios ... through simulations in game like interactions' can provide one way to bridge the 'abstraction level gap' (van Amstel and Hartmann 2011) thus allowing access to the specialist, tacit and practical knowledge of service-users, which designers are generally lacking (Garde 2013).

According to Bowen (cited in Better Services by Design 2015b) 'It's not so much that a design approach is a set of specific methods but as an attitude, a way of thinking about problems and solutions and being quite adaptive and adapting the approach according to a specific situation'. Better Services by Design (2015c) promote the use of a Double Diamond Design Process which has four consecutive phases.

Originally developed through research at the Design Council in 2005, the model provides a graphical way of describing the design process, with the shapes remaining generic, although they can be 'stretched and morphed depending on the project's characteristics' (Design Council 2007: 10). The phases are:

1 Discovery phase – identifies and questions what the focus of the project should be and this is where understanding of the needs of the service user is explored.
2 Define phase – important issues identified through the *discovery* phase provide a focus for defining and interpreting problems.
3 Develop phase – potential ways to solve the problems are explored through designing and testing possible solutions.
4 Deliver phase – this allows practical solutions to be implemented, enabling the service to be delivered.

(Better Services by Design 2015c)

The first three stages lend themselves to playful facilitation, particularly the discovery phase, which requires consideration of the needs of all those who will be using of the facility, service or product. This has been commendably demonstrated in the Patient and Family Advisor Partnership Program, which has contributed to the design of the UW Health at the American Center in Wisconsin (US). Gesler *et al.* (2004: 119) suggest that 'hospitals are behavior settings where there is a definite relationship between people (patients, staff, visitors) and the built forms of the hospital'. As such, all buildings 'are both shaped by people and capable of shaping occupants' behaviors and feelings' (Adams *et al.* 2010: 659). Sheehan (cited University of Wisconsin Hospitals and Clinics Authority 2015) states 'With a better understanding of our patients' perspectives and ideas, we're able to create a more welcoming, easy-to-navigate facility that not only meets their needs, but makes them true partners in their care experience'. The Patient and Family Advisors (PFA) also value the opportunity to engage in the process, stating: 'Patients' families have a unique perspective, they have insights that often don't cost anything but they make big changes' (Zimdars, cited in University of Wisconsin Hospitals and Clinics Authority 2015). Zimdars also notes that 'the openness of the whole experience seems to invite a collaboration – it just has a feeling of a humanness to it'.

Perhaps that 'humanness' derives from the spirit of social play (Gray 2009). In the Patient and Family Advisor Partnership Program, play has been used as a means of promoting cooperation, through the process of representation (Gray 2009), 'I was on a group to do a clinic floor, and so we built a clinic floor, from flat paper to little models' (Trachte, cited University of Wisconsin Hospitals and Clinics Authority 2015). This demonstrates how participatory design games have been developed to enable non-designers to take part in the design process, using turn-taking, rules and scenarios to engage the players' imagination (Garde 2013). Unlike

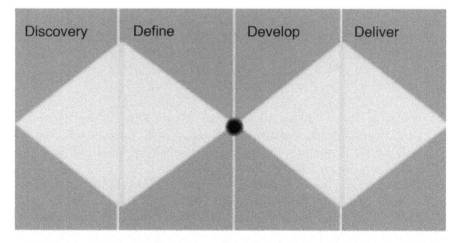

FIGURE 18.1 Double Diamond Design Process (Better Services by Design 2015c, based on work by the UK Design Council)

leisure games, design games have 'serious outcomes' that extend beyond the end point of the game and are often undertaken in small groups, whereby discussion between participants is an essential part of the creative process.

One of the key features of the Patient and Family Advisor Partnership Program was the commitment of the PFA and the willingness of the project team to capture and integrate their views and opinions into the whole design process. Waterworth (2014) uses the fable of the chicken and the pig to illustrate how user research feedback needs to be embraced by organizations, and how commitment rather than just involvement is essential.

> A chicken is having a meal in a restaurant with her friend, the pig.
>
> "We can cook better food than this," she says, "we should open our own restaurant."
>
> "Sounds good," says the pig, "what would we call it?"
>
> "I know," she replies, "how does Ham n' Eggs sound?"
>
> The pig thinks for a minute, "Sounds like I'd be committed, but you'd only be involved."

Waterworth (2014) extols the virtue of being a fully committed pig, 'soaking up background information, joining in discussions and continually adapting and refining … we do everything we can to make the insights we've gathered from users part of the team DNA'. This is the true meaning of participatory design with a significant role ascribed to play and playfulness in enabling and facilitating committed pigs to engage with the wider design process.

Design with play in mind

Two projects demonstrating how cultures of creativity can facilitate participatory healthcare design are explored in Box 18.1. Boex is an interior design and product agency based in Cornwall (UK) which has been involved in designing innovative healthcare settings for over ten years. What makes this company unusual, is the availability of their designs through their website, accompanied by images and narrative descriptions of how projects have been undertaken. Figure 18.1 (Image courtesy of Boex) is the result of a six-month project to design and refit a dementia ward and living space for an NHS hospital in England (Project A). It could be mistaken for a children's ward, with the use of bold, contrasting colors and an interactive sensory board (Figure 18.2) to promote stimulation and interactions with staff and family alike (Boex 2015a). Potential criticism of the perceived infantilization of the environment is addressed by providing a clear rationale for the choice of design features, from the use of teal blue walls to contrast against brown upholstery and ash wood, helping patients with impaired vision to recognize doors, windows and seating, to the use of color to improve orientation (Boex 2015a).

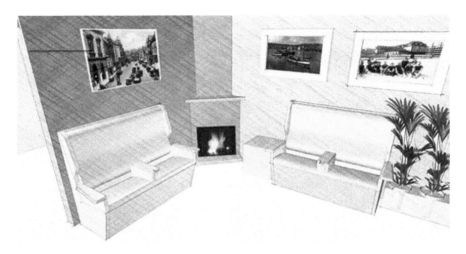

FIGURE 18.2 Design for the dementia lounge – a quiet space for patients, family members and staff (Boex 2015a)

Large images of natural landscapes provide a 'sense of place' whilst images of the local area from the 1920s promote reminiscence.

Although the final design of the ward contributes to the provision of a healing environment, perhaps one of the most intriguing points about this project is the way in which the design process was undertaken. The project began with meetings with staff to discuss the operational difficulties associated with the previous layout, followed by evaluative workshops with all the stakeholders, resulting in a collaborative process involving 'consultants, nurses, occupational therapists, hospital staff and patients' (Boex 2015a). An 'observational study of the ward during a working day' was also undertaken, which resulted in a mapping exercise to identify the use of different areas by staff and patients, as well as of underutilized space which subsequently became seating areas.

Project B is also the design of a ward for patients with dementia but this project is very different in terms of the final outcome for the project. The décor focused on the home environment and used visual cues that could be found in a domestic setting, such as bookshelves, a large kitchen table and cabinets, as shown in Figure 18.3 (Boex 2015b). This reassured patients as they were in an environment promoting safety and security. Wendy McCoy, who is a staff nurse on the ward commented '

> The farmhouse table has been wonderful, we've been playing games around it, and more people have come over and joined in. It feels like your kitchen table at home – the hub of everything – everyone gathered around the table enjoying each other's company
>
> *(Boex 2015b)*

In a conversation with Sam Boex (summarized in Box 18.1) it became clear that the ethnographic approach to the engagement process identified earlier is an integral part of the design methodology used by Boex for each of their projects. The two projects relating to the interior design of wards for patients with dementia were discussed and both suggest that Boex are 'fully committed pigs'.

BOX 18.1 SUMMARY OF A CONVERSATION WITH SAM BOEX EXPLORING THE DESIGN OF TWO DIFFERENT WARDS FOR PEOPLE WITH DEMENTIA

All projects begin with a workshop, during which the design team speak to everyone connected with the ward including patients, nurses and domestic staff. The workshops always include a play element, as it suggests comfort and familiarity, and this is tailored to the particular user-group and is especially important when working with older patients. If the project brief is to refurbish a space with a pre-existing function, the team immerses itself in that space to experience how it works and to explore how each person uses the space. This ensures that the design outcomes can be linked back to the immersed-engagement towards the end of the project. Specific features from two projects that emerged from an engagement process are now discussed. Project A: The use of interactive panels in this design (Figure 18.3) stemmed from engagement workshops with staff and patients and from spending time on the ward. Listening to their remarkable life-stories, it became apparent that many patients had previously been employed in manual jobs or trades and that the ward represented a restrictive environment to them. During time spent on the ward, the project team noted that some of these patients mimicked features of their previous employment. One patient would upturn a chair and fiddle with the springs; the team learned that he was previously a mechanic. Another patient would constantly knock things against the edge of the wall – he was previously a carpet fitter. Other actions, such as repeatedly turning a door handle, showed that patients both sought and found creativity in their own environment. These actions appeared to offer reassurance by giving the patient a sense of purpose linked to the physical space. The design mimicked some of these skilful actions through the development of a unique, interactive panel for each patient as an integral feature of the sensory board. This not only provides sensory stimulation but also generates a focal point for conversations between staff and families. Project B: This very different project was led by the ward manager. Patients tended to wander along an adjacent corridor but there was nothing to engage them or to help them find their way back to the ward. In this case, the design team explored the use of photographs for way-finding. The photos represented the play element of the engagement process in that it was designed to invoke reminiscence and to open-up conversations between patients, staff and the design team. The lounge area of the ward lacked logic and included several potentially confusing features. The goal of the design was to make the ward more visually comprehensible and functional in order that patients could 'locate themselves' with a purpose. This resulted in a design which emulated the kitchen of a home, with a big table and activities concentrated in that area (Figure 18.4). Learned experience and tacit knowledge are both important to a playful design process. Evidence-based practice demands that everyone who will use a particular space is involved in the design process. Sam Boex sums this up: 'space does not need to conform to a stereotype – it can be creative and you need to give people the ability to change and adapt'.

The University of Twente in the Netherlands provides two examples of work that has been published as part of PhD theses, both of which advocate the role of play as exploratory means of engagement. Amstel (2014) promotes the concept of *Expansive Design* as a 'practical approach to include activity as a subject of space'. Based on first-hand experience of how space is used, it shows how users will

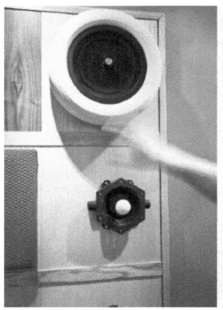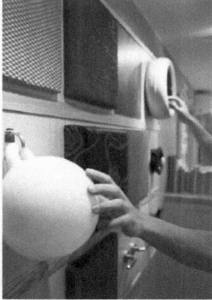

FIGURE 18.3 A sensory board featuring interactive panels which can be changed to reflect patients' individual life-stories (Boex 2015a)

Playful design **221**

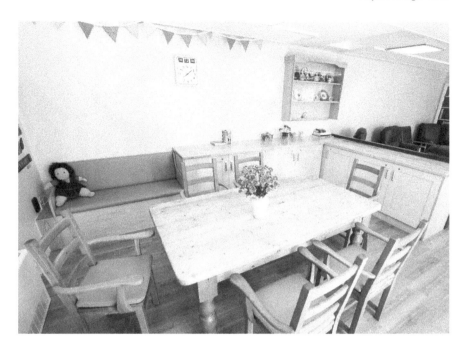

FIGURE 18.4 The large kitchen table 'providing lots of space for collaboration, activities and playing games' (Boex 2015b)

rearrange space by moving furniture or changing the function of a room to suit their own activities. However, this 'user perception' is seldom taken into account in the design of space usage, mainly due to economic reasons (Amstel 2014). Expansive design uses simple visualization tools such as the 'knitting game' to simply show the walking paths people follow when moving around the healthcare facility (Amstel 2014). This involves a map of the area and wool wrapped around certain points to show movement between spaces, which is then used to identify poor spatial layout resulting in unnecessary walking back and forth. This low tech tool can be replicated by a high tech version using dedicated software packages known as a 'walking paths BIM application' (Amstel 2014) as shown in Figure 18.5 (image courtesy of Boex).

Expansive design is a valid concept in the changing world of healthcare facilitation, especially with the dismantling of centralized services and the movement of healthcare services into the community (Taylor 2012). Van Amstel (2015) advocates the need to bring in the people who 'actually know how this activity happens – the shop floor of the hospital so to speak ... so they can join the discussion'. Van Amstel (2015) demonstrates the engagement process through a presentation that shows how healthcare professionals who are not design experts can be facilitated to engage in the planning process, which in turn enables them to think about how the activity itself can be expanded, enabling the adaptation that will be needed.

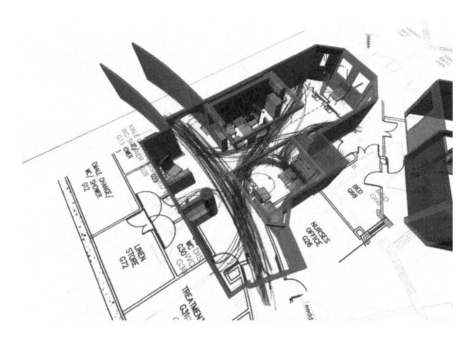

FIGURE 18.5 Mapping the flow of patients and staff: a high-tech version of the knitting wool game (Boex n.d.)

In order to disseminate the findings of his research to a broader audience, Amstel (2014) moved into 'serious gaming', through the design of a board game called the Expansive Hospital. The board game has been designed to enhance collaboration between construction and healthcare workers, following interviews with both sets of professionals. The key skill required by the game is 'negotiation', and the design problems inherent within the game must be worked out through social activity. Using the contradictions that exist in the design process, and which have been purposefully embedded in the game (van Amstel 2015), conflicts must be resolved by the players themselves. If they are not, 'patient satisfaction drops, together with the hospital income. Playing the game is an opportunity to learn the importance and the difficulties of designing for healthcare performance while having fun with the artificial conflict enactment' (Visico Center 2014). The game is demonstrated in the YouTube video 'The Expansive Hospital game walkthrough' (van Amstel 2014) as well as 'The Expansive Hospital serious game' (Visico Center 2014).

Garde (2103) also advocates the use of games for facilitating participation, noting that the design process needs to link all the differing elements associated with the healthcare environment and the activities that occur within it. In order to achieve this, 'practical knowledge and experience from the healthcare domain are essential' and Garde (2013: 3) focuses on bringing together healthcare practitioners through the use of design games to engage their participation in the design process.

The use of games can promote an informal atmosphere which is conducive to productivity and also 'levels the playing field', a crucial factor in considering the range and scope of the professional practice of the participants. In the context of Garde's approach to the design process, research is 'a playful activity in which one or more persons are given the assignment to achieve a specified design goal, means to use in achieving this goal and rules to play by' (Garde 2013: 45). Exploration of the differing methods and theoretical considerations are explored within Garde's PhD thesis, and those interested in a more theoretical exploration of how games and playful approaches to the design process can work in practice, can gain valuable insight from reviewing this work (Garde 2013).

Ultimately, the manipulation of the healthcare environment through the use of color, light, shape and form can reduce environmental stressors and thus enable people (both staff and service-users) to function flexibly within an environment which they can adapt to suit their changing needs (Boex 2015a). As van der Heide (2011) suggests:

> By appreciating the darkness when you design the light, you create much more interesting environments that truly enhance our lives.

References

Adams, A., Theodore, D., Goldenberg, E., McLaren, C. and McKeever, P. (2010) Kids in the atrium: comparing architectural intentions and children's experiences in a pediatric hospital lobby, *Social Science & Medicine*, 70: 658–667.

Amstel, F. (2014) *Expansive Design: Expanding Human Activity by Designing Space,* Online. Available at www.utwente.nl/ctw/visico/Living%20labs/Healthcare%20facilities/ Expanding%20Human%20Activity%20by%20Designing%20Space/expansive-design-visico-august2014/ (accessed 1 November 2015).

ArtCare (2014) *Robust Healthcare Design,* Salisbury: ArtCare.

Better Services by Design (2015a) *Lego Serious Play.* Online. Available at www.bsbd.org.uk/ cards/lego-serious-play/ (accessed 8 November 2015).

Better Services by Design (2015b) *Lessons Learned,* Online. Available at www.bsbd.org.uk/ lessons-learned/ (accessed 8 November 2015).

Better Services by Design (2015c) *Double Diamond Design Process,* Online. Available at www.bsbd.org.uk/double-diamond-design-process/ (accessed 8 November 2015).

Boex (2015a) *Dementia ward,* Online. Available at www.boex.co.uk/project/dementia-ward-design/ (accessed 21 November 2015).

Boex (2015b) *Healthcare Dementia Ward,* Online. Available at www.boex.co.uk/ project/healthcare-dementia-design/ (accessed 21 November 2015).

Cahnman, S. (2014) *Best Of 2014: Designing For The Patient Experience,* Online. Available at www.healthcaredesignmagazine.com/article/designing-patient-experience?page=3 (accessed 20 November 2015).

Design Council (2007) *Eleven Lessons: Managing Design in Eleven Global Companies: Desk Research Report,* London: Design Council.

Garde, J. (2013) Everyone has a part to play: Games and participatory design in healthcare, PhD Thesis, Universiteit Twente.

Gauntlett, D. and Thomsen, S. (2013) *Cultures of Creativity: Nurturing Creative Mindsets Across Cultures,* Billund: The Lego Foundation.

Gesler, W., Bell, M., Curtis, S., Hubbard, P. and Francis, S. (2004) Therapy by design: evaluating the UK hospital building program. *Health & Place,* 10: 117–128.

Gray, P. (2009) *Play Makes Us Human I: A Ludic Theory of Human Nature,* Online. Available at www.psychologytoday.com/blog/freedom-learn/200906/play-makes-us-human-i-ludic-theory-human-nature (accessed 8 November 2015).

Hunter, M. (2014) *The Link Between Design and Care,* Online. Available at www.design-council.org.uk/news-opinion/link-between-design-and-care (accessed 20 November 2015).

Lab4Living (2015a) *'State of the art' of Design in Health,* Online. Available at http://research.shu.ac.uk/lab4living/state-of-the-art-of-design-in-health (accessed 8 November 2015).

Lab4Living (2015b) *Art, Simulation and Surgical Humanities,* Online. Available at http://research.shu.ac.uk/lab4living/art-simulation-and-surgical-humanities (accessed 8 November 2015).

Lexicon/ft.com (2015) *Definition of a Wicked Problem,* Online. Available at http://lexicon.ft.com/Term?term=wicked-problem (accessed 8 November 2015).

Majzun, R. (2011) Coloring outside the lines: what pediatric hospitals can teach adult hospitals, *Pediatric Nursing,* 37 (4): 210–211.

Miller, W. (2014) *Definition of Design,* Online. Available at www.wrmdesign.com/Philosophy/Documents/DefinitionDesign.htm (accessed 31 October 2015).

Novotney, A. (2013) Despite what you've been told, you aren't 'left-brained' or 'right-brained', *The Guardian,* 16 November 2013. Online. Available at www.the guardian.com (accessed 1 November 2015).

O'Hara, J. and Isden, R. (2013) *Identifying Risks and Monitoring Safety: The Role of Patients and Citizens,* London: The Health Foundation.

Robinson, L. Smith, M. and Segal, J. (2015) *The Benefits of Play for Adults: How Play Can Improve Your Health, Work, and Family Relationships,* Online. Available at www.helpguide.org/articles/emotional-health/benefits-of-play-for-adults.htm. (accessed 1 November 2015).

Taylor, J. (2012) NHS reforms: moving care to the community, *The Guardian,* 20 June 2012 Online. Available at www.theguardian.com (accessed 21 November 2015).

Tonkin, A. (2015) *Exploring the Impact Environments have on Children and Young People's Experience of Healthcare: A Review of the Literature,* Online. Available at www.hpset.org.uk/environmentsofcare2015.html (accessed 8 November 2015).

Tsekleves, E. (2015) Co-designing playful urban park experiences for promoting community public health, *Design and Health, 11th World Congress and Exhibition,* Hong Kong, 16th July 2015.

University of Wisconsin Hospitals and Clinics Authority (2015) *Patient and Family Advisor Partnership Program: Better by Design: Engaging Patients In the Design of UW Health at The American Center,* Online. Available at www.uwhealth.org/patient-family-advisor/better-by-design-engaging-patients-in-the-design-of-uw-health-at-the-american-center/4264 1 (accessed 8 November 2015).

van Amstel, F. (2014) *The Expansive Hospital Game Walkthrough,* Online. Available at www.youtube.com/watch?v=eZ0tW60QBZ8 (accessed 21 November 2015).

van Amstel, F. (2015) *Expansive Design: Design with Contradictions,* Online. Available at https://vimeo.com/88862233 (accessed 21 November 2015).

van Amstel, F. and Hartmann, T. (2011) *Collaborative Planning for Healthcare Environments,* Online. Available at http://fredvanamstel.com/wp-content/uploads/2011/07/poster_bremen_meeting_vanamstel.pdf (accessed 8 November 2015).

van der Heide, R. (2011) *Why Light Needs Darkness,* Online. Available at www.ted.com/talks/rogier_van_der_heide_why_light_needs_darkness/transcript (accessed 21 November 2015).

Visico Center (2014) *The Expansive Hospital Serious Game,* Online. Available at https://vimeo.com/105001087 (accessed 21 November 2015).

Waterworth, J. (2014) From Chickens to Pigs, *Blog: User Research*, 15 July 2014, Online. Available at https://userresearch.blog.gov.uk/2014/07/15/from-chickens-to-pigs/ (accessed 8 November 2015).

19

PLAYING TOGETHER

Festivals and celebrations

Alison Tonkin and Shereen Jameel

This chapter provides an exposition of different cultural approaches to play, recreation and leisure in the context of their contribution to health and wellbeing. Celebrations and seasonal festivities lend themselves to the health of the community, with play being a significant feature of many celebrations. By embracing the potential for community celebrations to be seen within the healthcare arena, we recognize that emotional wellbeing and a sense of community can be utilized to enhance the holistic health of societies everywhere. This is neatly summarized in the statement 'Festivals ... all serve the purpose of bringing happiness to our lives, and strengthen our sense of community' (Hat Tours 2012).

Introduction

Throughout history, the role of play has been viewed as a central component of community-based cultural activities and practices and perhaps one of the best examples of this is the celebration of festivals. One of the outcomes of the recent global austerity agenda is that people tend to lead increasingly busy lives with less time for leisure and recreational activities (Target Study 2015). Celebrations, in the form of festivals, are a good way to break the monotony of work and to spend quality time with family and friends (Target Study 2015). They add rhythm and structure to our social lives and inspire recognition and acknowledgement of the important things and moments in life. Festivals reflect their cultural context, their main purpose being to promote peace, harmony and happiness as well as to strengthen our sense of community (Hat Tours 2012).

Al Aboud (2013) defines a festival as 'an event that is ordinarily staged by a local community that centers around and celebrates a unique aspect of that community'. Play as a feature of festivals offers the prospect of healthy rejuvenation, promotes communal harmony and leads to effective socialization. Festivals can be 'an organized set of special events' such as musical performances or food festivals (Cambridge University Press 2015) and play itself can be a focal point. For example, the Playful Arts Festival (2015) in the Netherlands is a bi-annual festival that celebrates the cross-over between 'art, play, technology, design and social interaction', whilst CounterPlay (2015) is an annual international festival 'exploring and challenging the role of games, play and playfulness in our jobs and our lives'. However, most festivals are traditionally associated with celebrating the memory of a religious event or covering a specific date or time period, with associated ceremonies, food and social activities (Cambridge University Press 2015). In this instance, festivals may not only bring people closer to spirituality, but may also enable them to understand and appreciate other cultures (Target Study 2015). By understanding the cultural characteristics of a group or community, health programs and services can be customized to meet the needs of members which can then have a direct and positive impact on their health and wellbeing (Kreuter and McClure 2004).

Wellness

The celebration of festivals can be framed within wellness, particularly in relation to their capacity to generate 'awe and wonder', both of which are defined as characteristics linked to spirituality. This aspect is addressed in detail in Chapter 20.

Chapter 8 includes an account of how the concept of wellness has emerged over the past 30 years as an 'alternative to the traditional, illness-based medical model for treatment of mental and physical disorders' (Myers *et al.* 2000: 251). Wellness emphasizes the integration of the mind, body and spirit, promoting a holistic approach to living life as fully as possible (wellness-research.org n.d.a). Wellness has a developmental focus, building on the strengths and assets of the individual to optimize growth across the lifespan (Myers and Sweeney 2008). Spirituality is considered to be a central feature of wellness (Meyers 2014) and is unique to each individual (Cashwell, cited in Meyers 2014). For many people, spirituality is interwoven with religion, although these are not equivalent concepts. Spirituality can be explored on an individual basis, simply by being in a quiet place with oneself, or through identification with a particular religious community (Meyers 2014). It is on this basis that the celebration of festivals can be seen to be a contributory factor to wellness 'by cultivating a sense of peace and hope' which are seen as 'antidotes to depression and anxiety' (Meyers 2014). Wellness has been conceptualized as a series of evolving models and these provide a useful framework within which to explore the potential role of play as an integral feature of festivals.

The wheel of wellness

This theoretical model was devised in the early 1990s by Sweeney and Witmer (Myers and Sweeney 2005) and was the first model based in counselling theory. Founded on Adler's Individual Psychology, it utilized 'cross-disciplinary research on

228 Alison Tonkin and Shereen Jameel

characteristics of healthy people who live longer and with a higher quality of life' (wellness-research.org n.d.b). It included five *'life tasks'* that are intertwined: spirituality, self-direction, work and leisure, friendship and love. As with many theoretical models, the wheel has evolved and Myers *et al.* (2000) extended the original seven subtasks to 12. Conceptualized as a circumflex, the core of the model is spirituality, as it was considered to be of central importance for a healthy person (wellness-research.org n.d.b). Although placing spirituality at the core of the model felt intuitively right, and had universal appeal with professional counsellors, the circumflex structure was not supported by statistical analysis, and placing spirituality as the central core could not be justified relative to other factors that contribute to wellness (Myers and Sweeney 2008).

The Indivisible Self

In 2003, Sweeney and Myers proposed an alternative, evidence-based model that could be used to view wellbeing across the lifespan. *The Indivisible Self* model of wellness proposes that it is a single, higher-order, 'indivisible factor', whilst also being a factor composed of many sub-components that can be identified as contributing to holistic wellness (wellness-research.org n.d.a). There are five second-order factors that comprise the Indivisible Self and each of these has further contributory third-order, wellness dimensions, summarized in Table 19.1.

TABLE 19.1 Components of the Indivisible Self Model (adapted from Myers and Sweeney 2008)

Second-order factor	Description	Third-order factors – wellness dimensions
Creative self	The combination of attributes that make us unique in our social interactions and allow us to positively interpret our world	Thinking, emotions, control, positive humor and work
Coping self	The combination of attributes that regulate responses to life-events and help us to cope with the negative effects of these events	Realistic beliefs, stress management, self-worth and leisure
Social self	Social support through connections with others, including intimate relationships, friendships and family ties	Friendship and love
The Essential Self	Existential meaning-making process relating to life, self and others	Spirituality, self-care, gender identity and cultural identity
Physical self	Physiological and biological processes that contribute to a person's functioning and development	Exercise and nutrition

Although these have been compartmentalized within Table 19.1, it should be noted that all components interact with one another and contribute to the holistic functioning of each individual (Wellbeing research.org n.d.a).

The 'Indivisible Self' model also acknowledges the role of contextual factors which are perceived ecologically and are reciprocal in nature. Contextual factors influence the individual which, in turn, results in the individual affecting their own context (wellness-research.org n.d.a). These contexts may be local, institutional, global or time-specific, although empirical studies linked to wellness have been limited to the beneficial effect of local contexts (Myers and Sweeney 2008). Barton and Grant (2006) position the community as a key determinant of health and wellbeing within local neighbourhoods, and festivals provide a powerful reflection of the ecosystem of the local human habitat. As social events that bring communities together, festivals can alleviate stress and are positively associated with health and wellbeing, due to the collective joy that is often generated (Al Aboud 2013). Festivals, and the playful elements within festivals, can be exemplified within each of the five second-order factors from the Indivisible Self model, showing how the celebration of festivals could be utilized and promoted for the enhancement of wellbeing within and across communities.

Creative self

'The Creative Self refers to the combination of attributes that each individual forms to make a unique place among others in his or her social interactions' (Adler 1954; Ansbacher and Ansbacher 1967). The five components of the 'Creative Self' are: thinking, emotions, control, positive humor, and work. Research and clinical experience suggest that our thought processes affect the emotions as well as the body. Enrichment of the ability to think clearly and creatively can help to decrease stress and, in turn, positively affect the immune system. Creative work and creative play are important elements of human experience which can enhance our capacity to live life to the full (Wellness-research.org n.d.a). This is beautifully demonstrated in the work of Garvald Edinburgh, which is explored in Chapter 13.

Rangoli is a traditional Indian art form dating back several centuries, which can be used to exemplify the concept of the 'Creative Self'. In India, *Rangoli* represent the origin of spirituality through art. The word *rangoli* derives from Sanskrit and means 'the expression of artistic vision through the joyful use of color or design in color' (Jansari Sevak Organization UK 2002). *Rangoli* is practiced on auspicious occasions at the entrance of a household or temple (mandirs), especially during Diwali, the 'festival of light', and is hence a welcoming gesture.

In the past, *rangoli* patterns were made with rice flour and grains. The origin of this idea was to feed the ants, birds and animals as a 'good deed for the day'. Nowadays, colored powders of various bright hues are most commonly used. *Rangoli* is not only aesthetically pleasing but also fundamentally therapeutic, since the colors are imbued with different meanings. White signifies purity, coolness and safety whilst red shows strength and energy. Yellow signifies richness, green implies harmony and balance, and blue denotes vastness, happiness and peace. Orange represents sacrifice (Jansari Sevak Organization UK 2002). *Rangoli* is claimed to have a calming effect, putting one at ease and generating feelings of comfort and joy. It is regarded as more than an art form and regarded as a 'science of vibration patterns', discovered by Indians thousands of years ago. The creative art of *rangoli* can thus be seen to have the potential to boost and enhance personal and communal health and wellbeing (Guruprasad's Portal n.d).

The Edinburgh International Festival is a three-week festival of music, dance, drama and opera held in August each year. Positive humor features heavily throughout the Festival and comedy is seen as an essential element of the 'Fringe' program. However, comedy can also be a means of therapeutic release and Simmons used his 'hour of clowning' as a vehicle for anecdotes about his childhood which included revelations about abuse (Merritt 2015). This represented an opportunity for Simmons to 'accomplish even serious tasks' (Myers and Sweeney 2008) whilst also enabling an appropriate expression of *emotions*.

A research study which supports the concept of the healing potential of the 'Creative Self' was conducted by Diane Crone and colleagues at the University of Gloucestershire (Crone *et al.* 2012). Patients suffering from a variety of conditions, including anxiety, stress, depression, chronic pain, illness and bereavement were referred to a ten-week arts program that included ceramics, words, drawing, mosaic and painting. They reported improvements in mood, a sense of increased recovery and, for a short time, relief from the symptoms of chronic pain. Patients also experienced an increase in confidence, a sense of achievement, as well as a feeling of renewed hope. Clinicians felt they were provided with a holistic, non-medical alternative to prescribing medicines for patients with mental health needs and a sense that arts intervention had the potential to reduce dependency. The study highlights the benefits of offering creative arts interventions within a primary care setting (Crone *et al.* 2012).

The first Global Health Film Festival took place in 2015. The festival provided a means of communication and of sharing peoples' stories on a global scale to 'stir emotions, to inspire, to encourage action and to redress inequities in health' (The Royal Society of Medicine 2015). One of the features at the festival was *Ping Pong,* a film about eight octogenarians who wanted to compete in the Over 80s World Table Tennis Championships, providing inspiration to the older generation to get actively involved in sport and thereby encouraging 'active aging to promote physical activity, active mind and social inclusion' (The Royal Society of Medicine 2015). As a consequence of the film, originally released in 2014, *The Ping Pong Care Campaign* was founded as a national health and wellbeing initiative. The film is used as a 'motivational starter' in older person settings, to challenge issues around aging and to promote the need for older people to 'keep your body healthy, keep your mind happy [and engage in] greater social interaction' (Ping Pong 2015).

Coping self

'Leisure is essential to the "Coping self" concept of wellness' (Wellness-research. org n.d.a). According to this model, learning to become totally absorbed in an activity such that time stands still, helps the individual not only to cope with, but to transcend, life's requirements (Csíkszentmihalyi 1990). Leisure opens pathways to growth on both spiritual and creative dimensions. The 'Coping Self' is 'composed of elements that regulate our responses to life events and provide a means for transcending their negative effects' (Wellness-research.org n.d.a).

This concept is manifest in Buddhist beliefs. According to Buddhism, it is possible to take responsibility for our own states of mind – and to change them for the better. Buddhism teaches that responsibility for one's own state of mind is the antidote to the personal sorrows, anxieties and general confusions that beset the human condition. Meditation is one way in which Buddhism encourages and develops the concentration, clarity, emotional positivity, and calmness necessary for personal transformation to occur. By engaging in meditative practices, the individual can learn the patterns and habits of the mind and cultivate new, more positive, ways of thinking and being (The Buddhist Centre n.d.).

'Peace in the Park – Festival of Spirit' is an event where individuals gather together to relax, create, play and dream. This is a widely accessible public occasion when an invitation to congregate in the interests of world peace offers the benefits of meditation in an atmosphere of playful unity. Music and the spoken word serve as vehicles to a higher level of consciousness of oneself and of one's place in the world community (Peace in the Park 2014).

Social self

The 'Social Self' focuses on friendship and love. Both of these components are considered as points on a continuum and have a strong association with reported health and wellbeing (Wellness-research.org n.d.a). At one end of the continuum, strong friendships and intimate relationships are known to enhance quality of life, active support networks across the lifespan being identified as the strongest predictor of positive mental health (Wellness-research.org n.d.a). At the other extreme, loneliness, isolation and separation from family and friends cause a range of detrimental health conditions, including premature death (Wellness-research.org n.d.a). The significance of friends, family and partners can be tested at times of illness, but this is often the time when these relationships are needed most – and the time when they are commonly ignored by those responsible for healthcare services (Relate 2015). Could celebrating festivals within the context of healthcare provide an opportunity for promoting relationships and the importance of social networks, particularly for those who have limited access to meaningful relationships?

Festivals provide communities with an opportunity to come together, usually to celebrate a theme of significance to that community (Small 2007). For the

232 Alison Tonkin and Shereen Jameel

members of the community, these festivals promote opportunities for social engagement and social networking, as well as entertainment and a sense of social cohesion (Small 2007). This entertainment usually incorporates an element of play as part of the celebrations, recognizing that 'play is a powerful force that can be leveraged for a multitude of purposes' (CounterPlay 2015).

The festival of Holi is a fun-filled, Indian Spring festival known as the 'Festival of Colors'. Bright colors of *'gulal'* (powder) fill the air and people take turns in pouring colored water and spraying colors on one another with their *'pichkaris'* (water guns). Songs, dance on the rhythm of *'dholak'* (drums) and mouth-watering Holi delicacies add to the flavour of the day (Society for the Confluence of Festivals in India n.d.). The significance of dancing in groups has been studied by the University of Oxford Department of Experimental Psychology, revealing that when people synchronize their body movements to the same musical rhythm and beat, they are drawn closer together, creating a sense of 'social cohesion' (Yau 2015). Physical activity, such as dance, releases endorphins which generate feelings of social cohesion and a sense to togetherness. An added benefit of dancing noted within the study was an increased tolerance to pain, which was attributed to 'bonding' over the same music, even when the synchronized movements were not exertive (Yau 2015).

Holi has a social significance in that it helps to bring the whole community together – the rich and the poor, Hindus and non-Hindus, friends and strangers. On this one day of the year, people do not differentiate and everybody celebrates the festival together in a spirit of camaraderie. The festival of Holi exemplifies the concept of the 'Social Self' as an element of wellness, through its expression of friendship and love, the exchange of gifts, sweets and greetings helping to revitalize relationships and strengthen emotional bonds (Society for the Confluence of Festivals in India n.d.).

The essential self

The 'Essential Self' integrates the four components of spirituality, self-care, gender identity, and cultural identity. According to Mansager (cited Myers and Sweeney 2005) 'spirituality, not religiosity, has positive benefits for longevity and quality of life'. It creates a sense of meaning, purpose, and hopefulness in life. Cultural identity acts as the filter through which life experiences are interpreted and understood. Both affect our 'meaning-making processes' in relation to life, self, and others (Myers and Sweeney 2005).

A project in which cultural references were used to reduce substance use among American Indian adolescents can be used to illustrate how cultural identification can lead to improvements in health and wellbeing. The *Storytelling for Empowerment Program* emerged from a cultural approach to social problems which began in the early 1970s, whereby community elders participated in the healing of their clients using a holistic approach drawing on cultural practices (Nelson 1999, cited Sanchez-Way and Johnson 2000). A storytelling intervention which incorporated cultural symbols was used as a way of helping young people deal with the 'social, cultural, and emotional factors faced in growing up amidst poverty in a minority community'. Its aim was to increase emotional strength and self-esteem as an accessory to reduced substance use. The study found that, as exposure to the story telling intervention increased over the course of a year, the use of drugs over the following months decreased (Sanchez-Way and Johnson 2000). The research suggests that strong cultural identification makes adolescents less vulnerable to risk factors for drug use and better able to benefit from protective factors than adolescents who lack this identification. The evidence indicates that American Indian adolescents who identify with their native culture are less likely to be involved in alcohol use than those who do not (Sanchez-Way and Johnson 2000).

Festivals have long been used as a means of expressing and celebrating lesbian, gay, bisexual and transgender (LGBT) culture, incorporating a diverse range of events that include theatre, music, comedy and dance (eFestivals 2015). Gay Pride has been described as 'amazingly wonderful, visually enticing and tantalizingly bright Mardi-Gras style carnival parades that take place annually in cities around the world' (Yosef 2006). The parades have a deep significance for the LGBT community in that they have been really successful in enabling 'ordinary-looking people without elaborate costumes, gay and straight, people of all races and all ages' to relax and have fun. As a means of promoting gender and cultural identity Gay Pride provides an opportunity to celebrate the essential self that goes beyond the immediate LBGT community. Yosef (2006) summarizes his experience of attending 'Pride Weekend' in Birmingham, stating: 'To have streets crammed with so many different people all enjoying themselves and accepting each other is, to me, what Pride represents' (Yosef 2006).

According to Public Health England (2015: 5), communities are 'the building blocks for good health', forming a bedrock for the development of health and wellbeing. Recognizing the importance of peer support and the sharing of lived experience for improving health (Public Health England 2015), Fenton and Varney (2015) identify how Pride marches and LGBT festivals can 'celebrate identity and social connectedness', providing an opportunity to address identified needs of the LGBT community. With issues such as discrimination and the health inequalities associated with being a member of a social minority, festivals and marches provide a visible demonstration of how the health and wellbeing of the whole community can be promoted through peer support and positive role modelling (Fenton and Varney 2015).

Physical Self

The 'Physical Self' consists of two components: exercise and nutrition. These are widely promoted but often over-emphasized to the exclusion of other, equally important, aspects of holistic wellbeing. Research points to compelling evidence for the importance of exercise and nutrition throughout the lifespan and shows that those who live the longest attend to both exercise and diet/nutrition (Myers and Sweeney 2005).

Beekun (2011), discussing how Muslims and non-Muslims can work more effectively together, describes how 1,400 years ago, the Holy Prophet (peace be upon Him) highlighted the importance of exercise by maintaining his own physical fitness and emphasizing the desirability of optimal health and fitness. Beekun (2011) states that 'Islam's holistic approach to life and thus health, offers us the ability to remain strong and healthy'. The Prophet Muhammad (peace be upon Him) advised his followers, 'to work, to be energetic, and to start their day early, all of which are conditions for a healthy body'. According to Islamic teaching, 'obesity or an inadequate diet, laziness and weakness are all afflictions for which we will be called to account' (Stacey 2008). The prevention of illness or injury is often not under personal control, but there are some conditions which are attributable to the failure to attend to diet and fitness. In Islam, food is associated with one's relationship with God and therefore carries great significance. Islamic teaching encourages a sense of responsibility for assuming a healthy lifestyle: Chapter 20, verse 81 of the Qur'an states: 'Eat of the good and wholesome things that We have provided for your sustenance, but indulge in no excess therein'. Fasting during the holy month of Ramadan teaches Muslims to practice moderation and to seek a spiritual path. A spiritual approach to food and nutrition is one that is grateful and appreciative of the food one gets (Department of Health 2007). In the Islamic calendar, the end of the month of fasting is celebrated in the festival of Eid ul-Fitr, one of the most significant days in the Muslim calendar. Beginning with prayers and breakfast, the day is spent feasting with friends and family, celebrating with gifts and decorating the home. Whilst emphasis is on the spiritual aspect of Ramadan, the added benefits for physical health can be significant (The Week 2015).

Throughout the world, the sharing of a meal is a form of celebration in itself and most celebrations and festivals incorporate the making and sharing of foods special to the occasion. In the US, the Mediterranean diet is celebrated through National Mediterranean Diet Month as a means of promoting the 'healthful pleasures of real food' (Minor 2011). This diet, endorsed by nutritional experts, also supports health promotion and the prevention of disease. Research into the traditional Mediterranean diet has demonstrated an associated reduction in the risk of heart disease and improvements in general health (Mayo Clinic 2013). An analysis of more than 1.5 million healthy adults demonstrated that adopting a Mediterranean diet reduced the risk of death from heart disease and cancer, as well as reducing the incidence of Parkinson's and Alzheimer's diseases (Mayo Clinic 2013). The Mediterranean diet consists of eating primarily plant-based foods, such as fruits and vegetables, whole grains, legumes and nuts; replacing butter with healthy fats, such as olive oil; using herbs and spices instead of salt to flavour foods; limiting red meat to no more than a few times a month; eating fish and poultry at least twice a week and drinking red wine in moderation. Using the Mediterranean Diet Pyramid as the focus of an education program that was delivered to one million homes (Minor 2011), this healthy eating regime serves as an example of how cultural influences can be celebrated, whilst promoting health benefits that can last a lifetime.

Conclusion

Public Health England (2015) have clearly identified the significance of using a community-based approach to health and wellbeing, utilizing the social networks, skills and community specific knowledge that are the foundations of good health. Festivals are a celebration of cultural identity that can be capitalized upon to encourage social cohesion, tolerance and diversity, using play as a means of engagement and fun. Healthcare providers could take advantage of the social nature of festivals, such as the potential for bringing people together, strengthening social relationships and facilitating the sharing of life experiences. Festivals represent a holistic approach to wellbeing with primary and secondary benefits for individuals, communities and society as a whole. As noted by Binder (2015): 'festivals promote diversity, they bring neighbours into dialogue, they increase creativity, they offer opportunities for civic pride, they improve our general psychological wellbeing. In short, they make cities better places to live' (Binder 2015).

References

Adler, A. (1954) *Understanding human nature,* New York: Fawcett Premier.

Al Aboud, K. (2013) Health hazards linked to festivals: an overview, *Journal of Public Health in Africa,* 4: e15.

Ansbacher, H. L. and Ansbacher, R. R. (1967) *The Individual Psychology of Alfred Adler: A systematic presentation in selections from his writings.* New York: Harper & Row.

Barton, H. and Grant, M. (2006) A health map for the local human habitat, *The Journal of the Royal Society for the Promotion of Health,* 126 (6): 252–253.

Beekun, R. (2011) Follow the sunna of the prophet (s): how exercise benefits the brain and overall performance, *The Muslim Workplace.* 1 December 2011. Online. Available at http://theislamicworkplace.com/2011/12/01/follow-the-sunna-of-the-prophet-s-how-exercise-benefits-the-brain-and-overall-performance/#comments (accessed 16 August 2015).

Binder, D. (2015) *David Binder Quotes,* Online. Available at www.brainyquote.com/quotes/authors/d/david_binder.html (accessed 3 December 2015).

Cambridge University Press (2015) *Festival,* Online. Available at http://dictionary.cambridge.org/dictionary/british/festival (accessed 28 July 2015).

CounterPlay (2015) *CounterPlay' 15,* Online. Available at www.counterplay.org/playful-organisations/ (accessed 28 July 2015).

Crone, D.M., O'Connell, E.E., Tyson, P.J., Clark-Stone, F., Opher, S. and James, D.V.B. (2012) 'It helps me make sense of the world': the role of an art intervention for promoting health and wellbeing in primary care – perspectives of patients, health professionals and artists, *Journal of Public Health,* 20 (5): 519–524.

Csíkszentmihalyi, M. (1990) *Flow: The Psychology of Optimal Experience.* New York: Harper and Row.

Department of Health (2007) *Ramadhan Health Guide – A Guide to Healthy fasting,* Online. Available at https://www2.warwick.ac.uk/services/equalops/resources/a_guide_to_healthy_fasting.pdf (accessed 29 November 2015).

eFestivals (2015) *Pride Events,* Online. Available at www.efestivals.co.uk/festivals/pride/ (accessed 2 December 2015).

Fenton, K. and Varney, J. (2015) LGB&T health – celebrating with pride, *Public Health Matters*, 26 June 2015 Online. Available at https://publichealthmatters.blog.gov.uk/2015/06/26/lgbt-health-celebrating-with-pride/ (accessed 3 December 2015).

Guruprasad's Portal (n.d.) *Why do Indians Draw Rangoli? Scientific Reason*, Online. Available at http://guruprasad.net/posts/why-do-indians-draw-rangoli-scientific-reason/ (accessed 2 December 2015).

Hat Tours (2012) *Festivals*, Online. Available at www.hattours.com/blog/festivals-2/ (accessed: 3 December 2015).

Jansari Sevak Organisation UK (2002) *Hindu Culture: Rangoli*, Online. Available at http://jansarisevak.org.uk/HinduCultureRangoli.htm (accessed 29 July 2015).

Kreuter, M.W. and McClure, S.M. (2004) The role of culture in health communication, *Annual Review of Public Health*, 25: 439–455.

Mayo Clinic (2013) *Mediterranean Diet: A Heart-healthy Eating Plan*, Online. Available at www.mayoclinic.org/healthy-lifestyle/nutrition-and-healthy-eating/in-depth/mediter-ranean-diet/art-20047801?pg=1 (accessed 28 November 2015).

Merritt, S. (2015) Edinburgh festival 2015 comedy review – heckling iPods, improve ballads and feminist rap, *The Observer*, 16 August 2015 Online. Available at www.theguardian.com (accessed 16 August 2015).

Meyers, L. (2014) *In Search of Wellness*, Online. Available at http://ct.counseling.org/2014/02/in-search-of-wellness/ (accessed 3 December 2015).

Minor, L. (2011) Celebrating Mediterranean diet month. *Examiner.com*, 20 May 2011, Online. Available at www.examiner.com/article/celebrating-mediterranean-diet-month (accessed 3 December 2015).

Myers, J. and Sweeney, T. (2005) The indivisible self: an evidence-based model of wellness, *The Journal of Individual Psychology*, 61 (3): 269.

Myers, J. and Sweeney, T. (2008) Wellness counselling: The evidence base for practice, *Journal for Counseling and Development*, 86 (3): 482–493.

Myers, J., Sweeney, T. and Witmer, J.M. (2000) The wheel of wellness counseling for wellness: a holistic model for treatment planning, *Journal of Counseling and Development*, 78 (3) 251–266.

Peace in the Park (2014) *Peace in the Park – Festival of Spirit*, Online. Available at www.peace intheparkfestival.org/ Accessed:28 July 2015

Ping Pong (2015) *About the Campaign*, Online. Available at http://pingpongfilm.co.uk/campaign (accessed 2 December 2015).

Playful Arts Festival (2015) *Playful Arts Festival*, Online. Available at http://playfularts-festival.com/ (accessed 15 August 2015).

Public Health England (2015) *A Guide to Community-centred Approaches for Health and Wellbeing: Full Report*, London: Public Health England.

Relate (2015) *The Best Medicine: Putting Relationships at the Heart of the NHS*, Online. Available at www.relate.org.uk/policy-campaigns/our-campaigns/best-medicine (accessed 2 December 2015).

Sanchez-Way, R. and Johnson, S. (2000) *Cultural Practices in American Indian Prevention Programs*, Online. Available at www.ncjrs.gov/html/ojjdp/jjnl_2000_12/cult.html (accessed 28 November 2015).

Small, K. (2007) Understanding the social impacts of festivals on communities, Unpublished PhD thesis, Western Sydney University.

Society for the Confluence of Festivals in India (SCFI) (n.d) *Holi Festival*, Online. Available at www.holifestival.org/holi-festival.html (accessed 2 December 2015).

Society for the Confluence of Festivals in India (n.d) *Significance of Holi*. Online. Available at www.holifestival.org/significance-of-holi.html (accessed 28 July 2015).

Stacey, A. (2008) *Health in Islam (part 4 of 4): Fitness and Exercise,* Online. Available at www.islamreligion.com/articles/1904/health-in-islam-part-4/ (accessed 13 November 2015).

Target Study (2015) *Importance of Festivals in Life,* Online. Available at https://targetstudy.com/articles/importance-of-festivals-in-life.html (accessed 3 December 2015).

The Buddhist Centre (n.d*.) What is Meditation?* Online. Available at https://thebuddhist-centre.com/text/what-meditation (accessed 28 July 2015).

The Royal Society of Medicine (2015) *Global Health Film Festival,* Online. Available at www.rsm.ac.uk/events/events-listing/2015-2016/groups/global-health/ghg01-global-health-film-festival.aspx (accessed 2 December 2015).

The Week (2015) Ramadan 2015: when does it end and tips for fasting, *The Week,* 13 July 2015, Online. Available at www.theweek.co.uk/ (accessed 3 December 2015).

wellness-research.org (n.d.a) *Wellness,* Online. Available at http://wellness-research.org/wellness/docs/wellness.htm (accessed 10 July 2015).

wellness-research.org (n.d.b) *The Wheel of Wellness: A Theoretical Model and the Wellness Evaluation of Lifestyle,* Online. Available at http://wellness-research.org/wellness/docs/wheel.html (accessed 15 August 2015).

Yau, J. (2015) Study reveals dancing in groups is good for your health. *YourEDM*, 5 November 2015, Online. Available at www.youredm.com/ (accessed 2 December 2015).

Yosef, A. (2006) *Pride – The real rainbow,* Online. Available at www.bbc.co.uk/birmingham/content/articles/2005/06/02/pride_the_real_rainbow_gay_village_feature.shtml (accessed 3 December 2015).

20

PLAYING FOR SPIRITUAL HEALTH

Catherine Hubbuck

This chapter aims to explore the intersection of spirituality and everyday human life. It will consider the impact of ill-health upon an individual's sense of spiritual wellbeing and how those involved in healthcare might recognize and respond to the spiritual needs of their patients. It will also consider the ways in which the experience of play may enhance or encourage spiritual growth and wellbeing. The discussion will specifically address the question of whether the use of therapeutic play techniques – such as those traditionally employed by Health Play Specialists (HPS) – may be used to uphold and safeguard the personal spirituality of adult patients within a variety of healthcare settings.

Introduction

There appears to be an innate drive within people to understand the essence of life, to achieve a state of wholeness and to find a sense of belonging and connectedness (Mental Health Foundation 2015). To describe this drive as 'innate' may jar with some readers – particularly with those who choose not to engage with any form of religious or spiritual belief or expression. However, the underlying premise of this chapter is that human beings appear to have been born with 'an inbuilt spiritual awareness' (Hay and Nye 2006) and that there is a spiritual aspect to all human experience. Upholding and prioritizing the expression and exploration of this spiritual dimension of life, as a basic human need and as a universal human right (United Nations 1948), is at the heart of this discussion.

Defining 'spirituality'

Any attempt to define what is meant and understood by the term 'spirituality' must respond to the challenge that spirituality means different things to different people who, in turn, express their spirituality in many and varied ways (Mental Health Foundation 2015). There runs the risk that the term 'spirituality', and an individual's choice to follow or identify with a certain religious system, are understood to be one and the same thing. It is important to separate the two concepts (spirituality and religion) and to accept that, whilst spirituality or a spiritual awareness may be inherent in all human beings (Hay 2007), the decision to express and explore this aspect through a particular faith system is a choice made by some individuals but certainly not by all.

The desire to provide a definition of something that is, by its nature, indefinable runs the risk of falling short in its intention to encompass all that is meaningful to all those for whom it holds significance. However, in the broadest sense, the term 'spirituality' can refer to the exploration by an individual of their own core identity – their essential humanity – and their desire to gain both an understanding *of* the world and of their place *within* the world (Hay 2007).

Defining 'play'

The value of play has been accepted as central to the facilitation of both practical skills and conceptual learning since the time of the ancient Greek philosophers, Plato and Aristotle (D'Anjour 2013). Children's play has been the subject of intense theoretical and practical study, particularly during the twentieth century. However, despite many and various historical attempts to study, theorize and gain an understanding of play and its role in development, there is a widespread consensus that it is virtually impossible to provide a concise definition of why human beings play (Hubbuck 2009). Despite an established understanding that play has multiple functions and that it underpins all aspects of development, there is still no concise or adequate definition that neatly conveys the depth and value of play.

Play, like spirituality, is experienced in many different ways. Its meaning differs, both in terms of the language used to describe the nature of play and in terms of the actual experience of playing. However, one definition that is widely accepted within the field of playwork is that 'play' refers to activities that are 'freely chosen, personally directed and intrinsically motivated' (Hughes 1982 cited in Hughes 2001). Given that the present discussion shifts the focus of play from child development to a consideration of the value of play throughout the lifespan, Hughes' definition, being non-specific to the age, location or state of the player, continues to provide a sound basis for how we think about the place of play through the life-cycle.

For the purposes of this chapter, the term 'play' is understood as encompassing an endless array of pleasurable, stimulating activities, undertaken with the potential for enjoyment by people of all ages. Play, in its many forms, allows those participating – the players – to engage in familiar activities, to acquire skills or to explore new challenges, to play alone or alongside others. Furthermore, by means of engaging with the enjoyment or challenge of playful tasks at a deep level – a psychological state known as 'flow' (Csíkszentmihalyi 1996 cited in Bateson and

240 Catherine Hubbuck

Martin 2013) – players may be enabled to experience or explore ways of understanding themselves or the world at a similarly deep level from within the safe familiarity of a task or environment. This is demonstrated in the case example in Box 20.1.

BOX 20.1 THE USE OF LEGO PLAY TO FACILITATE SAFE EXPLORATION OF FEELINGS THAT CANNOT BE EXPRESSED

At the age of 22 years, and nearing the completion of his degree in engineering, Paul experienced an episode of very deep, very bleak depression. Feeling unable to complete his studies, he left his university accommodation and returned to his childhood home and to the care of his parents. The state of his mental health left him almost unable to function or communicate about even ordinary everyday matters, let alone the depth of his current feelings of despair. He began a course of medication but hardly left his bedroom and his parents feared he was on the brink of a breakdown. One evening, an old school-friend from primary school paid Paul an unannounced visit. James brought with him a large box of Lego pieces and, over the course of the evening, the two friends sat and built models, broke them up, built more. During this activity, hardly a word passed between Paul and his childhood companion, yet his parents later reflected that during that evening they felt that Paul was the most relaxed he had been in months. In the weeks that followed, Paul's depression lifted sufficiently for him to speak to his parents about the struggles he had been experiencing and he agreed to see a counsellor. Paul later reflected that the evening spent building Lego models with James had provided him with a connection to a safe, happy point in his life. That evening proved to be the point from which he began to make sense of his near-overwhelming depression, which enabled him to return to his studies, graduating, a year later than his peers, with his degree.

Spirituality can be conceived, in broad terms, as a search or desire for wholeness and an understanding of oneself. Furthermore, key to spirituality is a need, a concern, or a longing to be connected to things, people or 'something more' than oneself – to live in community with others, in appreciation of one's surroundings and in acceptance of something transcendent, whether that is experienced as 'God' or as a mystery (Mental Health Foundation 2015). The search for understanding and for a feeling of connectedness which underpins the concept of spirituality reflects similar themes to those emerging from play theory. Play Scotland (2015) advocates the importance of play in these terms, stating 'it is through play that children understand each other and make sense of the world around them'.

Could it be that play and spirituality share a common core in their motivation for an understanding of the human predicament?

In seeking to consider both the importance of personal spirituality in the context of health and wellbeing *and* the ways that play can respond to a deep personal need for both pleasure and connection, this chapter is, in effect, an attempt to bring together two of the most indefinable and highly personal aspects of human experience. The value of both play and personal spirituality are practically impossible to measure in terms of beneficial outcomes from the perspective of the casual or external observer. The experience of connection with something beyond the self (whether that is God, a 'higher power', awe and wonder, or social bonding), like the pleasure or satisfaction that can be derived from playful activity, has a value in that it holds deep personal meaning for the individual. Both play and spirituality represent something different and personal for each individual, even when they arise from the same shared experiences, activities, and environment. No two individuals will receive, react or respond identically to an experience or set of circumstances but this does not diminish the significance of either concept to human development and wellbeing throughout the lifespan.

Healthcare: body, mind and spirit?

One difficulty with considering spirituality and the spiritual life of individuals within the context of modern healthcare is that 'conversations between spirituality and healthcare are conducted largely on healthcare terms' (Rumbold 2012). The western approach to healthcare is often dominated by a 'medical' or 'bio-medical' approach which is based on facts, knowledge and an aim to cure illness as the only perceived path to 'good health' (Finston 2015). The medical model does not encourage, or allow for, consideration of spiritual matters and regards these as a personal concern, external to the patient's physical condition and irrelevant to health-related discussion. In contrast, the rising popularity of social and bio-social models of health and illness (Rumbold 2012) hold other aspects of human life in higher regard and are more likely to recognize the important place of spirituality in the lives of some individuals and communities. As discussed in Chapter 17, the western approach to medicine has seen the divergence of mind and body as a unified system for at least the last century (Mantri 2008). Eastern and alternative approaches to health and wellness, however, have always advocated and acknowledged the need to consider each individual's emotional state alongside physical manifestations of illness or injury. With the advent of more 'person centred care' that reflects the spiritual needs of the individual for enhancing resilience and developing inner strength at difficult times, spirituality has acquired a more important role in healthcare (NHS Education for Scotland n.d.). Therefore, whilst the language of healthcare is still often focused on the physical state of health and the medicinal treatment of illness (Finston 2015), there is a gradual and continuing acceptance of the need to consider and uphold the social, emotional and spiritual needs of all those coming into contact with healthcare services.

It is worth noting that this recognition of the holistic needs of patients and others is taking place during a period of secularization and an apparent move away

242 Catherine Hubbuck

from organized religion in the main. This demands a certain boldness on the part of those advocating a place for spirituality in healthcare, if they are to retain legitimacy and kudos in an arena where the language of 'healthcare has the dominant voice' (Rumbold 2012).

Illness, healthcare environments and spiritual wellbeing

Early interest in the healthcare experiences of children identified 'two main dangers' – areas of vulnerability – as having the potential to affect a child's well-being in both the short- and long-term (Robertson 1958). These were classified as 'the traumatic' and 'the deprivational' and referred, in the first instance, to the challenges faced by children during a period of illness or hospital treatment and, in the second, to the effects of separation – specifically separation from the child's mother. Whilst much has been done to aid and ease children's experiences within healthcare settings, it is acknowledged that the risk of these two distinct 'danger areas' still exists (Care Quality Commission 2015; Vilas 2014; Tonkin 2014). It is valid to question whether these same potential risks or 'dangers' also apply to adults at the interface with modern healthcare systems.

The *traumatic* effects of being injured or becoming ill, or the experience of living with a chronic condition, will undeniably have an impact on a person's understanding of 'the self'. This relates to one's sense of self in the present, the past or the future, leading to either a crisis, a reconsideration, or an integration of a new set of circumstances (Falvo 2014; Kearney and Weininger 2012). Illness may lead to all three of these processes either partially, wholly, or in combination; clearly not everyone meets and responds to pain, sickness and suffering in the same way and 'for some, they're the making of character; for others its destruction' (Boyd 1980 cited Willows and Swinton 2000).

First-hand accounts offer the most affecting insight into the traumatic effects of illness and to their impact on a sense of self. In *The Diving Bell and the Butterfly*, Jean-Dominique Bauby, a French journalist who was almost totally paralysed by a catastrophic stroke, wrote of his experience of 'Locked-in Syndrome'. Bauby (1998) produced his memoir using eye-blinking in response to a sequence of letters being read to him. He tells of the agony, grief, bewilderment, frustration, and occasionally the macabre hilarity, of his experience of an altered state and of his attempts to re-establish who he is 'in himself' after his brain injury.

The *deprivational* effects of illness, disability or impairment, hospitalization, and eventual recovery or rehabilitation can be understood in terms of the impact of the resultant separations on an individual's sense of connectedness – to others and to the external world. Deprivation of faith practices and expressions of worship will represent both a personal loss and disconnection as well as a possible detachment from a cultural or national identity. Spiritual wholeness may be recovered in the physical space found in a place of worship as well as through the sense of community found therein. In secular life, reintegration and re-discovery of the self may take place in the home or workplace or anywhere there is space for the

Playing for spiritual health **243**

expression of shared interests, views, creativity or concern for each other's needs. The value of recognizing the celebration of festivals as a means of enabling this to happen is discussed in Chapter 19. Festivals often contain a spiritual element and Chapter 19 includes examples of how play and playfulness can provide focus and contribute to a mood of celebration, as well as how they provide a vehicle for conversation and opportunities to bring people together.

Memoirs can be equally insightful in their descriptions of the deprivational effects of illness on spiritual wellbeing and of the means by which individuals have understood and overcome these effects through their attempts to reconnect with their friends, family and beyond. Playful aspects appear to be helpful in providing a way back to reconnection in difficult circumstances. In a frank account of her experience of treatment for cancer, American playwright, author and activist Eve Ensler tells how, between undergoing surgery and commencing chemotherapy, she had an urge to paint and create. This had never been an activity she had enjoyed given that she perceived herself to be 'completely devoid of talent' (Ensler 2013). However, during the period of convalescence after surgery she would invite visitors to join her at the dining room table to draw or paint something. Fractured social connections were restored by this shared activity, despite some initial dismay on the part of her guests:

> 'People who came to visit were awkward. What was there to say? Right away I would ask them to draw or paint something with me. It worked like a charm. The idea of making art often traumatized them more than my cancer did ... They would start off grudgingly and terrified, but then they would get into it. I began to love this new way of communicating. My friends would sit by me and we would create together. It was quiet and communal. We were children. People began to paint images of my healing. Well, I asked them to.'
>
> *(Ensler 2013)*

Play and holistic care provision in healthcare

Within pediatric settings, qualified and registered Health Play Specialists (HPS) are employed to help children and young people manage the effects of illness and hospitalization. The role of the play specialist, working as part of the multidisciplinary team, is crucial to alleviating the potential distress and anxiety that can be associated with a healthcare experience. Creating and maintaining a space for play, the HPS aims to create a relationship of trust, a meaningful attachment by which the child can be helped to make sense of all they encounter in the strange new world of illness and its treatment.

The role of the HPS can be defined in terms of two main goals: to support optimal development and to facilitate positive coping in the face of challenging circumstances (Munn 2014). The healthcare play practitioner promotes the value of play and playfulness for the facilitation of making and maintaining connections – a central feature of a sense of personal spirituality.

A commitment to holistic care (which specifically includes the personal spirituality of all patients) is upheld by multi-faith chaplaincy services that are widely available throughout the NHS. Chaplains are professional staff, 'qualified and contracted to supply spiritual, religious and pastoral care to patients, service users, carers and staff' (Swift *et al.* 2015). In many cases, chaplaincy services are available 24 hours a day, seven days a week and respond to requests for support and input into patient care 'across the full range of clinical areas' (Swift 2015 *et al.*). Multi-faith chaplaincy services are available to those of all faiths and none and hospital chaplains will attend to anyone requesting their support.

It could be said that the services offered by Health Play Specialists and by chaplaincy services work in similar ways to enable individual patients to engage in activities that could be said to address their spiritual needs. Whilst these activities vary according to how much an individual seeks to explore or strengthen their personal faith or spirituality, the key is that help is available to enable patients to access whatever enhances their own sense of spiritual wellbeing. This process might include maintaining a sense of belonging to a faith tradition and taking part in rituals or symbolic acts of worship, reading or listening to scripture, engaging in prayer or meditation, disciplined reflective practices such as yoga, or simply spending time in nature. Other, more obviously play-based strategies, might include appreciation of the arts or participation in a creative endeavour or simply having the opportunity to socialize with other people (Royal College of Psychologists 2015).

At this point in the twenty-first century, there is a renewed acknowledgement that adults need to play and that, rather than detracting from the 'serious work' associated with maturity, playfulness and engaging in play activities actually enhance productivity, focus and mood (Brown 2010). Play in adulthood allows for a continuation of the exploration that begins and runs throughout childhood, – that of the self, of connections made with other people and, for some, with a higher power, a purpose in life or with God.

The Scout Association is the largest youth movement in the world and encouraging the spiritual development of its members is a principal aim (The Scout Association 2015). Stating that 'spiritual development is real [and] it is a step to being fully alive as a human being', the Scout Association (1996) has identified five principles that can facilitate spiritual development, all of which relate to everyday life. These principles are:

1   Develop an inner discipline and training
2   Be involved in corporate activities with others
3   Understand the world around them
4   Help to create a more tolerant and caring society
5   Discover the need for spiritual reflection (The Scout Association 2015).

Recognizing the need for caution when broaching such a personal and sensitive subject as spirituality in diverse communities, The Scout Association (2014: 28) has produced detailed guidance on how these five principles can be incorporated into the scouting program. A central theme of the guidance is the need to provide an appropriate environment that allows young people to 'reflect on life and the world around them'. These principles reflect the concept of spiritual healthcare as defined by the Royal College of Psychiatrists (2015), particularly in relation to finding meaning in life and to the importance of relationships. This refers, not only to the development of meaningful relationships with other people, but also to a connection with creation and nature. Play can facilitate both these aspects of spiritual exploration from the safety of a familiar platform.

What appears to be at the core of play in healthcare, and also central to the spiritual wellbeing of individuals, is the notion of 'exploring and making meaning' at times of challenge and struggle brought about by illness, hospitalization and having to accept one's own vulnerability or mortality.

Health Play Specialists (HPS) engage patients in activities that may help them to achieve an understanding of what has happened to them, what will be happening in the course of their treatment and, in many cases, what may happen to them in the future, with positive implications for their life-long development. In addition to the provision of free-play activities, this aspect of their work may be described as having an educational rather than purely exploratory purpose. Preparation and education resources used to help young patients understand what is happening to them, could find their counterparts in adult healthcare as a way of sharing health-related information with adults with a range of needs and capabilities. However, sometimes illness prompts a need to explore life's bigger questions (Nash *et al.* 2015). There may be a need or desire on the part of a patient to explore their personal circumstances, their state of health and perhaps some aspects of their spiritual life in relation to these. By establishing a relationship of trust with his or her patients, the HPS is in a strong position to assist the patient in this process. By being open-ended, creative and pleasurable, play in itself presents many unbounded possibilities as a medium for this exploration (Hubbuck 2009).

Traditional methods of preparation for treatment have been developed through the concept of *Co-creating Meaning* (Vilas *et al.* 2014). This is based in part on Victor Frankl's observation that coping in the face of stressful, even overwhelmingly traumatic circumstances, depends on 'the discernment of meaning and purpose' within an individual's life experiences and current circumstances and its integration into their 'mental maps' (McGrath 2012). It is interesting to note that Frankl's central concept, referred to as 'will to meaning', lent itself to the initial conceptualization of spirituality – that of 'meaning-centred' contexts for a more holistic approach to care (Davie and Percy 2012). It is this notion of meaning-centred care which laid the foundation for Dame Cicely Saunders' hospice movement.

Co-creating Meaning is an idea that relies on more open-ended, self-directed play and the use of 'loose parts', which is the term used to describe play materials that can be moved, carried, combined, redesigned, lined up, and taken apart and put

246 Catherine Hubbuck

back together in multiple ways (Kable 2010). Such materials, when used in play, empower creativity (Nicholson 1972) by virtue of having no specific set of directions. The exploration of abstract concepts is enabled by these somewhat 'unformed' playthings that can be used alone or combined with other materials. Within the field of play therapy it is acknowledged that play provides a safe space within which experimentation – with actual, tangible 'things' or with difficult or complicated concepts or relationships – can safely take place and new meaning can be created (Cattanach 2003). When this type of open-ended, creative play can be facilitated in a healthcare setting, play interventions can help to deepen a person's understanding of his or her own circumstances and to facilitate the integration of meaning into the implications of their immediate and longer-term health needs. The therapeutic play practitioner and patient may work together in an act of creativity (of a model, a representation, or a picture) that facilitates the exploration of a complex diagnosis, a confusing concept or an emotionally-charged set of circumstances from within the safe parameters of play. This creative process can be helpful to the individual in grasping, examining and understanding the circumstances they currently inhabit. It may also represent a safe means by which to process the life events (practical, physiological or spiritual) which have led up the present moment and to consider where the path of life may lead in the future.

Co-creating meaning seeks to 'empower the child [or patient of any age] to make his own meaning out of [their] diagnosis and treatment, as opposed to passively taking on an interpretation of [their] experience' by an appointed professional (Vilas 2014). Interactions of this kind may well 'create spaces, so that [an individual] may reveal something of their inner (spiritual) life' (Nash *et al.* 2015). To a greater or lesser extent this could also be said to be the role of the hospital chaplain or visiting faith leader, or indeed of any healthcare professional recognizing and seeking to support the spiritual needs of their patient. The role of pastor, when undertaken responsibly and sensitively, is not to tell people what to believe or how to conduct themselves, but rather to enable spiritual growth – through conversations, active listening and the facilitation (if sought) of worship or prayer (Lyall 2001). In this way, the roles of the facilitator of play and the facilitator of spiritual growth might be regarded as complementing one another.

Conclusion

Since the value of play and of personal spirituality sit so closely together with regard to their contribution to human development and wholeness, the provision of play within healthcare settings can undoubtedly enhance and support the spiritual wellbeing of all people, whatever their circumstance, condition, age or ability. The study of children has established that play is a powerful space for the exploration and consolidation of complex information. At a time of growing interest amongst adults in concepts such as mindfulness, it might reasonably be suggested that the provision of play in *adult* healthcare settings could offer equivalent benefits. Introducing tried-and-tested therapeutic play techniques, and a general encouragement of playfulness in the course of everyday interactions, could have a significant impact on efforts to address, to meet, and to uphold the spiritual needs of everyone involved in either using or delivering healthcare services.

References

Bateson, P. and Martin, P. (2013) *Play, Playfulness, Creativity and Innovation*, Cambridge: Cambridge University Press.

Bauby, J. (1998) *The Diving Bell and the Butterfly*, London: Fourth Estate.

Brown, S. (2010) *Play: How it Shapes the Brain, Opens the Imagination and Invigorates the Soul*, New York: Avery.

Care Quality Commission (2015) *Regulation 12: Safe Care and Treatment*, Online. Available at www.cqc.org.uk/content/regulation-12-safe-care-and-treatment#full-regulation (accessed 3 December 2015).

Cattanach, A. (2003) *Introduction to Play Therapy*, Brunner-Routledge.

D'Anjour, A. (2013) Plato and play: taking education seriously in Ancient Greece, *American Journal of Play*, 5 (3): 293– 307.

Davey, G. and Percy, M. (2012) The future of religion, in Cobb, M., Puchalski, C.M. and Rumbold, B. (eds), *Oxford Textbook of Spirituality in Healthcare*, Oxford: Oxford University Press: 481–486.

Ensler, E. (2013) *In the Body of the World: A Memoir of Cancer and Connection*, New York: Picador.

Falvo, D. (2014) *Medical and Psychosocial Aspects of Chronic Illness and Disability*, 5th ed., Burlington, MA: Jones and Barlett Learning.

Finston, P. (2015) *Why are Eastern and Western Treatments so Different?* Online. Available at http://acu-psychiatry.com/what-is-world-medical-wisdom/basic-differences-between-eastern-and-western-medicine/ (accessed 27 November 2015).

Hay, D. (2007) *Why Spirituality is Difficult for Westerners*, Exeter: Imprint Academic.

Hay, D. and Nye, R. (2006) *The Spirit of the Child*, London: Jessica Kingsley Publishers.

Hubbuck, C. (2009) *Play for Sick Children: Play Specialists in Hospital and Beyond*, London: Jessica Kingsley Publishers.

Hughes, B. (2001) *Evolutionary Playwork and Reflective Analytic Practice*, London: Routledge.

Kable, J. (2010) Theory of loose parts, *Let the children play*, 10 February 2010, Online. Available at www.letthechildrenplay.net/2010/01/how-children-use-outdoor-play-spaces.html (accessed 6 December 2015).

Kearney, M. and Weininger, R. (2012) Care of the soul, in Cobb, M., Puchalski, C.M. and Rumbold, B. (eds), *Oxford Textbook of Spirituality in Healthcare*, Oxford: Oxford University Press: 273– 278.

Lyall, D. (2001) *The Integrity of Pastoral Care*, London. Society for Promoting Christian Knowledge.

Mantri, S. (2008) Holistic medicine and the Western medical tradition, *AMA Journal of Ethics*, 10 (3): 177– 180.

McGrath, A. (2012) Christianity, in Cobb, M., Puchalski, C.M. and Rumbold, B. (eds), *Oxford Textbook of Spirituality in Healthcare*, Oxford: Oxford University Press: 25–30.

Mental Health Foundation (2015) *Spirituality*, Online. Available at www.mentalhealth.org.uk/help-information/mental-health-a-z/S/spirituality/ (accessed 6 December 2015).

Munn, E. (2014) Play with infants and toddlers: building coping capacities, *Child Life Council Bulletin*, 32 (1): 8– 9.

248 Catherine Hubbuck

Nash, P., Darby, K. and Nash, S. (2015) *Spiritual Care with Sick Children and Young People*, London: Jessica Kingsley Publishers.

NHS Education for Scotland (n.d.) *Spiritiual Care,* Online. Available at www.nes.scot. nhs.uk/education-and-training/by-discipline/spiritual-care.aspx (accessed 11 December 2015).

Nicholson, S. (1972) The theory of loose parts – an important principle for design methodology, *Home* 4 (2): 5–14.

Play Scotland (2015) *What is Play?* Online. Available at www.playscotland.org/what-is-play-playwork/what-is-play/ (accessed 11 December 2015).

Robertson, J. (1958) *Young Children in Hospital*, London: Tavistock Publications.

Royal College of Psychiatrists (2015) *Spirituality and Mental Health*, Online. Available at www.rcpsych.ac.uk/mentalhealthinfo/treatments/spirituality.aspx (accessed 27 November 2015).

Rumbold, B. (2012) Models of spiritual care, in, Cobb, M., Puchalski, C.M. and Rumbold, B. (eds), *Oxford Textbook of Spirituality in Healthcare*, Oxford: Oxford University Press: 177– 183.

Swift, C. in consultation with the Chaplaincy Leaders Forum (CLF) and the National Equality and Health Inequalities Team, NHS England (2015) *NHS Chaplaincy Guidelines 2015– Promoting Excellence in Pastoral, Spiritual and Religious Care,* London: NHS England.

The Scout Association (2014) *Rise to the Challenge: Exploring Spiritual Development in Scouting*, Chingford: The Scout Association.

The Scout Association (1996) *What is Spiritual Development? Fact Sheet 322021,* Online. Available at http://members.scouts.org.uk/documents/AdultSupport/AdultNetwork/fs322021.pdf (accessed 11 December 2015).

The Scout Association (2015) *Faith and Spiritual Development,* Online. Available at https://members.scouts.org.uk/supportresources/3136/faith-and-spiritual-development (accessed 11 December 2015).

Tonkin, A. (2014) *The Provision of Play in Health Service Delivery – Fulfilling Children's Rights under Article 31 of the United Nations Convention on the Rights of the Child. A Literature Review*, National Association of Health Play Specialists.

United Nations (1948) *Universal Declaration of Human Rights,* Online. Available at www.un.org/en/universal-declaration-human-rights/index.html (accessed 14 July 2015).

Vilas, D. (2014) Playing for the child who cannot play, *Child Life Council Bulletin*, 32 (3): 5, 10.

Vilas, D., Koch, C. and Passmore, L (2014) Co-creating meaning: loose parts in the 7th Dimension, *Child Life Council Bulletin,* 32 (1): 4–5.

Willows, D. and Swinton J. (eds) (2000) *Spiritual Dimensions of Pastoral Care*, London: Jessica Kingsley Publishers Ltd.

21

USING PLAY FOR LIFELONG LEARNING

Jeremy Weldon and Claire Weldon

The opportunity for play is as important for health-givers as for those they work with. This chapter is about enabling health-givers to acknowledge their own need to play and to find ways of incorporating play in their continuing professional development as a means of reducing stress and work-related burn-out.

Introduction

Play and playful activities can be used to enrich the continuing professional development of those working in healthcare with consequent positive implications for the patient experience. Recognizing play and playful activities as both a human need and a natural tendency offers a new perspective on the challenges inherent in work-related learning. The word 'play' often leads to misconceptions due to the widespread belief that play is only for children or that playing is easy. However, adults 'tend to engage in unusually challenging and difficult activities when we play, such as sports, music, hobbies and games like chess' (Csíkszentmihalyi 1990, cited in Rieber 1996). Learning in healthcare and continuing professional development can be anything but playful. This chapter will include case studies, from around the world, of innovative play-based learning and provides suggestions for a 'tool-kit' for optimizing learning through play.

The problem and possible solutions

Workplace stress is an issue in many work contexts and is reflected in high rates of sickness absence. According to the Health and Safety Executive (n.d.) 'the total number of cases of work-related stress, depression or anxiety in 2014/15 was 440,000'. This is equivalent to 9.9 million working days lost, averaging 23 days per case. The occupations reporting the highest number of stress-related cases were health professionals, health and social care associate professionals and teaching and education professionals. NHS Staff Survey results showed significant and disappointing health and wellbeing results (NHS Staff Survey 2014). Only 43 per cent of respondents said that their organizations took positive action on health and wellbeing. Of particular concern is the fact that 65 per cent of staff said they had attended work in the last three months despite not being well enough to perform their duties, although this proportion had reduced in comparison to the previous year. Work-related illness was another worrying factor, with 39 per cent of staff reporting having felt unwell in the preceding 12 months as a result of work stress.

In 2009 an independent review was commissioned by the Department of Health to investigate the health and wellbeing of its staff. The central finding of this review was the significance of the connections between staff health and wellbeing, productivity, and the quality of services provided to patients (Boorman 2009). It is estimated that a reduction in NHS staff sickness absence by one-third would increase the number of NHS staff days available by 3.4 million, the equivalent of 14,900 full-time staff, with an estimated cost saving of £555 million (Boorman 2009).

Caregiver wellbeing and patient experience

In 2011 the Department of Health produced the document *Healthy Staff, Better Care for Patients*. This promoted the idea that a healthy workforce is a pre-requisite of 'safe, effective and efficient patient care' (Department of Health 2011).

Patient experience is taken as a valuable indicator of quality in the assessment of healthcare services, which are increasingly being scrutinized. Perhaps less well recognized or examined is the link between caregiver wellbeing and the experience of patients. An examination of different areas of healthcare systems can help increase understanding of some of the unique effects that good or poor caregiver wellbeing can have on the patient experience. Powell *et al.* (2014) studied three years' worth of NHS Staff Survey data against various human resources measures, patient satisfaction, and infection and mortality rates. They found that 'staff experience is clearly linked to outcomes, especially intermediate outcomes such as absenteeism' and that individual employee satisfaction was a precursor to, rather than a consequence of, poor patient outcomes and experience. In order to achieve improvements in the area of staff experience, the study recommends an investment in leadership and supervisor support, such as the time-management of staff and the monitoring of health and wellbeing (Powell *et al.* 2014). Maben *et al.* (2012a) examined the effects of staff coping-mechanisms on the experiences of elderly patients. Nursing staff struggling to provide high quality care created an environment characterized by the differentiation between 'Poppets and Parcels'. Patients seen as difficult or as having complex needs were referred to as 'parcels' and given less personalized care than those who evoked staff sympathy or engagement, who were referred to as 'poppets'. Maben *et al.* (2012a) cite investment in staff wellbeing and in the ward climate as dual means to the delivery of consistent high quality care for older people.

Using play for lifelong learning **251**

In a qualitative study, also by Maben *et al.* (2012b), the effects of staff motivation and wellbeing on the patient experience were assessed. A data collection model which used various methods of patient experience feedback identified specific indicators for poor quality care in a ward environment providing care for the elderly. Emergent themes included: a lack of personalized care; poor response times to calls for assistance; patients being referred to by a bed number; the dehumanising effect of being rushed; perceived interference of relatives; and lack of assistance with basic functions.

Another important theme in relation to staff wellbeing was the team dynamic. The researchers noted significant differences between team environments perceived as 'weak' and 'strong'. This is reflected in the following staff responses, quoted in the report.

> I think the whole team tends to work as a ward, there's a high degree of professionalism in that you know if you're struggling or somebody else is struggling, I think we all try and help each other out.

> I think they (patients) enjoy the friendliness of us all, because we work well as a team, I think they pick up on that.
>
> *(Maben et al. 2012b)*

In contrast, poor team environments were characterized by distinctions between staff grades, perceived negative effects of multicultural and multi-ethnic staff, and bullying or incivility.

The use of humor

The use of humor in healthcare is nothing new, however there is new debate about its appropriate use. Many authors have found a link between the use of humor as a coping strategy for caregivers in emotionally demanding caring roles (Dean and Major 2008; McCreaddie and Wiggins 2008; Smyth 2011). Differentiation between the use of humor with patients and humor between staff, is important. Humor has been shown to have significant value in inter-professional and team dynamics, 'If you argue with her she won't help you out …You're off the list …So if you can joke with her, she will be there to help you out' (Dean and Major 2008). There are many examples, across various health settings, of humor being used to support team-delivered care and emotional health in demanding and stressful workplaces, and McGhee (n.d.) notes that access to humor makes people more resilient. Hospital humor is recognized as being 'different' from other types and when asked to use a single word to define hospital humor, 90 per cent of the time doctors and nurses use the descriptor 'sick' (McGhee n.d.). Renowned for being inappropriate and insensitive outside the hospital context, hospital humor provides a coping mechanism that allows healthcare professionals to deal with the 'extreme emotional stress' that can result from facing serious illness, injury, death and dying on a daily basis (McGhee n.d.). Appropriately used humor is an obvious example of a play-based skill that can be learnt, developed and embedded in the everyday practice of health teams.

There is a growing body of evidence to link both patient experience and clinical outcomes with caregiver wellbeing. In the light of this, NHS England has initiated a drive to promote staff wellbeing. According to NHS England Chief Executive Simon Stevens,

> NHS organizations will be supported to help their staff to stay well, including serving healthier food, promoting physical activity, reducing stress, and providing health checks covering mental health and musculoskeletal problems – the two biggest causes of sickness absence across the NHS.
>
> *(NHS England 2015)*

A number of different strategies are available, and already in use in some areas, to improve staff health and wellbeing. The next part of the chapter will identify and discuss some of the play-based strategies that can help caregivers deliver a high quality of care, either individually or as part of a team. It also explores, describes and develops other play-based activities that healthcare workers can employ when undertaking continuing learning.

Choirs

Many NHS Trusts have established workplace choirs. Lewisham and Greenwich NHS Trust Choir were featured in a BBC documentary series which highlighted the importance of workplace choirs. The benefits included building relationships across disciplines and departments, developing confidence as well as identifying a method for reducing stress (Lewisham and Greenwich NHS Trust 2015).

The Walton Centre Case Study

An example of a playful approach to the management of stress and ill-health is provided by the Walton Centre. A recent report from the British Broadcasting Corporation (BBC) demonstrated how the Walton Centre in Liverpool, a specialist NHS hospital treating injuries to the brain, spine and nervous system, dealt with the issues of high sickness rates (Hughes 2015). This NHS Trust has established activity and exercise classes including netball,

> a staff football team, a running club, Pilates classes, massage and aromatherapy, weight management programs and a host of other schemes and activities. All are designed to increase physical activity, relieve stress and improve the health and wellbeing – physical and mental – of staff.
>
> *(Hughes 2015)*

Using play for lifelong learning **253**

The benefits of physical play and recreation have been described in Chapter 7.

Staff sickness affects patient care and also has financial implications for the employer. Play-oriented interventions have the potential to influence sickness rates with benefits for patients, staff and the organization and at a relatively low financial cost. Staff sickness rates in 2010 averaged 7 per cent of the 1,300 workforce, which was higher than average, and could be even higher at certain times of year such as during an outbreak of flu. These rates fell to 4 per cent in 2015, which is on a par with the rest of the NHS (Health and Social Care Information Centre 2012), suggesting a link with the implementation of the staff activity and exercise program.

Schwartz Rounds

Another example of an approach that contributes to the wellbeing of staff is the concept of Schwartz Rounds (The Point of Care Foundation n.d.). Schwartz Rounds were developed by the Schwartz Center for Compassionate Healthcare, Boston USA. Set up in 1995, this not-for-profit organization focuses on the importance of the relationship between the patient and caregiver. Ken Schwartz was a healthy 40 year old non-smoker who developed, and later died from lung cancer. During his ten-year battle with the disease, he 'came to realize that what matters most during an illness is the human connection between patients and their caregivers'. He also 'reminds caregivers to stay in the moment with patients' and how 'the smallest acts of kindness' make 'the unbearable bearable' (The Schwartz Center n.d.).

Schwartz Rounds were developed in order for staff to develop a deeper understanding of the emotional issues that arise when caring for patients. Schwartz rounds are multi-disciplinary meetings that focus on the emotional aspects of working with cancer patients. These hour-long meetings usually take place on a monthly basis and represent an opportunity for team members to reflect on issues arising in the course of their work. This can help to strengthen a multi-disciplinary approach and to improve team-work. A valuable difference between Schwartz Rounds and other meetings is that they are not intended for problem-solving and nor do they have a pre-determined outcome. 'Playing with' thoughts and feelings in an atmosphere of safety and acceptance is a recognized route to creative development and change (Power 2011).

Raso (2009) states that patients often 'don't care what you know' but 'want to know that you care'. It is therefore crucial that staff are provided with opportunities to explore and develop the emotional, caring aspects of their practice. Participants in Schwartz Rounds report the positive effects of just talking about the difficult issues that arise when caring for the needs of complex patients (Goodrich 2012). 'Everyone else has benefited from doctors talking about the emotional impact on them. It is not part of the culture of medicine to talk about the emotional content, and these are senior consultants talking too. It is important for staff to hear it' (Goodrich 2014). The 'serious play' involved in such meetings is radically different from other clinical, business or organizational meetings and this is reflected in the effects on participants and on clinical teams. Humor and light heartedness are not forbidden and are perhaps even to be encouraged as a coping mechanism (McGhee n.d.). As a means of changing the 'modus operandi' of a healthcare setting, Schwartz Rounds provide an interestingly different approach to care.

Education

Continuing Professional Development (CPD) has become a compulsory learning and development tool for most professions. The Health and Care Professions Council (HCPC) state that CPD is 'a range of learning activities through which health and care professionals maintain and develop throughout their career to ensure that they retain their capacity to practice safely, effectively and legally within their evolving scope of practice' (HCPC n.d.) Rather than being perceived as a positive part of working practice, CPD is often regarded as a chore and can become a source of work-related stress.

CPD is vital to maintaining quality and safe practice but it is intended to be an enjoyable experience. 'CPD can initially appear daunting. However, it can, and should be an enjoyable aspect of developing yourself and your professional practice' (Sibson 2015). Although some CPD is mandatory, the remainder of an individual's CPD can be self-selected and, if considered carefully, can be enjoyable (and playful!).

There has been much research into learning styles. Honey and Mumford (2006) developed a learning styles questionnaire, based on the work of Kolb, to enable individuals to establish the way they learn best so that they can become better all-round learners as well as understanding the learning needs of others. Honey and Mumford (2006) state that:

> Learning is your most important capability simply because it is the gateway of every other capability you might wish to develop. Whether you become fluent in another language, and/or become better at winning friends and influencing people, and/or become better at surfing the web, and/or better at football, learning is the key. The process of learning underpins *everything*.

Individuals will be drawn to activities that interest them and this will usually link to their preferred learning style. It is important to remember that, as individual learning styles vary, so will an individual's perception of 'enjoyable' activities. Therefore, when considering CPD activities, what is enjoyable for one person may not be for another. For example, comics and toys may be used as a means of both peer and patient engagement, as discussed in Chapter 14.

Just as humor has both its advocates and critics, alternative learning resources need to be carefully introduced and applied in order that the novelty factor does not diminish the message being conveyed.

Active learning is considered by many experts to be the best way to learn. According to Prince, (2004) 'Active learning is generally defined as any instructional method that engages students in the learning process. In short, active learning requires students to do meaningful learning activities and think about what they are doing'. This could include any activity where the individual participates in, and engages with, the learning process rather than being the passive recipient of information, which results in better recall and understanding as well as enjoyment. It can also promote specific skills such as the use of all available evidence, not just that which appears to be more obvious or more appealing (Tonkin 2009).

Innovation in health education

A recommendation of the Francis Report (2013) was to improve education, particularly with regards to patient safety. Ensuring that those working in health environments achieve and maintain competency, requires the identification of new methods of delivery. Rapidly-changing healthcare organization, funding arrangements, patient age demographics, disease profiles and worldwide migration all place increasing demands on those delivering healthcare. A rapidly-changing model of healthcare demands parallel changes in working practice, raising the importance of innovative educational strategies.

A review of play-based initiatives featured in the education theory literature suggests subtle changes in the way nursing and midwifery education is being delivered (Baid and Lambert 2010).

Drawing on the work of Dearnley *et al.* (2013), *Innovation in Teaching and Learning in Health Higher Education* examines and reviews new teaching methods, the influence of technology and cultures of innovation. The document reviews primary and secondary research for medical, nursing and allied health professions and there follows a discussion of the various topic areas, highlighting some of the resources available. By definition, some innovative practices are difficult to assess and research formally; however, in presenting the full range we hope to enthuse, to stimulate further ideas, and to promote discussion of the potential for playfulness in health education.

Web-based resources

The use of simulation in medical training has a long history and has been extended by the application of modern technology.

In the Netherlands, medical students have recorded consultations with a simulated patient onto a web-based platform (Hulsman and van der Vloodt, 2015). The value of the web-based method proved to be an effective tool for self-evaluation and for the continually increasing requirements of peer-feedback.

Students in the United Kingdom have used simulation sessions, in conjunction with online video records and feedback, to gain CPR skills (Bowden *et al.* 2012). Both students and teachers reported benefits of online recording and feedback.

Students were able to use them for the purposes of revision, aiding retention of information, and teachers found that the assessment and delivery of feedback was also easier. There can be even greater benefits when simulations use games as part of the process, which enables skills to be practiced and also understood (Pelletier and Kneebone 2015).

Smartphone resources

The mobile nature of health makes the use of smartphones an obvious next step for clinicians, for patient education and for patient monitoring (Mosa *et al.* 2012). The availability and usage of phone apps continue to increase year on year. The investigation of their potential integration with electronic patient records, and with monitoring devices, would further enhance smartphone and mobile application use.

In Taiwan, an environment where smartphone technology has some of highest population usage in the world, Wu *et al.* (2011) showed that nursing students favoured smartphone learning systems over conventional methods. The researchers also showed that the acquisition of knowledge about the respiratory system was improved using smartphone technology when compared to a control group. Students showed a tendency for accessing information using mobile devices since they were integral features of their everyday experience. The researchers also planned to extend the learning activity to involve the sharing and exchange of ideas. This research is included to show the potential and actual crossover from the use of mobile technology for leisure and play-oriented activity to its use in learning and skill-sharing. This crossover phenomenon also applies to the use of social media which are now widely used to both access and convey health-related information, as discussed in Chapter 15 and elsewhere in this book.

Gaming resources

The use of gaming in nurse education can provide 'a useful, educationally sound addition to the teaching repertoire' for achieving learning outcomes when integrated with other learning methods (Peddle 2011). McLafferty *et al.* (2010) reported that students found gaming workshops preferable to more formal teaching styles for learning the skills involved in the care of older people.

In Brazil, a team of clinicians, academics and programmers devised a game to help teach physicians the fundamentals of insulin therapy (Diehl *et al.* 2013). The creation of the game using a team approach, was described as 'effective' and, with the increased use of technology in education and web-based distribution, the future use of games such as these is considered to be secure. This particular approach was compared with other more traditional distance-learning methods and considered to be both more interesting and more successful. Both learner engagement and successful learning itself were considered important. The value of gaming as a playful learning tool has been clearly demonstrated in this context.

According to research by Knox *et al.* (2015) students found that practical learning was easier to understand, was an important part of the learning process, and helped to hold their attention. In a joint study between North America and the UK, two games using experiential learning were developed to raise awareness of cultural difference. Evaluated by Graham and Richardson (2008), the first game was similar to a traditional card-game and the second game was an exercise in which the participants had to learn by practising the rules of another culture. Students found that both games challenged their views of other cultures and experienced heightened emotions while participating.

The use of gaming resources can help to develop skills in a specific area of health education whilst also making the activity more interesting and enjoyable. Play and playfulness have long been recognized as effective learning tools in the field of childhood education (Moyles 2010) and current research shows that adults also learn new tasks better when it is presented in a playful and enjoyable way. Play can help to stimulate the imagination, encourage adaptation and develop problem-solving skills (Robinson *et al.* 2015) all of which are key features of successful learning.

Digital and innovative technical resources

The active and interactive nature of digital and innovative technological resources mimics some of the characteristic features of play and can tap-into the individual's natural tendency for pleasure-seeking to provide a useful alternative to standard teaching methods.

Emerging data from Australia regarding student preferences for accessing differing learning resources, suggests subtle changes in the way people interact with educational material. This study examined the experiences and regularity of usage of students accessing an online physiotherapy database (Maloney *et al.* 2013). Participants likened accessing the educational resource online to general online experiences and made direct comparisons with commercial search engines. Importantly there was also evidence that this type of resource supported lifelong learning as well as academic achievement. Again this illustrates how technology originally used in a personal, recreational capacity is finding application in the educational context.

In Ireland, an artificial intelligence tool for assessing hand hygiene techniques against World Health Organization standards, showed comparable results to assessment by human assessors. The tool also offers real-time feedback using a traffic light system and is therefore useful for both training and assessment (Ghosh *et al.*, 2013).

Acting, role-play and debating resources

Hall (2011) showed the effects of debating on the communication skills and critical thinking exhibited by allied health professionals in the USA. Debating demonstrated students' abilities to gather and use evidence to form a coherent argument, to actively listen and to convey information clearly and succinctly. Additional benefits to the students included increased confidence and a respect for other viewpoints. The focus of debating as a learning tool revolves around presenting an argument, listening to counter argument and on communication in general. However, in this example, debates were competitive and therefore bore a resemblance to sporting contest. Emphasis on the skills gained from debating, rather on the debate itself, helped to focus participants on the important areas for relevant learning. Several students preferred the debating format to traditional lectures as they were considered more engaging.

In a similar study in Finland, medical students used three different methods to teach communication skills: theatre in education; simulated patient interviews using actors; and peer role-play (Koponen *et al.* 2011). The results were overwhelmingly positive with respondents rating the various methods between 80 per cent and 90 per cent in terms of suitability. 'In general, all three methods aroused more positive than negative emotional reactions, and all methods were considered pleasant and fun' (Koponen *et al.* 2011). As an example of a near universally successful playful approach to learning, the findings from this study have potentially widespread application in the field of medical education.

In the USA, actors have been used to aid the development of empathetic communication skills in medical students. This innovative approach, using trained actors to engage participants in fun, observational and role-play type games aimed to improve empathetic communication (Reilly *et al.* 2012). The success of this initiative was judged by feedback from teaching staff, the actors and participants and showed a degree of disparity as encapsulated in the following comment by one participant; 'It was an entertaining session but I don't know how effective it was in teaching empathy. For sheer entertainment value, it was highly worthwhile' (Reilly *et al.* 2012). The enjoyment of an activity does not necessarily indicate that it has learning potential but, as a play-based approach, drama and role-play offer well-established routes to the achievement of mutual and empathetic understanding.

In Australia, Warland and Smith (2012) used an online role-play discussion method to teach communication and collaboration skills to midwifery students. This particular method combines a number of the playful techniques already discussed and is validated by this study. Communication and collaboration are common threads running through the quoted examples. The recorded success levels of active and interactive approaches to learning, whether traditional or derived from the use of modern technology, suggest that a playful approach to learning contributes to the achievement of educational outcomes.

Whose Shoes?

It is perhaps fitting to end this chapter with one of the most innovative and engaging CPD engagement tools that has recently been developed – with play and playfulness at its heart. *Whose Shoes* is a 'Putting People First board game – a

Using play for lifelong learning **259**

learning and development tool designed to help people make progress with the personalisation agenda in health and social care and the wider community' (WhoseShoes 2010). The game was designed and developed by Gill Phillips (2015) as a means of discussing personalization, providing a vehicle for visualizing and understanding the 'Putting People First' (HM Government 2010) vision and commitment.

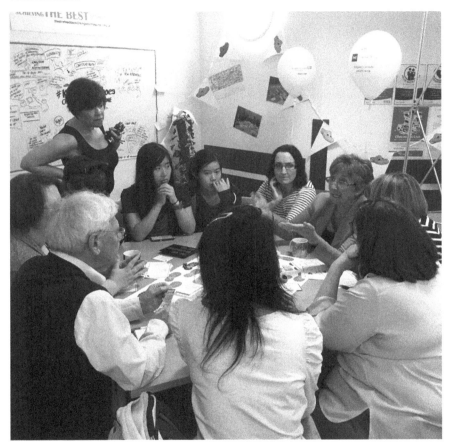

FIGURE 21.1 Playing 'Whose shoes?'

Philips (cited WhoseShoes 2010) describes the game, stating: 'Whose Shoes has been developed ... to help you to understand the key concerns and opportunities involved in personalisation, from a range of perspectives'. The game was designed to facilitate a collaborative approach enabling the discussion of key issues, through the use of color-coded resources, that allow participants to 'build the path to personaliation'. The game can be played as an individual or in teams, and this flexible approach also allows the game to be played in a manner that best serves the needs of those who are playing. Five years on, there is 'now an electronic version of the game, developed in partnership with [the] "Think Local' Act Personal"' (TLAP) National Coproduction Group.

Conclusion

This glimpse into changes in worldwide health education shows that the educational map is being re-drawn to incorporate what we know about the value of play-based learning. Play-based activities are now seriously challenging traditional teaching methods, not only as a user preference, but also in terms of outcomes. Technology using simulation, the internet and smartphones are blurring the boundaries between recreation and education and challenge the traditional conception of work and play as two distinct entities.

References

Baid, H. and Lambert, N. (2010) Enjoyable learning: the role of humour, games, and fun activities in nursing and midwifery education, *Nurse Education Today*, 30 (6): 548–552.

Boorman, S. (2009) *NHS Health and Well-being: Final Report*, Online. Available at http://web archive.nationalarchives.gov.uk/20130107105354/www.dh.gov.uk/prod_consum_dh/gro ups/dh_digitalassets/documents/digitalasset/dh_108907.pdf (accessed 16 December 2015).

Bowden, T., Rowlands, A., Buckwell, M. and Abbott, S. (2012) Web-based video and feedback in the teaching of cardiopulmonary resuscitation, *Nurse Education Today*, 32 (4): 443–447.

Dean, R.A.K. and Major, J.E. (2008) From critical care to comfort care: the sustaining value of humour, *Journal of Clinical Nursing*, 17 (8): 1088–1095.

Dearnley, C., McClelland, G.T. and Irving, D. (2013) *Innovation in Teaching and Learning in Health Higher Education,* London: The Higher Education Academy.

Department of Health (2011) *Healthy Staff, Better Care for Patients,* Leeds: Department of Health.

Diehl, L.A., Souza, R.M., Alves, J.B., Gordan, P.A., Esteves, R.Z., Jorge, M. L.S.G. and Coelho, I.C M. (2013) InsuOnline, a serious game to teach insulin therapy to primary care physicians: design of the game and a randomized controlled trial for educational validation, *JMIR Research Protocols,* 2 (1): e5.

Francis, R. (2013) *The Mid-Staffordshire NHS Foundation Trust Public Enquiry: Executive Summary,* London: The Stationery Office.

Ghosh, A., Ameling, S., Zhou, J., Lacey, G., Creamer, E., Dolan, A. and Humphreys, H. (2013) Pilot evaluation of a ward-based automated hand hygiene training system, *American Journal of Infection Control*, 41 (4): 368–370.

Goodrich, J. (2012) Supporting hospital staff to provide compassionate care: Do Schwartz Center Rounds work in English hospitals? *Journal of the Royal Society of Medicine*, 105 (3): 117–122.

Goodrich, J. (2014). Compassionate care and Schwartz Rounds: the nature of the work – acknowledging it is hard, *Nurse Education Today*, 9 (34): 1185–1187.

Graham, I. and Richardson, E. (2008) Experiential gaming to facilitate cultural awareness: its implication for developing emotional caring in nursing, *Learning in Health and Social Care*, 7 (1): 37–45.

Hall, D. (2011) Debate: innovative teaching to enhance critical thinking and communication skills in healthcare professionals, *International Journal of Allied Health Sciences and Practice*, 9: 16–19.

Health and Care Professions Council (HCPC) (n.d.) *Continuing Professional Development (CPD)*, Online. Available at www.hpc-uk.org/registrants/cpd/ (accessed 12 September 2015).

Health and Safety Executive (n.d.) *Work Related Stress, Anxiety and Depression Statistics in Great Britain 2014/15,* Online. Available at www.hse.gov.uk/statistics/causdis/stress/ (accessed 23 November 2015).

Health and Social Care Information Centre (2012) *Sickness Absence Rate among NHS Workers Falls to 4.12 per cent,* Online. Available at www.hscic.gov.uk/article/2421/Sickness-absence-rate-among-NHS-workers-falls-to-412-per-cent (accessed 17 December 2015).

HM Government (2010) Putting people first: a shared vision and commitment to the transformation of adult social care, Online. Available at http://webarchive.national archives.gov.uk/20130107105354/http:/www.dh.gov.uk/prod_consum_dh/groups/dh_ digitalassets/@dh/@en/documents/digitalasset/dh_081119.pdf (accessed 2 April 2016).

Honey, P. and Mumford, A. (2006) *The Learning Styles Questionnaire 80-item Version: Revised Edition*, Maidenhead: Perter Honey Publications Limited.

Hughes, D (2015) *Exercise Classes Help Cut NHS Staff Sickness Rates,* Online. Available www.bbc.co.uk/news/health-33571422 (accessed 09 September 2015).

Hulsman, R. L. and van der Vloodt, J. (2015) Self-evaluation and peer-feedback of medical students' communication skills using a web-based video annotation system. Exploring content and specificity, *Patient Education and Counseling*, 98 (3): 356–363.

Knox, S., Cullen, W., Collins, N. and Dunne, C. (2015) First evaluation of CPD advanced paramedic teaching methods in Ireland, *Journal of Paramedic Practice*, 5 (1): 29–35.

Koponen, J., Pyörälä, E., and Isotalus, P. (2011) A comparison of medical students' perceptions of three experiential methods, *Health Education*, 111 (4): 296–318.

Lewisham and Greenwich NHS Trust (2015) *The Trust Choir*, Online. Available at www.lewishamandgreenwich.nhs.uk/the-trust-choir (accessed 17 December 2015).

Maben, J., Adams, M., Peccei, R., Murrells, T. and Robert, G. (2012a) 'Poppets and parcels': the links between staff experience of work and acutely ill older peoples' experience of hospital care, *International Journal of Older People Nursing*, 7 (2): 83–94.

Maben, J., Peccei, R., Adams, M., Robert, G., Richardson, A., Murrells, T. and Morrow, E. (2012b) *Exploring the Relationship between Patients' Experiences of Care and the Influence of Staff Motivation, Affect and Wellbeing, Final Report*. Southampton: NIHR Service Delivery and Organization Programme.

Maloney, S., Chamberlain, M., Morrison, S., Kotsanas, G., Keating, J.L. and Ilic, D. (2013) Health professional learner attitudes and use of digital learning resources, *Journal of Medical Internet Research*, 15 (1).

McCreaddie, M. and Wiggins, S. (2008) The purpose and function of humour in health, health care and nursing: a narrative review, *Journal of Advanced Nursing*, 61 (6): 584–595.

McGhee, P. (n.d.) *Part IV: Humor and Mental Health: Using Humor to Cope with Stress*, Online. Available at www.nurseslearning.com/courses/nrp/NRPCX-W0009/html/body. humor.page7.htm (accessed 16 December 2015).

McLafferty, E., Dingwall, L. and Halkett, A. (2010) Using workshops to prepare nursing students for caring for older people in clinical practice. *International Journal of Older People Nursing,* 5 (1): 51-60.

Mosa, A.S.M., Yoo, I. and Sheets, L. (2012). A systematic review of healthcare applications for smartphones, *BMC Medical Informatics and Decision Making*, 12 (1): 67.

Moyles, J. (2010) *Thinking about Play: Developing a Reflective Approach*, Maidenhead: Open University Press.

NHS England (2015) *Simon Stevens Announces Major Drive to Improve Health in NHS Workplace,* Online. Available at www.england.nhs.uk/2015/09/02/nhs-workplace/ (accessed 07 December 2015).

NHS Staff Survey (2014) Briefing note: issues highlighted by the 2014 NHS Staff Survey in England, Online. Available at www.nhsstaffsurveys.com/Caches/Files/NHS%20staff% 20survey_nationalbriefing_Final%2024022015%20UNCLASSIFIED.pdf (accessed 16 December 2015).

Peddle, M. (2011) Simulation gaming in nurse education; entertainment or learning? *Nurse Education Today*, 31 (7): 647–649.

Pelletier, C. and Kneebone, R. (2015) Playful simulations rather than serious games medical simulation as a cultural practice, *Games and Culture,* doi: 1555412014568449.

Petty, G. (2015) *Active Learning,* Online. Available at http://geoffpetty.com/for-teachers/ active-learning/ (accessed 09 September 2015).

Phillips, G. (2015) *LinkedIn: Gill Phillips*, Online. Available at www.linkedin.com/in/ whoseshoes (accessed 17 December 2015).

Powell, M., Dawson, J., Topakas, A., Durose, J. and Fewtrell, C. (2014) Staff satisfaction and organisational performance: evidence from a longitudinal secondary analysis of the NHS staff survey and outcome data, *Health Service and Delivery Research,* 2 (50).

Power, P. (2011) Playing with ideas. The affective dynamics of creative play, *American Journal of Play,* Winter: 288–323.

Prince, M (2004) Does active learning work? A review of the research, *Journal of Engineering Education,* 93 (3): 223–231.

Raso, R. (2009) Improving practice with Schwartz rounds; the DNP degree, *Nursing management,* 40 (8): 56.

Reilly, J.M., Trial, J., Piver, D.E. and Schaff, P.B. (2012) Using Theater to Increase Empathy Training in Medical Students, *Journal for Learning through the Arts*, 8 (1), Online. Available at http://escholarship.org/uc/item/68x7949t (accessed 22 February 2016).

Rieber, L. P. (1996) Seriously considering play: Designing interactive learning environments based on the blending of microworlds, simulations, and games. *Educational Technology Research and Development*, 44(2): 43–58.

Robinson, L., Smith, M. and Segal, J. (2015) *The Benefits of Play for Adults,* Online. Available at www.helpguide.org/articles/emotional-health/benefits-of-play-for-adults. htm (accessed 27 November 2015).

Sibson, L. (2015) An introduction to CPD for paramedic practice, *Journal of Paramedic Practice,* 1 (2): 73–75.

Smyth, D. (2011) Black humour in health care: a laughing matter? *International Journal of Palliative Nursing*, 17 (11): 523.

The Point of Care Foundation (n.d.) *Schwartz Rounds*, Online. Available at www.pointof-carefoundation.org.uk/Schwartz-Rounds/ (accessed 17 December 2015).

The Schwartz Center (n.d.) *Our Story and Mission,* Online. Available at www.theschwartz-center.org/about-us/story-mission/ (accessed 23 November 2015).

Tonkin, A. (2009) *Promoting the Use of Evidence through a Teddy Murder Mystery*, Online. Available at http://www2.rcn.org.uk/__data/assets/pdf_file/0005/271076/2.1.3_Sure_ start_community_childrens_nursing.pdf (accessed 17 December 2015).

Warland, J. and Smith, M. (2012) Using online roleplay in undergraduate midwifery education: a case-study. *Nurse Education in Practice*, 12 (5): 279–283.

WhoseShoes (2010) *Whose_Shoes_Intro.mp4,* Online. Available at www.youtube.com/ watch?v=W2XRmmsyZos (accessed 17 December 2015).

Wu, P.H., Hwang, G.J., Tsai, C.C., Chen, Y.C. and Huang, Y.M. (2011) A pilot study on conducting mobile learning activities for clinical nursing courses based on the repertory grid approach, *Nurse Education Today*, 31 (8): e8–e15.

22
PLAYING POLITICS

Carol Sullivan-Wallace and Alison Tonkin

This chapter explores how politics can be used to develop and promote play-based strategies within healthcare provision. It will review the role of policy for developing innovative practice and how, in times of global fiscal restraint, play-based techniques have been used as a positive means of engaging people with the current health agenda at local, national and international levels.

Introduction

The term playing politics is defined as the 'use of a situation or the relationships between people for your own advantage' (Cambridge Dictionaries 2015). The Urban Dictionary (2015) provides an equivalent, if blunter, definition of 'politics' as:

> Poli – many Tic(k)s – blood sucking creatures = many blood sucking creatures

This exemplifies the negative impression many people have of modern politics, with personal advantage often being sought at the expense of others (MindTools 2015).

These perceptions appear to be a far cry from the original roots of human politics associated with the Greek philosophers such as Plato and Aristotle (Farrelly 2013). Originating from the Greek word *politikos* which means pertaining to 'the polis' or 'city state', cities such as Athens and Sparta were relatively small, cohesive units in which political, religious and cultural concerns were intertwined (Miller 2011). Aristotle, who died in 322 BCE, travelled extensively and his experiences are thought to have heavily influenced his political thinking. Aristotle viewed politics as a practical science 'since it is concerned with the noble action or happiness of the citizens' (Miller 2011). Aristotle believed that all things should lead to human good and that political science should be used to facilitate this through 'good governance'

(Farrelly 2013), by politicians and statesmen. This governance should occur through the development of laws and customs for the citizens of the city states, including the maintenance and reform of laws and customs where necessary to protect the integrity of the political system (Miller 2011).

Within the United Kingdom, the desire of the nation to care for people 'at the point of need' rather than according to the ability to pay, necessitates a political agenda that conforms to the collective will of the people (Tempest 2015). The NHS is funded on the principle that 'good healthcare should be available to all – regardless of wealth' (NHS Choices 2015) and as a result, the health ecosystem (as described in Chapter 2) impinges on all our lives (Tempest 2015). This democratic process exemplifies Dewey's (1916) assertion that democracy is more than government and relates to a means of 'associated living [and] communicated experience'. With democracy comes active participation by citizens in the decision-making process, which means political parties seek to advance their position by reaching out to the electorate in an effort to capture their votes. Farrelly (2013: 487) proposes that this type of 'democratic political activity can be conceived of as social and imaginative explorative play' which has a significant developmental function. Play is known to promote skill acquisition, enabling the development of new strategies and behaviors in a safe and secure environment. Farrelly (2013: 490) goes on to suggest that these strategies, instead of being defined as play, but rather as democratic politics, 'ensure the polity can flourish in unpredictable and challenging environments'.

The fragile state of adult health

Healthcare is a political 'hot potato' (Tempest 2015). In the UK, the NHS is financially under strain and is unlikely to meet its challenges unless additional funding is identified (The Kings Fund 2015).

People are living for longer, resulting in more long-term health issues with obvious cost implications for health service provision. The Royal College of Physicians (2012) note that two thirds of hospital admissions are of patients over the age of 65 years and that neither hospitals nor clinicians are equipped to treat the complex needs of an aging population. AgingCare.com (2015) list the 11 most common health issues exacerbated by age, of which the first three are heart problems, dementia and depression. As noted in earlier chapters, all three conditions can benefit from the provision of play-related activities. Worldwide improvements in healthcare and a fast growing elderly population are now reflected in the increased number of dementia sufferers, although dementia is more prevalent in developing countries (Alzheimer's Disease International n.d.). In the UK, it is reported that the estimated number of people with dementia is in excess of 850,000 with an annual cost of £26 billion (Alzheimer's Society 2015). Dementia may be a growing health problem but it is not the only health issue facing our aging population and dementia is not purely a problem of the elderly. With an increased demand on services, partly due to the growth of an aging population and partly to the number of people accessing emergency care, the NHS finds itself in serious difficulties. Many political commentators suggest that the NHS is itself too sick to survive in its present state (Toynbee 2014). Change is essential if the NHS is to continue to deliver the range and depth of services it currently provides and, without change, it is predicted that services will worsen and that the NHS will slide into a 'managed decline' (Nicholson 2014). Sir David Nicholson (2014), the former Chief Executive of NHS England, clearly advocates the need for change, noting that 'we need to be shoulder to shoulder in these changes and tackle the politics'.

The NHS is not alone in its current predicament, with health systems across the globe facing considerable financial pressures. This is particularly noticeable in most low-economy countries which have insufficient access to even the most basic resources (World Health Organization 2010). Health inequalities are a global issue and poor health systems themselves are known to be part of the problem (Institute of Public Health in Ireland 2015). The World Health Organization (WHO) (2015a) states that all countries, irrespective of whether they are low-, middle- or high-income economies, have 'wide disparities in the health status of differing social groups'. For example, in the wealthier part of London, men's life expectancy can vary by up to 17 years: men living in the affluent ward of Kensington and Chelsea have a life expectancy of 88 years, whilst in Tottenham Green ward, one of London's poorest wards just a few kilometres away, the life expectancy for men is just 71 years (Marmot 2010). This demonstrates the implications of health inequalities for individuals and society as a whole. Health inequalities result in a loss in productivity and income from taxes, as well as higher welfare and healthcare costs. In the European Union (EU) this is estimated to be 1.4 per cent of the gross domestic product (GDP), equating to almost the entire EU defence budget of 1.6 per cent GDP (World Health Organization 2015a).

The instability of social, economic and political factors, as well as an aging population, all contribute to a re-distribution of health-related risk factors, which have left adult health in a state of fragility (World Health Organization 2015b). Politics has a role to play and the World Health Organization (2015a) clearly identifies the unfairness of health inequalities and state that these 'could be reduced by the right mix of government policies'. This suggests that politics can be both a causative factor of poor health and a protective factor against poor health, the latter being the focus of the remainder of this chapter.

Using politics to enhance adult healthcare

The burden of unhealthy life choices has serious consequences for individuals and for society as a whole, particularly in relation to the development of chronic health conditions which significantly reduce 'disability free life expectancy'. The impact of chronic ill-health is set out in the first half of Chapter 7 and the likelihood of developing a chronic illness is known to follow the social gradient (Marmot 2010). Marmot (2010: 32) identifies the need to 'strengthen the role and impact of ill-health prevention' through policy intervention and recommends that ill-health prevention and health promotion should be prioritized across all government departments. Chapter 14 discusses the role of health literacy as a key strategy in health education and promotion. In 2001, Whitehead *et al.* stated: 'our contention is that it is possible to challenge health inequities with purposeful public policy. Such a challenge is long overdue' (Whitehead *et al.* 2001: 309). Public policy is known to be a powerful driver for change and identifying macroeconomic policies as the 'key policy entry points in the promotion of health equity' enables public policy to promote 'purposeful national action' (Whitehead *et al.* 2001: 314).

Using sport and recreation as an example, Cox (2012) collated an evidence base to support the claim that 'sport and recreation are good for you. This statement feels instinctively right. After all what could be better for you than fresh air, exercise, teamwork, nature, camaraderie?' (Cox 2012: 5).

Sport offers physical and mental health benefits (Conn 2015) and leading a more active lifestyle produces personal and societal gain (Cox 2012). Cox (2012: 6) also points out that this will only happen 'if the government ensures this is their priority'. Evidence to support this claim followed the staging of the 2012 Olympic Games in London. Increased public participation in sport was always framed as a key legacy from the Games and, from the 2005 announcement that London was to host the Games in 2012, contrary to initial indications that numbers participating in sport were on the increase, numbers have gradually declined, particularly among those from poorer socioeconomic groups. Those in poorer socioeconomic groups are disproportionately represented in the total 1.2 million people who do not participate in any kind of sport (Perraudin 2015) with 75 per cent of people in poorer economic groups not involved in regular sporting activity (Conn 2015). Conn (2015) identifies that 'sport always reflects the culture it is played in, and sadly the latest figures expose an unequal, mostly sedentary nation'. Interestingly, Conn (2015) cites research which shows that hosting a televised mega sporting event does not encourage *regular people* to do more exercise. So, despite massive political intervention and financial investment in present systems, it still seems that alternative means of engaging the population in an active, healthier lifestyle will be necessary.

Chapter 17 explores an alternative approach to the promotion of a healthy lifestyle through the use of complementary healthcare techniques to facilitate play, recreation and leisure. A central focus of the chapter is Traditional Chinese Medicine (TCM), which has been fully institutionalized in China through the support of the Chinese government and plays an integral role in the healthcare system of modern China, 'which is good for the health of the nation' (Ho 2015). The status of this alternative healthcare approach in China contrasts starkly with attitudes in the UK, where debate continues around the efficacy of alternative and complementary medicine and whether or not it should be available on the NHS, despite 'large proportions of British people' genuinely believing it could be effective (Dalhgreen 2015).

Linking behavioral politics to health and wellbeing

The global move towards health promotion (Campbell *et al.* 2015), and the endorsement of preventative treatments (NHS England 2014), are noted as being essential steps forward in healthcare. Government intervention in the lives of its citizens is usually undertaken to make society better (Dolan *et al*. 2010) and Farrelly (2013: 495) states that 'an account of the good society is predicated upon an understanding of what it is to be human'. Playful behavior is a manifestation of what it is to be human and it follows that this natural predisposition could be used as a means of enhancing individual and societal health and wellbeing. Dewey (1916) was aware of this innate human drive to play and noted that the enjoyment of recreational leisure and play was the responsibility of education 'not only for the sake of immediate health, but still more if possible for the sake of its lasting effect upon habits of mind'.

Health-related habits are established in early childhood and these early attitudes will often determine our behavior throughout adulthood (Bruce *et al*. 2010). It is therefore essential to challenge behavior that is not conducive to a healthy lifestyle, although this needs to be done sensitively and with care.

The complex nature of behavior change is fundamental to Bandura's Social Learning Theory, which 'addresses both the underlying determinants of health behavior and methods of promoting change' (Ontario Health Promotion Resource System n.d.). Due to its complexity, Bandura's theory has no overarching framework, but the key elements are described within Table 22.1.

TABLE 22.1 Key elements of Bandura's Social Learning Theory (Allen and Gordon 2011)

Reciprocal determinism	Our thinking, behavior and the environment are constantly interacting and changing the way we think and feel. This means that what, how and where we do things are linked together and each will affect the other
Self-efficacy	This describes how an individual personally perceives and responds to differing situations. It links observational learning, social experience and reciprocal determination to define the individual's own beliefs as to how well they can manage and succeed on any given task
Role-modelling	Most human behavior is learned through observation, which can lead to imitation. The stages leading to imitation are attention (see it), retention (remember it), reproduction (use it) and motivation (have reason to use it)

Behavioral economics utilizes insights from science and behavioral theory to address policy challenges. These have resulted in some noticeable successes, such as reducing the incidence of drink-driving or the abolition of smoking in enclosed public places (Dolan *et al*. 2010) although other behaviors, such as a lack of exercise, have been resistant to policy initiatives.

The British Nutrition Foundation (2012) has identified ten key facts relating to behavior change, the first one being 'before trying to change behavior it is vital to try to understand the nature of the behavior you want to change in a real-life context'. Bandura's theory suggests that this is not a simple task.

268 Carol Sullivan-Wallace and Alison Tonkin

The Foundation noted that only a small proportion of our food choices are under conscious control (about 14 out of 200), suggesting that 'interventions that encourage change on a conscious level will be limited by the fact that so many of these choices are made on an unconscious level'. This applies equally to most other decisions relating to behavioral choice. Dolan *et al.* (2010) have identified nine elements (using the acronym *MINDSPACE)* that operate largely in the 'automatic system', meaning that cognition or rational thought have a limited influence on how we behave.

TABLE 22.2 MINDSPACE elements (Dolan *et al.* 2010)

Messenger	We are heavily influenced by who communicates information
Incentives	Our responses to incentives are shaped by predictable mental shortcuts such as strongly avoiding losses
Norms	We are strongly influenced by what others do
Defaults	We 'go with the flow' of pre-set options
Salience	Our attention is drawn to what is novel and seems relevant to us
Priming	Our acts are often influenced by sub-conscious cues
Affect	Our emotional associations can powerfully shape our actions
Commitments	We seek to be consistent with our public promises, and reciprocate acts
Ego	We act in ways that make us feel better about ourselves

MINDSPACE and the politics of play invite consideration of numerous examples of how these theoretical concepts apply to healthcare and wellbeing.

Messenger

The potential for intergenerational message exchange has always been present in families and nowadays children and young people are being actively encouraged to engage with the older generation through formalized sharing events. Chaudhari (2014) reports on a fortnightly program between Turton School sixth formers and local pensioners who meet up to share their skills. The program, now in its tenth year, enables young people to learn how to knit and to play traditional games like dominoes, whilst the elderly participants learn about new technology such as apps and tablet computers. This open communication and sharing of life-skills promotes messages relevant to health and wellbeing that are applicable to both parties, although it is unlikely that either party are aware of this. In terms of promoting respect and understanding, the program, in the words of one sixth former, 'is important because it makes the older generation more approachable and they are fun' (Dunkerley, cited Chaudhari 2014). The form and delivery of health-related messages is covered in detail in Chapter 14.

Incentives

Incentives can be understood as cause-and-effect motivation, which links to the Model of Intentional Change by Boyatzis (2006). The model outlines a five step process that can be followed in order to achieve lasting personal change (Mindtools 2015). One example is the incentivization approach utilized by 'diet clubs' which are popularly attended by people of all ages. These work on the premise that members are offered an incentive in the form of either a reward or the avoidance of loss. Morris (2012) suggests that the reason slimming clubs worked for her, was because of the mixture of motivational fear and being part of a group of people who shared the same needs and issues. Dolan *et al.* (2010) suggest that smaller, quicker rewards are preferable to larger ones that take longer to attain, and confirm the value of weekly weigh-ins in the presence of a group of people who either congratulate or commiserate with members, depending on desired weight-loss. Within the group sessions, food-themed games are played as a means of learning and facilitating social interaction, and these playful elements provide a safe environment in which sensitive topics can also be addressed (Gray 2009).

Norms

Dolan *et al.* (2010) suggest that social norms 'can spread rapidly through social networking or environmental clues about what others have done'. A recent example of this 'social spread' of ideas is the 'ALS Ice Bucket Challenge' which originated in the US in 2014. Amyotrophic Lateral Sclerosis (ALS) is a progressive neuro-degenerative disorder which strikes rapidly and at random (ALS Association 2015a) and the Ice Bucket Challenge represents a hugely successful attempt to raise awareness of this invariably fatal medical condition.

The Challenge demands that individuals accept and then dump a bucket of ice-cold water over their heads, an escapade which is videoed and then uploaded onto social media, along with an invitation to others to take-up the challenge. The Ice Bucket Challenge is a fund-raising initiative which has become a global phenomenon, with over 17 million people uploading their Challenge videos onto Facebook, and it is now set to become an annual event (ALS Association 2015b). One simple playful activity became a socially accepted norm that has done a huge amount of good in advancing research into this debilitating and cruel disease.

For the past 50 years, Health Play Specialists have applied the concept of 'normalization' to help children and young people manage a hospital stay or course of treatment. By 'bringing the outside in' to the hospital or other healthcare setting, play is used to facilitate communication, reduce fear and anxiety and promote resilience. Environmental normalization can be used to similar effect with other population cohorts, including the elderly and those living with dementia. In the Netherlands, a village complex has been designed to give its elderly residents a secure but seemingly free environment, with clubs, shops and, most importantly, opportunities for choice and for fun (Henley 2012). This village community is expertly designed to focus on what residents remain capable of, rather than on their limitations. By maintaining the focus on the familiar, residents exhibit less confusion and are consequently less reliant on medication, whilst remaining active for longer. This approach to residential care may be costlier than traditional alternatives, but it can be argued that savings from lower rates of prescribing and reduced hospital admissions would recover those costs.

Defaults

A default is considered to be a 'pre-set option' that is triggered when no active choice is taken to do otherwise. This can be linked to habitual behavior, which is seen as 'easy, comforting and rewarding' particularly when it does not require you to reason with yourself in terms of what is the best thing to do (Behave n.d.). Frieden (2010: 592) identifies how changing the environmental context can enable healthy choices to become the default option, suggesting that 'individuals would have to expend significant effort not to benefit from them'. Walking is considered to be the most popular form of exercise in the world and provides benefits to both physical and mental health (C3 Collaborating for Health 2012). Using public policy to promote walking as a safe and enjoyable form of exercise is key to making it a viable default option. Schemes such as car-free zones, as well as limited parking or expensive car park charges, increase the likelihood of walking. These are strategies which have transformed Copenhagen in Denmark, over the course of 50 years, from a traffic-dominated city to a pedestrian-orientated space.

Salience

People are more likely to hear and personalize messages and change their attitudes and behaviors accordingly, if they believe the information contained therein is relevant to them (Advocates for Youth 2008). Promoting salience is particularly important for men, who are less likely to visit their GP than women and are therefore more likely to need emergency care (netdoctor 2012). It has been shown that men are more likely to take note of health messages if the information is playful as well as targeted specifically at them. Accepting the notion that sex is a form of adult play, and noting the popularization of so-called 'sex toys', health messages about safe sexual practices naturally invite a playful approach. A health charity in Norway recently employed a young man to dress as a giant penis and to spray couples with gold confetti in a bid to educate people on safer sex in an attempt to reduce the incidence of chlamydia (*Daily Telegraph* 2015). The *Daily Telegraph* (2009) featured 15 funny adverts from around the world highlighting the need for safe sexual practice. The underlying message is that sex is fun – but the results of unsafe sex are not. This is discussed in more detail in Chapter 14.

Priming

The principle behind priming is defined as 'the potential for Behavior B to be affected by activity or environment A, where A precedes or is linked' (Healthier Choices 2015). Pena and Kim (2014) undertook research that manipulated the appearance of self and opponent avatars as part of an exergame that mimicked physical activity in real life. The research demonstrated that when the self and opponent avatar were obese (A), physical activity levels decreased (B) and conversely, when the self and opponent avatars were 'normal', the physical activity levels were at their highest. This simple example demonstrates how priming used within exergames can influence physical activity levels and demonstrates how games can be used to prime health-related behavior.

Affect

Play is an effective way of modifying emotions (affect) and as such, fits this element of the MINDSPACE model really well. For example, Gordon (2014) looks at the ethical questions behind 'doll play' as a means of calming older patients and asks if it is demeaning to give an older person a doll to hold in a caring way. Interestingly, Gordon (2014) notes that the ethics of using therapy dolls as opposed to the efficacy and outcomes of their use is often highlighted, ignoring 'the multiple benefits to the general emotional wellbeing of the individual'. Pet Dogs have been considered as therapeutic benefit for stroke suffers for many years (Pets as Therapy 2012) and sensory environments have been designed for both their calming and stimulating effects with older people. Tea dances have been reported to help older people make friends and to raise happiness levels (Arts for Health Cornwall and Isles of Scilly 2010). The Elevate Program offers vintage tea parties on two of the wards at Shaftesbury's Westminster Hospital. 'As one of our musical "hostesses" says: "The tea party transports people from the hospital environment to a happier place full of smiles, cupcakes and music – what magic!' (ArtCare 2011). There are organizations that will supply free sessions … Britain reportedly has the loneliest population in Europe (Bingham 2014), with one in six people in living in residential care facilities (NHS England 2014) and it may be that fun is the one thing lacking in the lives of the lonely and infirm. Play knows no boundaries and has many benefits for both physical and mental wellbeing. It should be embraced, encouraged and enjoyed as a cost effective tool for the treatment of older people.

Commitments

Making a commitment to change behaviors that are detrimental to health and wellbeing can be difficult, with many of us delaying a decision to change our behavior, despite the long-term benefits change may bring (Dolan *et al.* 2010). Political commitment on the part of the government can have a significant effect on the potential success of a change program. For example, Change4Life was publicly launched in 2009 with a television and print campaign, a website presence and information line (Department of Health 2009). The government committed substantial public funds to the campaign – £75 million over three years (Department of Health 2009: 55) – recognizing the need to 'encourage individuals and families to desire, seek and make healthier choices but also to create an environment in which those choices become easier' (Department of Health 2009: 3).

The marketing strategy for the Change4Life project used the behavior-change funnel to show how short-term commitment to change is easier than long-term commitment, and therefore, the use of personal commitment devices will need to be employed to enhance the chances of success (Dolan et al. 2010).

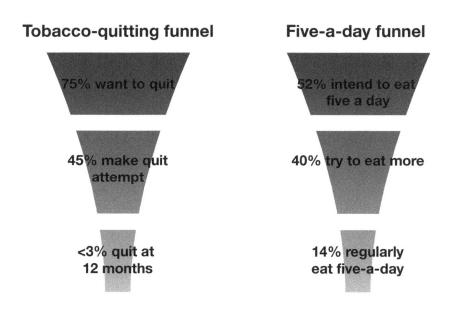

FIGURE 22.1 Comparing behavior change funnels for tobacco quitting and eating five portions of fruit and vegetables a day (Department of Health 2009: 30)

Making commitments public is known to increase effectiveness (Dolan et al. 2010) and this is promoted as one of '12 weird and wonderful ways to help you stop smoking' (Kelly 2014). Play-based strategies feature in three of the suggested tips, ranging from taking up a new hobby or playing a new sport, undertaking activities that keep your hands busy or rewarding yourself 'with a treat or something fun' (Kelly 2014).

Ego

We may respond better to health messages when they are delivered by our peers (Winstead-Derlega et al. 2012). Although this is mainly applicable to young people, it is also becoming true of older people (Peel and Warburton 2009), especially through the use of video as a means of sharing experiences. The Scout Association (2015a) has launched a Community Impact Campaign called 'A Million Hands' that aims to 'mobilise half a million people in support of four social issues chosen by young people'. The campaign features a video clip entitled 'A million hands – dementia' (The Scout Association 2015b) in which a couple share their experience of living with dementia and offer a message of hope for those who may be in similar situations. The video also shows how going-out and undertaking recreational activities has therapeutic benefits – a powerful message with cross-generational appeal.

Conclusion

An informed awareness of the concept of 'habits of mind' suggests that the enjoyment of recreational play and leisure should be adopted as a means of encouraging healthier lifestyle choices. Political backing in the form of a bold commitment to explore alternative approaches to health and wellbeing is crucial to the implementation of play-based policies. Policymakers have the political tools to enable citizens to lead healthier and more prosperous lives and the 'play and politics' analogy has much to offer those responsible for the commissioning and delivery of healthcare services. Governmental promotion of play-based health strategies demonstrate how politics, as envisaged by Aristotle, can be organized for the 'noble action or [health and] happiness of the citizen'.

References

Advocates for Youth (2008) *Peer Education: Promoting Healthy Behaviors*, Online. Available at www.advocatesforyouth.org/publications/publications-a-z/444-peer-education-promoting-healthy-behaviors (accessed 22 November 2015).

ALS Association (2015a) *This Infographic Answers the Question: What is ALS?* Online. Available at www.alsa.org/fight-als/what-is-als.html (accessed 22 November 2015).

ALS Association (2015b) *ALS Ice Bucket Challenge – FAQ,* Online. Available at www.alsa.org/about-us/ice-bucket-challenge-faq.html (accessed 22 November 2015).

ArtCare (2011) *Elevate Programme,* Online. Available at www.artcare.salisbury.nhs.uk/elevate.htm (accessed 23 November 2015).

Arts for Health Cornwall and Isles of Scilly (2010) *Dancing for Older Peoples' Health and Wellbeing Toolkit,* Online. Available at www.artsforhealthcornwall.org.uk/wpcontent/uploads/2010/10/AFHC_Dance_Toolkit.pdf (accessed 6 April 2015).

Alzheimer Disease International (n.d.) *Dementia statistics*, Online. Available at www.alz.co.uk/research/statistics (accessed 22 February 2016).

Alzheimer's Society (2015) *Dementia UK: Update*, Online. Available at www.alzheimers.org.uk/dementiauk (accessed 22 February 2016).

Behave (n.d.) *Habitual Behaviour*, Online. Available at www.cres.gr/behave/framework_theory_2.htm (accessed 22 November 2015).

Bingham, J. (2014) Britain the loneliness capital of Europe, *Daily Telegraph*, 18 June 2014. Online. Available at www.telegraph.co.uk (accessed 23 November 2015).

Boyatzis, R. (2006) An overview of intentional change from a complexity perspective, *Journal of Management Development*, 25 (7): 607–623.

British Nutrition Foundation (2012) *Behaviour Change Conference – 10 Key Facts*, Online. Available at www.nutrition.org.uk/nutritionscience/behaviour/behaviour-10-key-facts (accessed 15 August 2015).

Bruce, T., Meggitt, C. and Grenier, J. (2010) *Child Care and Education*, 5th ed., London: Hodder Education.

C3 Collaborating for Health (2012) *The Benefits of Regular Walking for Health, Wellbeing and the Environment*. London: C3 Collaborating for Health.

Cambridge Dictionaries Online (2015) *English Definition of 'Play'*, Online. Available at http://dictionary.cambridge.org/dictionary/british/play (accessed 30 March 2015).

Campbell, J., Kesetebirhan, A., Soucate, A. and Tlou, S. (2015) Maximizing the impact of community-based practitioners in the quest for universal health coverage. Online. Available at www.who.int/bulletin/volumes/93/9/15-162198.pdf?ua=1 (accessed 22 February 2016).

Chaudhari, S. (2014) Young and old teach each other new skills, *The Bolton News*, 8 February 2014, Online. Available at www.theboltonnews.co.uk/news/bolton/10997281. Young_and_old_teach_each_other_new_skills/ (accessed 22 November 2015).

Conn, D. (2015) Britain's Olympic legacy is a sedentary nation, *The Guardian*, 15 June 2015. Online. Available at www.theguardian.com/commentisfree/2015/jun/15/britain-olympic-legacy-london-2012 (accessed 6 August 2015).

Cox, S. (2012) *Game of Life: How Sport and Recreation Can Help Make Us Healthier, Happier and Richer*, Sports and Recreation Alliance.

The Daily Telegraph (2009) *15 Smart and Funny Safe Sex Adverts that Don't (really) Mention sex*, 22 October 2009, Online. Available at www.telegraph.co.uk (accessed 23 November 2015).

Dalhgreen, W. (2015) *Many Believe Alternative Medicines are Effective*, Online. Available at https://yougov.co.uk/news/2015/03/06/many-believe-alternative-medicine-effective/ (accessed 22 November 2015).

Department of Health (2009) *Change4Life Marketing Strategy*, London: DH Publications.

Department of Health (2011) *Start Active, Stay Active: A Report on Physical Activity from the Four Home Countries' Chief Medical Officers*, London: Department of Health.

Dewey, J. (1916) *Democracy and Education*, Online. Available at www.gutenberg.org/files/852/852-h/852-h.htm#link2HCH0015 (accessed 4 August 2015).

Dolan, P. Hallsworth, M. Halpern, D. King, D. and Vlaev, I. (2010) *MINDSPACE: Influencing Behaviour through Public Policy*, London: Institute for Government.

Farrelly, C. (2013) Play and politics, *Journal of Political Science & Education*, 9 (4): 487–500.

Frieden, T. (2010) A framework for public health action: the health impact pyramid, *American Journal of Public Health*, 100(4): 590–595.

Gordon, M. (2014) *More Than Child's Play: Ethics of Doll Therapy in Dementia*, Online. Available at www.annalsoflongtermcare.com/blog/michael-gordon-doll-therapy-dementia (6 August 2015).

Gray, P. (2009) *Play Makes Us Human I: A Ludic Theory of Human Nature*, Online. Available at www.psychologytoday.com/blog/freedom-learn/200906/play-makes-us-human-i-ludic-theory-human-nature (accessed 8 November 2015).

Healthier Choices (2015) *About the Healthier Choices Pilot*, Online. Available at www.healthier choicespilot.com/ (accessed 23 November 2015).

Helpguide.org (2015) *The Benefits of Play for Adults*, Online. Available at www.help guide.org/articles/emotional-health/benefits-of-play-for-adults.htm (accessed 4 April 2015).

Henley, J. (2012) *The Village Where People Have Dementia – and Fun,* Online. Available at www.theguardian.com/society/2012/aug/27/dementia-village-residents-have-fun (accessed 29 March 2015).

Ho, M. (2015) *Traditional Medicine in Contemporary China,* Online. Available at www.i-sis.org.uk/GCM3.php (accessed 22 November 2015).

Institute of Public Health in Ireland (2015) *Health Inequalities: Global,* Online. Available at www.publichealth.ie/healthinequalities/healthinequalitiesglobal (accessed 6 August 2015).

Kelly, V. (2014) 12 Weird and wonderful ways to help you stop smoking, *Sofeminine Health and Fitness,* 11 October 2014 Online. Available at www.sofeminine.co.uk (accessed 3 December 2015).

Marmot, M. (2010) *Fair Society, Healthy Lives.* The Marmot Review.

Miller, F. (2011) *Aristotle's Political Theory,* Online. Available at http://plato.stanford.edu/cgi-bin/encyclopedia/archinfo.cgi?entry=aristotle-politics (accessed 1 August 2015).

MindTools (2015) *Dealing With Office Politics: Navigating the Minefield,* Online. Available at www.mindtools.com/pages/article/newCDV_85.htm (accessed: 29 July 2015).

Morris, L. (2102) Slimming clubs are a 'straitjacket'? No, *The Guardian,* 28 January 2012. Online. Available at www.theguardian.com (accessed 21 October 2015).

Netdoctor (2012) *Dodging the Doctor – Are You Man or Mouse?* Online. Available at www.netdoctor.co.uk/menshealth/feature/ma (accessed 21 October 2015).

NHS Choices (2015) *The NHS in England,* Online. Available at www.nhs.uk/NHSEngland/thenhs/about/Pages/overview.aspx (accessed 4 August 2015).

NHS England (2014) *Five Year Forward View,* Online. Available at www.england.nhs.uk/wp-content/uploads/2014/10/5yfv-web.pdf (accessed: 29 March 2015).

Nicholson, D. (2014) *Change Is the Key to NHS Survival,* Online. Available at www.england.nhs.uk/2014/03/03/nhs-survival/ (accessed 3 August 2015).

Ontario Health Promotion Resource System (n.d.) *Social Learning Theory,* Online. Available at www.ohprs.ca/hp101/mod4/module4c7.htm (accessed 15 August 2015).

Peel, N. and Warburton, J. (2009) Using senior volunteers as peer educators: what is the evidence of effectiveness in falls prevention? *Australasian Journal on Ageing,* 28 (1): 7–11.

Pena, J. and Kim, E. (2014) Increasing exergame physical activity through self and opponent avatar appearance, *Computers in Human Behavior,* 41: 262–267.

Perraudin, F. (2015) Government launches consultation to tackle fall in sport participation, *The Guardian,* 4 August 2015. Online. Available at www.theguardian.com/uk-news/2015/aug/04/government-consultation-sport-participation-fall (accessed 6 August 2015).

Pets As Therapy (2012) *Lottery Funded 'Stroke and PAT' Project,* Online. Available at www.petsastherapy.org/general/stroke-and-pat (accessed 4 April 2015).

Tempest, M. (2015) Healthcare: political hot potato or key to electoral success? *Civitas Newblog.* 14 January 2015 Online. Available at http://civitas.org.uk/newblog/2015/01/healthcare-political-hot-potato-or-key-to-electoral-success/ (accessed 3 August 2015).

Telegraph Video (2015) *Giant Glitter-spraying Penis Stars in Norwegian Sex Education Advert,* 25 June 2015, Online. Available at www.telegraph.co.uk/ (accessed 23 November 2015).

The Scout Association (2015a) *A Million Hands,* Online. Available at www.amillionhands.org.uk/ (accessed 22 November 2015).

The Scout Association (2015b) *A Million Hands – Dementia,* Online. Available at www.facebook.com/scoutassociation/videos/10152991829728021/ (accessed 22 November 2015).

The Kings Fund (2015) *Is the NHS Heading for Financial Crisis?* Online. Available at www.kingsfund.org.uk/projects/verdict/nhs-heading-financial-crisis (accessed 28 march 2015).

The Royal College of Physicians (2012) *Hospitals on the Edge? The Time for Action*, Online. Available at www.rcplondon.ac.uk/sites/default/files/documents/hospitals-on-the-edge-report.pdf (accessed 4 April 2015).

Toynbee, P. (2014) The NHS is on the brink: can it survive till May 2015? *The Guardian*, 9 May 2014, Online. Available at www.theguardian.com/ (accessed 3 August 2015).

Urban Dictionary (2015) *Politics*, Online. Available at www.urbandictionary.com/define.php?term=politics (accessed 1 August 2015).

Whitehead, M. Dahlgren, G. and Gilson, L. (2001) Developing the policy response to inequities in Health: a global perspective, in, Diderichsen, F. Bhuiya, A. and Wirth, M. (eds.) *Challenging Inequities in Health Care: from Ethics to Action*. New York: Oxford University Press: 309–322.

Winstead-Derlega, C., Rafaly, M., Delgado, S. Freeman, J., Cutitta, K., Miles, T. Ingersoll, K. and Dillingham, R. (2012) A pilot study of delivering peer health messages in an HIV clinic via mobile media, *Telemedicine Journal and e-Health*, 18 (6): 464–469.

World Health Organization (2010) *The World Health Report: Health Systems Financing; The Path to Universal Coverage*. Geneva: World Health Organization.

World Health Organization (WHO) (2015a) *10 Facts on Health Inequities and their Causes*, Online. Available at www.who.int/features/factfiles/health_inequities/en/ (accessed 6 August 2015).

World Health Organization (WHO) (2015b) *World Health Report: Overview*. Online. Available at www.who.int/whr/2003/overview/en/index3.html (accessed: 19 July 2015).

23

PLAYING FOR HEALTH, WEALTH AND HAPPINESS

Julia Whitaker and Alison Tonkin

Introduction

Much can be determined about a society by the health of its citizens. The relationship between the way in which we deliver health services, the health of individuals and the wealth of society is a complex one, 'but the three are inextricably linked so that investing cost-effectively in health systems can contribute to the ultimate goal of societal wellbeing' (Figueras *et al.* 2009; McKee *et al.* 2009, cited in Figueras and McKee 2012). The World Health Organization has re-stated the value of health as a fundamental human right (WHO Regional Office for Europe 2008) and health is also now widely regarded as a key indicator of social development and wellbeing as well as a means to increasing social cohesion (Figueras and McKee 2012).

The way in which we organize, manage and deliver healthcare services is under constant review in the light of changing economic circumstances, societal expectations and the prioritization of needs. Increasing attention given to the social determinants of health (Commission on Social Determinants of Health 2008) demonstrates that the physical environment, education and transport systems can have an even greater influence on a nation's health than health systems in isolation. This book has recognized 'health and wellbeing' to mean much more than the physical health status of individuals and incorporates, within the definition of health, the notions of quality-of-life and self-fulfilment. We have addressed the issue of equity and accessibility in service delivery ... as well as the spiritual aspects of life and health.(Chapter 20).

Where have we come from and how did we arrive at this place?

Alphonse de Lamartine, the nineteenth century French poet, writer and politician stated: 'History teaches us everything, even the future' (cited Mokosso 2007).

Looking back over the evolution of play in healthcare offers us the opportunity to reflect on the past in order to inform the future – a future where play for all is seen as an integral part of routine healthcare provision.

In 1959 Robert Platt drew government and public attention to the predicament of children in hospital when illness or injury separated them from everything that was familiar. The report *Welfare of Children in Hospital* (Ministry of Health 1959) recognized the short- and long-term implications of a health system that, in the course of performing its duty, caused unintentional emotional harm to the next generation. It made a number of recommendations relating to the non-medical aspects of children's hospital care, including the need for children to have access to play and recreation to reduce the negative effects of separation from the family, the disturbance of routine, and a lack of specialist knowledge regarding their psychological needs. The Platt Report marked the birth of the Hospital Play movement which has been at the forefront of promoting play as an essential component of pediatric health and healthcare for over 50 years (National Association of Health Play Specialists 2012). Hospital Play (now referred to as Healthcare Play) affords young patients in the UK the recognition of play as a right (Tonkin 2014); as an innate motivator (Reddy 2010); as a form of communication (Zeedyk 2011) and as a therapeutic intervention (White and Epston 1990). Professionally trained and registered Healthcare Play Specialists are employed throughout the NHS and beyond, in hospitals, hospices and community teams, by reason of the fact that those responsible for pediatric healthcare provision know, from clinical evidence and experience, that professionally organized and delivered play services reduce the length of hospital stays (Glapser *et al.* 2016); minimize the need for analgesic and sedative medicines (Winskill and Andrews 2008); and contribute to an overall improved patient experience (Tonkin 2015). Child Life Specialists occupy a similar role in pediatric healthcare in the United States and Canada and Healthcare Play Specialists, Hospital Play Specialists and Child Life Therapists are recognized professions in Japan, New Zealand and Australia respectively.

However, there can be no room for complacency. In 2010, the UK government published the Kennedy Report, in an attempt to address the fact that 'Many people who work in and use the NHS would agree that the services provided [still] do not measure up to the needs of children and young people. They are not good enough in a number of ways' (Kennedy 2010: 4). This report is notable in that it concentrated on understanding the role of *culture* in healthcare systems and focused on identifying cultural barriers to change and improvement. In Chapter 3, we have discussed how cultural perceptions of health and healthcare are inextricably linked to the way in which services are delivered and received and to the conceptualization of play as a feature of health. Kennedy emphasized the critical role of policy in driving change in attitudes and behavior (discussed in Chapter 22); the importance of collaborative working between different services and aspects of the same service (Chapter 21); the promotion of positive health (Chapters 14 and 15); and the need to challenge historical practices in order for change to occur.

Whilst Kennedy was reporting in the context of health services for children and young people, his approach invites parallel consideration of the way in which adult services are organized and delivered – for all citizens but in particular for the most vulnerable groups in society: the elderly, those with additional access needs, and those whose lifestyle choices contribute to poor health outcomes.

In 2013 the publication of the Francis Report into the failings at the Mid-Staffordshire Foundation Trust (Francis 2013) re-stated in the adult context, what Kennedy had alluded to in relation to children and young people three years earlier. It found a healthcare system that was complacent in its self-evaluation, resistant to change and which failed in the attention given to the patient experience. The recommendations of the Francis Report are summarized thus: 'The patients must be the first priority in all of what the NHS does. Within available resources, they must receive effective services from caring, compassionate and committed staff, working within a common culture, and they must be protected from avoidable harm and any deprivation of their basic rights' (Francis 2013).

In December 2015, as this book was in its final stages of preparation, the BBC revealed the findings of a report into a series of unexplained deaths of vulnerable patients in the NHS Southern Health Trust, one of the UKs largest mental health trusts providing services to over 450,000 people (Buchanan 2015). The report found that the likelihood of an unexpected death being investigated by the Southern Health Trust depended on the type of patient concerned. The report found that the average age at death of those with a learning disability was 56 years compared with a national average of 81 years, and that just 1 per cent of these deaths were investigated. For those aged over 65 years with a mental health diagnosis, the figure was just 0.3 per cent. Criticisms in the report again focused on the culture of care at the Trust where care systems were described as 'chaotic' and organized more around staff than patient needs (Buchanan 2015).

In this book we advocate a healthcare culture which recognizes its users as people before patients, a culture which values the right of every individual to aspire to satisfy the desire for self-fulfilment and completeness and to be supported in this undertaking. A 'caring, compassionate and committed' (Francis 2013) healthcare system is one in which both patients and staff are valued for who they are and one which engages its users on manifold levels.

Play as a facilitator and enabler

In Chapter 2, play was conceptualized within a biopsychosocial framework, using Barton and Grant's (2006) Health Model. The significance of this health-specific ecological model is the explicit identification of play as an activity that determines health and wellbeing. The content of this book has provided numerous examples to substantiate the inclusion of play as a determinant of health, along with other activities such as working, shopping, moving, living and learning (Barton and Grant 2006). Chapter 2 also discusses the role of human motivation, showing how the evolution and adaptation of theory over time can be used to explore and develop ideas, generating new areas for debate and discussion. This was Maslow's (1943) original intention when his seminal article 'A theory of human motivation' was published in 1943. Maslow (1943: 371) lamented 'the very serious lack of sound data in this area …due primarily to the absence of a valid theory of motivation' and proposed that the publication of his own theory filled a conceptual void. However, Maslow only ever intended his own work to be a catalyst, proposing that it 'must be considered to be a suggested program or framework for future research … researches to be done, researches suggested perhaps, by the questions raised in this paper' (Maslow 1943: 371). Over 70 years after the original publication of 'A theory of human motivation', Maslow's notion of a hierarchical framework of needs which determine human motivation is as relevant today as it ever was (Chapman 2014). Maslow (1943) identified the ultimate human need as the 'desire for self-fulfilment' – the need for self-actualization. Maslow (1943: 382) famously stated, 'what a man can be, he must be' and that 'a musician must make music, an artist must paint, a poet must write, if he is to be ultimately happy'. This is exemplified in Chapter 18 (Box 18.1) which describes how locked-in memories of their previous occupations, such as that of mechanic or carpet-fitter, led patients with dementia to mimic familiar activities from their former lives by adapting features of the present environment in order to satisfy a deep-rooted need.

Originally described by Goldstein (Maslow 1943), self-actualization is understood to refer to the process through which an organism or person reaches their full potential. Boa (2004: 118) identifies the need for courage in order for this process to persist in the face of adversity, when the need to seek 'safety and self-protection in the face of pain [and] fear of the unknown' can be overwhelming. It is when adverse factors overwhelm, that play has much to offer. Just as children in the hospital setting know instinctively how to operate in a playful environment in order to achieve a sense of control and normality (Tonkin 2015), adults also deploy playful strategies to achieve similar ends, although these may not always appear obvious.

Recognizing individual patient needs and designing health services that revolve around the 'patient as person' lie at the heart of this book. Patients are always more than their diagnosis or their 'type' and healthcare which recognizes, respects and responds to the patient as an individual, a family member and part of a social community – regardless of age or circumstance – is care that addresses holistic health and wellbeing needs, including the human tendency for play and playfulness as essential to personal growth and development (as discussed in Chapters 4, 8 and 17). We have become bashful in the west about using the word 'play' in relation to adult activity. Suggestions have been made that its use in the healthcare context represents the infantilization or devaluing of adult recreational and creative activities. We make no apology in this regard, offering the counter argument that to call what we choose to do in the pursuit of pleasure anything other than play, is to suggest an unwarranted shamefulness in the pursuit thereof.

When Plato spoke of play (*pleida*) in the fourth century BC he did not shy away from naming the subject of his attention and acknowledged the association between the 'playful' and the 'serious'. In discussing Plato's philosophy of play,

Ardley (1967) writes that 'Fecundity, genuine seriousness, real understanding, are to be found only in aerial flights of play', expressing with far greater eloquence than most, the intersection of play and matters of serious personal and public concern.

The compartmentalization of the playful and the serious is certainly a common feature of contemporary life, although not exclusively so. Yet play at work need not be seen as a contradiction in terms. Starbuck and Webster (1991) suggest that distinctions between work and play are becoming increasingly blurred, with more jobs demanding expertise in a particular area and more people working from home and using modern technology. Webster (1989 cited in Starbuck and Webster 1991: 2) found that many people talked about deriving enjoyment from using computers at work and playful behaviors have also infused many aspects of traditional forms of employment (Roy 1960; Garson 1977).

Nonetheless, the work/play divide persists, most notably in the affluent west where play is regarded as reward or respite from the material substance of everyday life; play is what we do when we are not working and therefore to be justified or excused. We can learn much here from other societies who would find such a dichotomy bewildering and nonsensical. In tribal societies, work is often infused with rituals and customs that incorporate the creative and the playful and endow it with pleasurable qualities (McLean *et al.* 2014). We have read in Chapter 13 of how the social therapy model, arising from Steiner's interpretation of Schiller's philosophy of play, revives the conjunction between work and play to great effect, a feature that is being re-discovered and replicated throughout contemporary creative industries (Stewart 2013).

> Advertising agents, creative writers, designers, planners, and social theorists use fantasy and imagination. Athletes compete. Consultants and researchers explore. Mathematicians solve puzzles. Therapists may use therapeutic play. Such people cannot work without playing.
>
> *(Starbuck and Webster 1991: 87)*

Taking a creative approach to healthcare delivery does not imply the abandonment of reason and logic. Information gathering and evidence-based analysis are critical features of the creative process – as well as imagination. 'To get to innovative ideas and solutions, we have to constantly toggle between analysis and synthesis, or between reality and possibility' (Robertson 2013). Children are the experts in the creative domain because they are curious about possibilities and are not afraid to get things wrong – capacities that we can lose with maturity and a growing awareness of the negative consequences of making mistakes. This was demonstrated by Zabelina and Robinson (2010) in a controlled study which confirmed the benefits of thinking like a child for subsequent creative originality. It is the lack of child-like courage which prevents systems from seeking and implementing innovative alternatives to historical practices because of the fear of sanction or loss-of-face but, in the words of Robinson (2006), an expert in creativity: 'If you're not prepared to be wrong, you'll never come up with anything original'.

282 Julia Whitaker and Alison Tonkin

There have been recent bold moves by some healthcare providers, in the UK and elsewhere, to integrate play into the serious business of looking after people's health.

Chapters 9, 10, 11 and 12 offer insights into the use of music and the creative arts as playful health interventions aimed to enhance quality and to achieve measurable improvements in targeted outcomes. Whilst the synthesis of the evidence for the use of the Arts to improve the healthcare experience presents certain challenges, due to the diversity of interventions and lack of evaluative standardization, it is clear is that 'bringing visual, performance and participatory arts into hospitals for the benefit of staff and patients has become common practice' (Royal Society for Public Health 2013). Chapter 10 describes one innovative small-scale project which illustrates music's demonstrable impact on social, psychological and physical health outcomes.

In 2011, in an article entitled 'What pediatric hospitals can teach adult hospitals', Mazjun posed a challenge to those working in adult healthcare, inviting them to 'embrace the emotional nature of the work' (Mazjun 2011) in the drive to foster an empathic culture of care that nurtures connections between patients and staff and between members of professional teams. We have learned from the aforementioned crises in the NHS (Francis 2013; Buchanan 2015) that it is the ownership of this emotional connection that is frequently found to be lacking when systems implode.

Mazjun (2011) stresses the importance of patients being able to connect with each other in the isolating hospital environment but this also applies to the loneliness that can accompany a life-long health condition. The demonstrable benefits of peer-identification and peer-support surface throughout the preceding chapters, whether in reference to Men's Sheds (Chapter 7), integrated sporting facilities (Chapter 16), or the celebration of festivals (Chapter 19). Chapters 15 and 21 have examined the widespread application of gaming technology to the achievement of health-related goals, both in health promotion and engagement and in the training and professional development of health service personnel.

Mazjun (2011: 211) writes that, 'Grown-ups need play, too. It reduces stress by taking patients out of the mental space of being sick' and advocates the use of playful distraction as a means of helping patients to cope with painful and distressing medical treatment interventions. Increasingly, Health Play Specialists employed by children's services in the UK are being invited by colleagues in adult health to assist with the distraction and medical preparation of adult patients. At University College Hospital in London, play specialists have worked with a number of young adults to facilitate their coping during scanning and other procedures, using tried-and-tested distraction techniques. Distraction and relaxation techniques used with children have already found widespread application in the field of dentistry (Corah et al. 1979). Adult service users are often made anxious or ill-at-ease by their interface with medical services, particularly if their communication and accommodation skills are compromised by cognitive or sensory impairment (Chapter 5). A playful approach to environmental design (Chapter 18), including way-finding and the creative presentation of printed material (Chapter 14) convey positive messages of acceptance, welcome and belonging with measurable benefits for engagement and treatment compliance.

However, it is not the intention of this book to make the case for play only as a feature of healthcare intervention, although that is important. The essence of play is that it is much more than merely a means to an end; although it is clearly functional, it is not its functionality that establishes the concept of play as worthy of further exploration and discussion. Asma (2015) writes:

> The stakes for play are higher than we think. Play is a way of being that resists the instrumental, expedient mode of existence. In play, we do not measure ourselves in terms of tangible productivity (extrinsic value), but instead, our physical and mental lives have intrinsic value of their own. It provides the source from which other extrinsic goods flow and eventually return.
>
> *(Asma 2015)*

If we consider play in terms only of its 'usefulness' – in the pursuit of wellness or otherwise – then we diminish both the act of 'playing' and the player. To play (whether in music, dance, sport, art, or with Lego) is to find fulfilment in the very act of seeking it (Asma 2015). When we engage in playful activity, purely for the pleasure therein, we are open to possibilities of 'wellness' in every sense of the word. Sandelands and Buckner (1989) have said that for an activity to be playful it must generate both immediate pleasure and involvement. It is the co-existence of involvement and immediate pleasure that make play inherently engaging for the player, both motivating and focusing that engagement.

Csíkszentmihalyi (1975) contends that a player feels pleasure and involvement when the play's challenges balance their own capabilities. Insufficient challenge creates boredom or anxiety whilst excessive challenge creates worry or anxiety. When capabilities and challenges are well-balanced, the player experiences a state of total pleasure and involvement which Csíkszentmihalyi calls 'flow'.

> Players shift into a common mode of experience when they become absorbed in their activity. This mode is characterized by a narrowing of the focus of awareness, so that irrelevant perceptions and thoughts are filtered out; by loss of self-consciousness; by a responsiveness to clear goals and unambiguous feedback; and by a sense of control over the environment …. It is this common flow experience that people adduce as the main reason for performing the activity.
>
> *(Csíkszentmihalyi 1975: 72)*

Immediate pleasure and involvement are consistent features of play (Sandelands and Buckner 1989), and Starbuck and Webster (1991) relate these to five inter-related consequences:

1 Emphasis on immediate reinforcement;
2 Emphasis on means rather than ends;
3 Emphasis on short-term goals;
4 Concentration;
5 Persistence.

(Adapted from Starbuck and Webster 1991: 8)

Conclusion

When people judge playful activities to be appropriate, they adopt them readily and are motivated to continue doing them. The relevance of play to adult health is that play itself offers fulfilment whilst at the same time fulfilling a health need. We become involved in play because of how it makes us feel in the here-and-now and its reinforcement of those pleasurable feelings focuses our energies and motivates us to continue in our play to unknown ends. Until we play, we do not know what we are capable of, what possibilities life holds in store for us: 'Play energizes us and enlivens us. It eases our burdens. It renews our natural sense of optimism and opens us up to new possibilities' (Brown and Vaughan 2009). Play is at the core of being who we are: of 'wellbeing' and of 'being well'.

References

Ardley, G. (1967) The role of play in the philosophy of Plato, *Philosophy*, 42 (161): 226–244.
Asma, S.T. (2015) Reclaiming the power of play, *New York Times*, 27 April 2015, Online. Available at http://opinionator.blogs.nytimes.com/2015/04/27/reclaiming-the-power-of-play/?_r=0 (accessed 15 December 2015).
Barton, H. and Grant, M. (2006) A health map for the local human habitat, *The Journal of the Royal Society for the Promotion of Health*, 126 (6): 252–253.
Boa, K. (2004) *Augustine to Freud: What Theologians and Psychologists Tell Us about Human Nature (And Why it Matters)*, Nashville, TN: B&H Publishing Group.
Brown, S. and Vaughan, C. (2009) *Play, How in Shapes the Brain, Opens the Imagination and Invigorates the soul*, London: Penguin.
Buchanan, M. (2015) *NHS Trust 'Failed to Investigate Hundreds of Deaths'*, Online. Available at www.bbc.co.uk/news/health-35051845 (accessed 14 December 2015).
Chapman, A. (2014) *Maslow's Hierarchy of Needs*, Online. Available at www.businessballs.com/maslow.htm (accessed 9 December 2015).
Commission on Social Determinants of Health (2008) *Closing the Gap in a Generation: Health Equity Through Action on the Social Determinants of Health: Final Report of the Commission on Social Determinants of Health*, Geneva: World Health Organization.
Corah, N.L., Gale, E.N. and Illig, S.J. (1979) The use of relaxation and distraction to reduce psychological stress during dental procedures The use of relaxation and distraction to reduce psychological stress during dental procedures The use of relaxation and distraction to reduce psychological stress during dental procedures, *Journal of the American Dental Association*, 98 (3): 390–394.
Csíkszentmihalyi, M. (1975) *Beyond Boredom and Anxiety*, San Francisco, CA: Jossey-Bass.

Figueras, J., Lessof, S., McKee, M. *et al.* (2009) *Health Systems for Health, Wealth and Societal Well-being.* Copenhagen: WHO Regional Office for Europe on behalf of the European Observatory on Health Systems and Policies.

Figueras, J. and McKee, M. (eds) (2012) *Health-systems, Health, Wealth and Societal Wellbeing,* Maidenhead: McGraw Hill. The use of relaxation and distraction to reduce psychological stress during dental procedures The use of relaxation and distraction to reduce psychological stress during dental procedures.

Francis, R. (2013) *The Mid Staffordshire NHS Foundation Trust Public Enquiry: Executive Summary,* London: The Stationery Office.

Garson, B. (1977) *All the Livelong Day,* New York: Penguin Books.

Glapser, E.A., McEwing, G. and Richardson, J. (eds) (2016) *Oxford Handbook of Children's and Young People's Nursing,* 2nd ed., Oxford: Oxford University Press.

Kennedy, I. (2010) *Getting it Right for Children and Young People. Overcoming Cultural Barriers in the NHS to Meet their Needs,* Online. Available at www.gov.uk/government/uploads/system/uploads/attachment_data/file/216282/dh_119446.pdf (accessed 14 December 2015).

McLean, D., Dayer-Berenson, L., Seaward, B.L., Hurd, A. and McLean, D. (2014) *Kraus' Recreation and Leisure in Modern Society,* Boston, MA: Jones and Bartlett.

Maslow, A. (1943) A theory of human motivation, *Psychological Review,* 50 (4): 370–396.

Mazjun, R. (2011) Coloring outside the lines: what pediatric hospitals can teach adult hospitals. *Pediatric Nursing,* 37(4): 2010–2011

Ministry of Health (1959) *The Welfare of Children in Hospital, Platt Report,* London: Her Majesty's Stationery Office.

Mokosso, H.E. (2007) *American Evangelical Enterprise in Africa: The Case of the United Presbyterian Mission in Cameroon 1879–1957,* New York: Peter Lang Publishing.

National Association of Health Play Specialists (2012) *National Association of Hospital Play Staff Milestones,* Online. Available at http://nahps.org.uk/index.php?page=history (accessed 15 December 2015).

Reddy, V. (2010) *How Infants Know Minds,* Cambridge, MA: Harvard University Press.

Robertson, S. (2013) *Why You Should Have a Child-like Imagination (and the Research which Proves It!),* Online. Available at www.ideastogo.com/the-science-of-imagination (accessed 15 December 2015).

Robinson, K. (2006) *Do Schools Kill Creativity? TED 2006,* Online. Available at www.ted.com/talks/ken_robinson_says_schools_kill_creativity (accessed 15 December 2015).

Roy, D.F. (1960) 'Banana time': job satisfaction and informal interaction, *Human Organization,* 18: 158–168.

Royal Society for Public Health (RSPH) (2013) *Arts, Health and Wellbeing Beyond the Millennium: How Far Have We Come in 15 Years?* Online. Available at www.rsph.org.uk/en/policy-and-projects/areas-of-work/arts-and-health.cfm (accessed 16 December 2015).

Sandelands, L.E., and Buckner, G.C. (1989). *Of Art and Work: Aesthetic Experience and the Psychology of Work Feelings,* in, Cummings, L.L. and Staw, B.M. (eds), *Research in Organizational Behavior, Vol. 11.* Greenwich, CT: JAI Press: 105–131.

Starbuck, W. H. and Webster, E. J. (1991) When is play productive? *Accounting Management and Information Technologies,* 1: 71–90.

Stewart, J. B. (2013) Looking for a lesson in Google's perks, *New York Times,* 15 March 2013 Online. Available at www.nytimes.com/2013/03/16/business/at-google-a-place-to-work-and-play.html?_r=0 (accessed 14 December 2015).

Tonkin, A. (2014) *The Provision of Play in Health Service Delivery Fulfilling Children's Rights under Article 31 of the United Nations Convention on the Rights of the Child: A Literature*

Review, Online. Available at http://nahps.org.uk/uploads/Final_full_report_NAHPS_. pdf (accessed 16 December 2015).

Tonkin, A. (2015) *Exploring the Impact Environments Have on Children and Young People's Experience of Healthcare: A Review of the Literature,* Online. Available at www.hpset.org.uk/ environmentsofcare2015.html (accessed 8 November 2015).

White, M. and Epston, D. (1990) *Narrative Means to Therapeutic Ends,* New York: W.W. Norton.

Winskill, R. and Andrews, D. (2008) Minimizing the 'ouch' – A strategy to minimize pain, fear and anxiety in children presenting to the emergency department, *Australasian Emergency Nursing Journal,* 11 (4): 184–188.

WHO Regional Office for Europe (2008) *The Tallinn Charter: Health Systems for Health and Wealth. Copenhagen: WHO Regional Office for Europe,* Online. Available at www.euro. who.int/document/E91438.pdf (accessed 15 December 2015).

Zabelina, D. and Robinson, M. D. (2010) Child's play: facilitating the originality of creative output by priming manipulation, *Journal of Aesthetics,* 4: 57–65.

Zeedyk, S. (2011) *The Connected Baby,* produced by Suzanne Zeedyk and James Robertson (DVD).

INDEX

abnormality 102–3
Abrahams, Caroline 92
accessing healthcare services: challenge of communication 71–5; dementia sufferers 73; engagement and communication, contrasting approaches to 75–81; online 73
accommodation 19
acting 258
active learning 255
Acton, G.J. and Malathum, P. 76
acupuncture 202–3, 205; Traditional Chinese Acupuncture 206–7
Acupuncture Points Functions Colouring Book, The (Hutchinson) 207
adaption 14, 34
adaptive practices 106
addiction: alcohol 89–90; drug 90–1
Addiction to Medicines (National Treatment Agency) 91
Adler's Individual Psychology 227
adolescence 53–5; lifespan period 33
Adorno, T. 129
adult coloring 107
adult health 264–5
adult healthcare 265–73
adult world: exploring play in 5–7
adventure playgrounds 26
After-School Clubs 26
age: as a categorising framework 33–4

Ainsworth, M.D.S. and Bowlby, J. 49
Al Aboud, K. 226
Albinal 90
alcohol 89–90
Alcohol Concern 89
Aldridge, C. 124
Alexander Technique 205, 207–8
Alnorthumbria Veterinary Group 203
alternative medicine *see* complementary and alternative medicines (CAM)
Alzheimer's disease: pillars of prevention 88–9; *This is me* tool 168
Alzheimer's Research UK 88
Alzheimer's Society: fact-sheets 167
Alzheimer's UK 121
Ambiguity of Play, The (Sutton-Smith) 7
Amstel, F. 220, 221, 222
Amyotrophic Lateral Sclerosis (ALS) 269
anaesthetics 121
Ancient Greece: infirmaries 144
Ancient Greeks 115–16
animals: and acupuncture 203
anthroposophy 39–40, 76, 157
anti-depressive medication 23
anxiety 73
anxiety disorders 105
Apollo 116
apps: diabetes 179; health and wellness 178–80
Arabic medicine 117

288 Index

Aristotle 101, 116, 263–4
aromatherapy 205
art 61
ArtCare 119, 213
art for health 143–9; benefits for family
   members 146, 147; Craft Café project
   145–6; focus of initiative 144; Gallery
   Social initiative 146, 147; purpose of
   initiative 144
Art for Health report 147
Art Nouveau 152
Art of Health program 40
Arts4Dementia 125
Arts and Crafts 152
Arts and Health Diamond 144
art therapy 13, 65
Asma, S.T. 283
Aspire/Aspire Leisure Centre 189–90; case
   study 196–7; dance studio 192; exercise
   classes 192; fitness studio 192;
   InstructAbility 193; integration 190;
   non-judgemental environment 191;
   parasports 193; promotion of health and
   well-being 191; rehabilitation and sport
   193; services 190; sports hall 192;
   swimming pool 191–2
assimilation 19
asylum era 118
Australia 258
autism 62, 71, 74
Autistic Spectrum Disorders (ASD)
   79–80
Avicenna 117
Axline, Virginia 27
Ayurveda 40

Bach Flower Remedies 205
baking bread 9–10
balance 115–16, 168, 177, 203, 204, 206,
   208, 209
Bandura, A. 20, 35, 267
Barbakoff, A. 12
Barch, G.R. 138
Barrett, R. 21–2
Barthes, Roland 129
Barton, H. and Grant, M. 19, 229
Basu, S. 11
Bauby, Jean-Dominique 242
Bebbington *et al.* 100
Beekun, R. 234

behavioral theory 267
behavioural perspective 35
being active 12; mental wellbeing 109
Benedict, Ruth 37
Bennett, Alan 166–7
Bennett *et al.* 25
Bergen, D. and Pronin Fromberg, D. 23
Bergson, Henri 42
Berthoud, R. 101
Better Services by Design 215–16
Betts Adams' *et al.* 94
Bidna Capoeira 38
Big Pharma 105
Biller, H. 85, 86
Binder, D. 235
Bioecological Theory of Human Development
   (Bronfenbrenner) 19
biofeedback games 178
biopsychosocial models 162
Block *et al.* 92
blood glucose levels 87
blue gym research 66
blue space 11
Boa, K. 280
bodily organs 206, 207
body image 66
body language 166
Boex 217–20
Bowen (cited in Better Services by Design
   2015b) 215
Bowen Technique 205, 208
Boyd, D. and Bee, H. 20
Boyer, E. 128
brain development 25
brain studies 46
breath play 201
British Nutrition Foundation 267–8
Brocklesby, R. 118
Bronfenbrenner, Urie 19; contextual
   perspective 36
Browne, R. 115
Brown, F. 25
Brown, S. and Lomax, J. 24
Brox *et al.* 177
Bruce, T. and Meggit, C. 60
Buchanan, R. 174
Buddhism 231
Building Better Healthcare 75

cancer 202

Index **289**

CandoCo 192
capabilities and challenges 283
capacity 72
Capello, P.P. 140
capoeira 38
Capoeira for Peace 38
caregiver wellbeing 250–1, 252
CARROR fit app 179
cartoons 169
catharsis 27
cave drawings 6
celebrations 226
Celsus 117
chamber music: being connected 130; Indian harmonium 132; interaction of musicians 129–30; level playing field 127; musicians with dementia 125–7, 130, 131–2; personal musical sensibility of musicians 129; players 128–9; space of play 130–1, 131; students 126; workshops 125–6, 128, 130, 132
Change4Life campaign 90, 271–2
chaplaincy services 244
Chasen, L.R. 136, 139
Chaudhari, S. 268
childhood play 41
Child Life Specialists 278
Child Life Therapists 278
child-raising 51
child-rearing 48
children: categories of development 34
China: importance of play 41–2
Chinese Herbal Medicine 205, 208–9
choirs 252
Chopped (game) 207
chronic illness 85, 86–9
chronic pain 202
Clappison, J. 207–8
classical conditioning 35
climbing 9–10
clown doctors 8
Co-creating Meaning 245–6
cognitive perspective 36
collaboration skills 258
coloring books, therapeutic 107
comedy 230
comics 169
Comic-strip Conversations 74, 75
commitment 271–2
communication: approaches to 75–81;

challenge of 71–5; and health literacy 165–6
communication skills 258
community identity 159
community institutions: and spiritual health 64
complementary and alternative medicines (CAM) 199–201; Alexander Technique 205, 207–8; Bowen Technique 205, 208; Chinese Herbal Medicine 208–9; differences with Western approach 200; essential role of relationships 203–4; range and breath of therapies 204–5; Traditional Chinese Acupuncture 206–7; underlying concepts 201–5; see also Traditional Chinese Medicine (TCM)
conception 47–8
conceptualizing play 18; play deprivation 22–6; playing for health and wellbeing 26; play therapy 26–7; social ecology of health 18–20; using play as a motivational tool 20–2
Confucius 41
Conn, D. 266
Connected Baby, The 53
connectedness 12
connect, mental wellbeing 109
contexts 229
contextual perspective 36
coping mechanisms 251
coping self 228, 231
coronary heart disease (CHD) 88
'Couch to 5k' project 60–1
Coulter, N. and Rushbrook, S. 204
CounterPlay 227
Cox, S. 266
CPD (continuing professional development) 254–5
craft-based learning/work 152, 156
Craft Café project 145–6
Crawford et al. 52
creative self 228, 229–30
creativity 78; cultures of in playful design 214–17; enhancement through play 213; mental health 65; right-brain/left-brain dominance 212
Cripples Olympiad 187
Crone et al. 230
cross-generational change 37–9

290 Index

Csíkszentmihalyi, M. 54, 283
cultural identity 232–3, 235
cultural relativism 102–4, 104
culture: mental illness 103–4; mourning
  rituals 103, 106; play as 37; view of self
  and reality 103
Curry, N.A. and Kasser, T. 107
Cuypers *et al.* 145

Dahlgren, G. and Whitehead, M. 19
dance: functions of 135; personal
  development 136; significance of 232;
  therapeutic role of 138–40; *see also*
  drama
Dance Dance Revolution game 176
Dance Mat (PlayStation One) 176
dance studio, Aspire Leisure Centre 192
Darwin, Charles 36
da Vinci, Leonardo 144
day centers 63
daydreaming 5
day services 63
Deaflympics 187
deafness 72
debating resources 257–8
Debong, Fredrik 180
deep play 8, 24
defaults 270
define phase, Double Diamond Design
  Process 215, 216
Definitive Guide to Play (Sissons) 186
deliver phase, Double Diamond Design
  Process 215, 216
dementia 71; age-related 1; clinical features
  of 124; cognitive effects of music 124–5;
  communicating messages 166–7;
  familiarity of music 131–2; lifestyle
  trends 88–9; A Million Hands campaign
  273; and music 121; psychological and
  emotional barriers 73; TimeSlips project
  168–9; *see also* chamber music; Gallery
  Social; Museum of Modern Art
  (MOMA)
democracy 264
Department of Health 12, 144; *Healthy
  Staff, Better Care for Patients* 250; staff
  health and wellbeing review 250
Department of Work and Pensions 55
depression 100, 105, 145; physical activity
  108

deprivational danger 242
design *see* playful design
Design Council 212
destiny, play as 7
developmental niche 37
develop phase, Double Diamond Design
  Process 215, 216
de Vries, Kets 5–6, 6, 11
Dewey, John 128, 264, 267
diabetes 1, 86–7; apps for 179
Diabetes UK 62, 87
Diagnostic and Statistical Manual of
  Mental Disorders (DSM) 102–3, 104
diagnostic over-expansion 104
diet clubs 269
digital and innovative technical resources
  257
digital immigrants 174
digital natives 174
dimensional approach, mental health 105,
  106
disability: attitudes about integration
  188–90; in the UK 188; *see also* Aspire
  Leisure Centre
disability sport 187–8
discovery phase, Double Diamond Design
  Process 215, 216
disposition for play 38–9
Diving Bell and the Butterfly, The (Bauby)
  242
Djembe drumming 120
Dobbins and McLane (cited Wahowiak
  2014) 169
dogs 271
Dolan *et al.* 268, 269
doll play 271
doodles 178
Doodles, Sue 178
dot.com companies 11–12
Double Diamond Design Process 215–16
drama: functions of 135; personal
  development 136; power of, as play
  136–7; role of play in 136; therapeutic
  role of 138–40; *see also* dance
dreams 154
drugs: illegal 90–1; psychotropic 104
DSM-5 104
DSM-5 Task Force 105
DSM (Diagnostic and Statistical Manual of
  Mental Disorders) 102–3, 104

dying with dignity 64

early adulthood: lifespan period 33
early-onset alcohol problems 89
Ecominds project 109
economic deprivation 25
economic wellbeing 110
eco-therapy 110
Edinburgh International Festival 143, 230
Edinburgh Social Union 144
education: health, innovation in *see*
  innovation in health education; lifelong
  learning 254–5
ego 272–3
Eid ul-Fitr 234
Elderflowers program 21
Elevate Program 119–20, 271
Ellis (cited in Ellens) 48
embodiment 138
emerging adulthood 33
emotional care: cancer treatment 202
emotional health 61–2, 191
engagement: approaches to 75–81; positive
  153
English Chamber Orchestra Ensemble
  (ECO Ensemble) 125, 127
Ensler, Eve 243
environmental health 65–7
epigenetics 34
Epilepsy Action 62
EPR model 138
Equality Act (2010) 71
Erikson, Erik 5, 35; sideways movement 6
ESOL (English for Speakers of Other
  Languages) courses 169
essential self 228, 232–3
ethical healthcare 70
eurhythmy 40
European Centre for Environment and
  Human Health 11
European Health Literacy Survey 163
Evans, A.B. and Sleap, M. 66
Evans, Kath 182
Evening Play Centre Committee (EPC) 26
evolutionary perspective 36
Ewles, L. and Simnett, I. 21
exam stress 23
exercise: physical self 233–4; walking 270;
  see also physical activity
exercise patterns 86

exercise referral schemes 93
exergames 176–8
expansive design concept 220–2
Expansive Hospital (boardgame) 222

Facebook 174, 181
fairytales 157
FA Mars Just Play sessions 10
family, creating and growing a 45–7;
  adolescence 53–5; arrival of babies
  48–51; family life under stress 55–6;
  playful parenting 51–3; sowing the seed
  47–8
family life-cycle 46
family systems theory 46
Faragher, Meg 147
Farrelly, C. 264, 267
fasting 234
fate, play as 7
feedback loops 46
Feldman, R.S. 35
Fenton, K. and Varney, J. 233
festivals 156–9, 226–7, 229; cultural
  identity 232–3, 235; Eid ul-Fitr 234;
  Holi 232; LGBT 233; sharing food 234;
  social self 231–2
field-theoretical approach 18–19
Finland 258
Fire Element (Traditional Chinese
  Medicine) 201
Fitbit mobile app 180
Fitness City 181
fitness studio, Aspire Leisure Centre 192
flash-cards 206–7
flow 54–5, 239–40, 283
Foresight Mental Capital and Wellbeing
  Project 108, 109
fotonovelas 169
Frances, A. 104
Francis Report 255, 279
Frankl, Victor 245
Freeman, C. 21
Freud, Anna 27
Freud, Sigmund 5, 35
Frieden, T. 270
frivolous, play as 7
Froebel, F. 6
Fruit Basket (exergame) 177
fun 8
fundraising initiatives 63

292 Index

Furedi, Frank 51, 107–8

Gadamer, H.G. 38, 157, 159
Galen 117
Gallery Social 146, 147
game-playing 170
gamification, of healthcare 178–81
gaming resources 256–7
Garde, J. 215, 222–3
Garvald approach 75, 76, 76–8
Garvald Edinburgh 75–9, 152; Social
    Charter 79; *see also* Glass Studio
Gauntlett, D. and Thomsen, S. 215
Gay Pride 233
General Health Questionnaire 111
Gentile's taxonomy of motor skills 177
GIANTmicrobes® 164
Gilles, R. 129–30
giving, mental wellbeing 109
giving to others 12
Glasser (cited Buck 2013) 102
Glass Studio 153, 154–6, 157
Global Health Film Festival 230
Goethe, Johan Wolfgang von 156–7
Goldstein, J. 173
Gomez, Gina 80
Goodall, Jane 24
Google: workplace 65
Gordon, M. 271
Gould, S.J. 106
Graphic Medicine 169
Gray, Carol 74
Gray, Millie 148
Gray, P. 213, 214
Gray, Peter xiii
Greek Medicine 115–16
Green, A. 25
green environments 65–6
'The Green Snake and the Beautiful Lily'
    157
green space 110
grief 61–2
Grondin, J. 157
Groos, K. 5
growing up 24
Grywacz, J. and Fuqua, J. 19
Gu, S. 209
Guttmann, Ludwig 187
gyms: outdoor 11, 66

Halhuber, C. and Halhuber, M. 88
Hall, D. 257–8
happiness 41, 49, 78, 101, 102
Hartogh *et al.* 127
Hat Tours 223
health: benefits of play for 9–13; definition
    70; exploring play in an adult world
    5–7; physical play for 10–11; play and
    mental wellness 11–13; playing to learn
    and learning through play 14–15; play
    within healthcare 13–14; social ecology
    of 18–20; and wellbeing 59–67; *see also*
    art for health
health adaption 70
Health and Care Professions Council
    (HCPC) 254
healthcare: areas of vulnerability for
    children 242; evolution of play in
    278–9; gamification of 178–81; play and
    holistic care provision 243–6; and
    spirituality 241–2
healthcare environment 75
Healthcare Play movement 278
Healthcare Play Specialists 278
healthcare services: accessibility 70;
    adaption and change 70–1; in Scotland
    72; *see also* accessing healthcare services
Health Development Agency 147
health inequality 265
health literacy 160–1; communicating
    messages 165–6, 166–7; defining 161–3;
    ESOL 169; health promotion strategies
    164, 166; laughter 167, 168; narrative
    graphics 169; picture stories 169; in
    practice 163–70; skills and knowledge
    163; storytelling 168–9; supermarket
    checkout 167; use of humor 163–4,
    167, 167–8
Health Play Specialists 74
health professionals 72
health promotion 266–7
health services: interface with 73
Healthy Staff, Better Care for Patients 250
hearing impairments 72
heart attacks 88
Heart Burned™ Mini Microbe Box 164
Heart Warming™ Mini Microbe Box 164
herbal remedies 208
Herbal Think-TCM (game) 208–9
Hessenberg, C. and Schmid, W. 130–1

hierarchy of needs 21, 105, 280
Hill, Octavia 26
Hoffenaar *et al.* 48
Hogan, K. and Stubbs, R. 72
Holi, festival of 232
holistic approaches 15
holistic care 199; provision in healthcare 243–6
holistic healthcare design 214–15
holistic wellbeing 65
Holmes, R.M. 37
homoeopathy 205
Honey, P. and Mumford, A. 254
hospital humor 251–2
Hospital Play movement 278
Hospital Play Specialists 278
HPS (Health Play Specialists) 49–50, 243–4, 245, 269, 278, 282
Huber *et al.* 70
Hughes, B. 23–4, 25, 239
Huizinga, Johan 38
human development 19; *see also* lifespan development
humanistic perspective 36
human motivation 21
humor 21, 153; in health literacy 163–4, 167, 167–8; hospital 251–2; lifelong learning 251–2; self-deprecating 168
Hurd, A. and Anderson, D. 9
Hutchinson, R. 207
Huxley, Aldous 45

Ibn Hindu 117
Ice Bucket Challenge 269
identity, play as 7
I Heart Guts 164–5
illegal drugs 90–1
illness 242–3
Ilyas, S. and Moncreiff, J. 104
imaginative world 39
Impact Arts 145
Improving Access to Psychological Therapies (IAPT) 105
incentives 269
individual needs 20–2
indivisible self model of wellness 228–9; coping self 228, 231; creative self 228, 229–30; essential self 228, 232–3; physical self 228, 233–4; social self 228, 231–2

infancy: lifespan period 33
infertility treatment 47
inner-child work 27
innovation in health education 255; acting, role-play and debating resources 257–8; digital and innovative technical resources 257; gaming resources 256–7; smartphone resources 256; web-based resources 255–6; *Whose Shoes* boardgame 258–60
Innovation in Teaching and Learning in Health Higher Education 255
Inspire Leisure Centre 189
InstructAbility 193
International Classification of Diseases (WHO) 79
International Creativity and Ageing Study 145
International Silent Games 187
International University of Laughter Yoga 40–1
internet 173; impact on healthcare 174
Internet of Things (IoT) app 180
Invictus Games 14, 188
iPads 175
Irish Men's Sheds Association 95
Islamic teaching 234

Japan: family bonds 45; suicide rates 24–5
jingyan 203–4
Jones, P. 138
joy 201
joyfulness 40–1, 76
Jung, Carl 28
J. Walter Thompson Advertising 163–4

Kaddish 106
Kaksawadia, A. 160
Kate (cited Graham 2015) 178
Keeton, Meredith 94
keizu 45
Kelsey, Tim 73
Kennedy Report 278–9
Kennedy Shriver, Eunice 188
Kenny, C. 130
Killick, J. 54
The Kings Fund 85
Klein, Melanie 27
knitting 94; therapeutic 106
Knitting Equation 94

294 Index

Knox *et al.* 257
Konig, Karl 76
Kummervold *et al.* 73
Kuschner, D. 9
Kyle *et al.* 72
Kyrle Society 144

Lab4Living 213
Laberge, M. 34
Lamartine, Alphonse de 277
Langley, D. 136
late adulthood: lifespan period 33
late-onset alcohol problems 89
laughter 41, 167, 168, 201
laughter yoga 40–1
Lazar, Wendy Bryan 164–5
learning 12; through play 14–15
learning, mental wellbeing 109
Lee, D. and Nazroo, J. 91
Lego-based therapy 75, 79–81
LeGoff, D. 80
Lego Learning Institute 80
Lego Serious Play 213–14
Lego toys 79–80
leisure 9; definition 9
Lerner, R. 53
Lewin, Kurt 18–19, 20
Lewis, J.L. 38
LGBT festivals 233
life balance 201–2, 203
A Life like Other People's (Bennett) 166–7
lifelong learning 249; caregiver wellbeing
   and patient experience 250–1; choirs
   252; education 254–5; innovation in
   health education *see* innovation in
   health education; problem and possible
   solutions 249–54; Schwartz Rounds
   253–4; use of humor 251–2; Walton
   Centre case study 252–3
lifespan development 32–3; approaches 39–
   42; categorising 33–5;
   cross-generational change and the
   perception of play 37–9; developmental
   process of play 37; theoretical considerations 35–7
lifestyle trends 85–6; alcohol 89–90;
   chronic health conditions and illnesses
   86–9; coronary heart disease (CHD) 88;
   dementia 88–9; diabetes 86–7; exercise
   referral schemes 93; factors detrimental

to health 89–92; knitting 94; Men's
   Sheds 95; obesity 86; play as relaxation
   93–6; promoting play 92–3; sexual
   health 91–2; social networking 95;
   sporting activities 93; strokes 87–8;
   substance misuse 90–1
lighting 75
Living with Dementia 166
Lofton (cited Urist 2014) 180
Logbook app 180
London College of Music (LCM) 125
London Paralympic Games (2012) 187
loneliness 94, 95, 145, 271
Lorenz, Konrad 36
love needs 21
Lyons *et al.* 176

Maben *et al.* 250, 251
Macmillan Cancer Support 63
mahjong 41–2
malaria 163
Male Cancer Awareness Campaign 164
Manaka, Y. and Urquhart, I. 206
maqamat 117
Margolis, R. and Myrskyla, M. 49
Maslow, Abraham 20–1, 105, 280;
   humanistic behaviour 36
maternal bliss 48–9
Maughan, D. 109
Mazjun, R. 282
McCoy, Wendy 218
McGee, P. 168
McLafferty *et al.* 256
Mead, Margaret 37, 55
medical model of disability 188–9
medical model of healthcare 241
medication, costs of 71
medicine: music as 115–22; *see also*
   complementary and alternative
   medicines (CAM); modern medicine
meditation 231
Mediterranean diet 234
Mehrabian, Professor Albert 166
memoirs 242, 243
Men's Sheds 95
Mental Health Foundation 99, 108,
   110–11
mental illness 22, 100–1, 102; prescribing
   of drugs for 104–5; treating conditions
   of 104–8

mental wellness 11–13, 99, 191; and culture 103–4; differences with mental wellbeing 107; dimensional approach 105, 106; enhancing for all 108–12; five a day concept 108, 109; mental health and the impact of cultural relativism 102–4; Mental Health Foundation practical tips 110–11; mind-state of the nation 99–102; treating mental health conditions 104–8; *see also* wellbeing
message exchange 268
'Messy Church' 64
metaphor 52
Meyers, L. 61
Michelangelo 144
middle adulthood: lifespan period 33
military re-enactment 5
Miller, Michael 41
A Million Hands campaign 273
Mind 109
mind/body dualism 200
MINDSPACE 268
Mitchell *et al.* 110
Mobility, Mood and Place project 110
Model of Intentional Change 269
modern medicine 200
Monkeys without Play (Suomi and Harlow) 24
Moor, J. 79
Morris, C. 11
Morris, L. 269
Morris, William 156
mother-infant attachment 49
motivation 21, 35
motivational tool, play as 20–2
mourning rituals, cultural variations 103, 106
Moya, M.C. 32
Moyels, J. 14
Moyle, W. 73
Mozart effect 119
Mueller *et al.* 63
Museum of Modern Art (MOMA) 146–7
museums of madness 118
music 62; as a social process 127–8; *see also* chamber music
musical performance 129
music as medicine 115; across the lifespan 118–21; ancient beginnings 115–16; awakenings of evidence for musical medicine 117–18; cross-cultural, international concept 120; musical evolution 116–17
music therapy 117, 118, 120, 125; familiarity 131–2
Myers *et al.* 228
mySugr app 179–80

Nachmanovitch, S. 47
narrative graphics 169
National Institute for Play 59
National Leisure and Culture Forum 71
National Mediterranean Diet Month 234
National Wellbeing Measures 100, 101
Natural Environment White Paper 76
natural green environments 65–6
natural landscapes 66
natural selection 36
nature/nurture debate 34–5
needs: hierarchy of 21, 105, 280; individual 21
Nei Ching Su Wen 206
nerve-energy potential 206
neuroplasticity 25, 106–7
NHS Choices 12, 175
NHS (National Health Service) 70; adult health, fragile state of 264–5; principle of 264; staff sickness 250, 253
NHS Scotland 161
NICE (National Institute for Health Care Excellence) 93, 105; back pain advice 193
Nicholson, Sir David 265
normalization concept 269–70
Norton *et al.* 80–1
nurse education 257
nurture *see* nature/nurture debate
nutrition: physical self 233–4

obesity 1, 86
older people: alcohol misuse 89, 90; sexual health problems 91–2; substance misuse 90–1; *see also* Craft Café project
Old Testament 117
Olowokure *et al.* 92
operant conditioning 35
organs, bodily 206, 207
Orwell Arts 75, 76–9
Ottawa Charter 161

296 Index

Our Invisible Addicts (Royal College of Psychiatrists) 90
outdoor gyms 11, 66
outdoor play 71
outdoor recreation 71
Owens *et al.* 80
Owens, G. and LeGoff, D. 80
Oxford Brookes University 148

Pact mobile app 179
palliative care 64
Palmer, J. 203–4
Panksepp, J. 112
Papworth Trust 188
Paralympic Games 187–8
Paralympic Summer Games 188
parcels, patients as 250
parent education 51
Parkes *et al.* 103
Parkinson's disease 61
Park Nicollet Women's Center 214
participatory design 215, 217, 218–20
passports, Aspire Leisure Centre 193
pastors 246
Patient and Family Adviser Partnership Program 216, 217
patient experience 75, 250–1
patients 250
patient support groups 62–3
Peace in the Park – Festival of Spirit 231
pediatric healthcare 74
Pena, J. and Kim, E. 271
perceptions of play 37–9
personal approval 76
personal fulfilment 152
personal growth and development 6
personality 34
personas 214
person centred care 241
Pestalozzi, Johann Heinrich 6
pet dogs 271
Peterson, A.C. 53
Phillips, Jill 259
physical activity 10; benefits of 71; and coronary heart disease (CHD) 88; and diabetes 87
physical health 60–1, 191
Physically Handicapped and Able Bodied (PHAB) clubs 194
physical play 10–11

physical rehabilitation 13–14
physical self 228, 233–4
physics play 108
physiological needs 21
Piaget, Jean 5, 19, 36
picture cards 75
picture stories 169
Ping Pong (film) 230
Pitkala *et al.* 94
Plato 136, 280–1
Platt, Robert 278
play: communal living and social cohesion 186–7; as culture 37; definitions 5, 8–9, 239–41; as a facilitator and enabler 279–84; holistic care provision in healthcare 243–6
play bias 23–4
play deprivation 22–6
play-element 38–9, 40
Playful Arts Festival 227
playful design 212–14; Amstel concept of expansive design 220–2; Boex projects 217–20; concept of 213; cultures of creativity 214–17; dedicated facilitation 215; participatory design 215, 217, 218–20; service user input 215; transforming healthcare 213; use of games for facilitating participation 222–3
playful learning 14–15
playfulness 8, 21, 153; therapeutic relationship 204; *see also* art for health; Glass Studio
playful parenting 51–3
playful pedagogy 14
playful teaching 15
playground equipment 10–11
playing politics 263–4, 273; adult health 264–5; commitments 271–2; defaults 270; ego 272–3; enhancing adult healthcare 265–73; incentives 269; linking behavioural politics to health and wellbeing 266–8; message exchange 268; play 271; priming 271; public policy 266; salience 270; social norms 269–70
'Playing to Get Well' 79
Play Scotland 240
play theorists 6
play theory 7

play therapy 26–7
PlayZone 11
pleasure 24
politics *see* playing politics
Pomerantz, A. 103
poppets, patients as 250
pornography 47
positive engagement 153
positive health 13, 59–60
positive parenting 55
positive psychology 54, 76
Powell *et al.* 250
power, play as 7
prana 206
pre-assessment visits 74
pregnancy 47–8; health challenges 48;
    physical activity and social participation
    48
pre-natal: lifespan period 33
Prensky, M. 174
pre-potency concept 21
pre-school period: lifespan period 33
prescriptions (drugs) 104–5
Preti, C. and Boyce-Tillman, J. 119
priming 271
Prince, M. 255
Prodehl, Caroline 209
progress, play as 7
projection 138
psychodynamic perspective 35
psychosocial health 100
psychotropic drugs 104
Public Health England 233, 235
pure play 14
Putting People First 259

Qi 103, 201–2, 203, 206
quality of life, enhancing 86

rangoli 229–30
Raso, R. 253
Read (cited in Danson and Trebeck 2013)
    143
reciprocal determinism 20, 34
recreation 9; benefits of 266; definition 9;
    therapeutic 91
recreational therapists 87
reflexology 205
Register of Chinese Herbal Medicine
    (RCHM) 208

rehabilitation, Aspire Leisure Centre 193
Reiki 205
Relate 21, 47
relationship continuity 73–4
relationships 45–6
relationships, essential role of 203–4
relaxation: play as 93–6; ways of 107–8
religion 239
Remploy 194
Renaissance 117
Rennie, S. 27
representation of the imaginary, play as 7
Rhythmic Auditory Stimulation (RAS)
    121
Richman *et al.* 78
Ringham, L. 72
risk-averse society 24
Rocky Mountain Herbal Institute
    (RMHI) 208
Rogers, Carl: humanistic behaviour 36
role play 136, 138, 258
Roma children 25
Rosenzweig, M.R. 25
Rousseau, Jean-Jacques 6
Royal Botanic Gardens 148
Royal College of Physicians 264
Royal College of Psychiatrists 91
Royal National Orthopaedic Hospital
    (RNOH) 190–1, 193
Rubin, S. 139
Ruskin, John 156
Ruud, E. 131
Ryall *et al.* 39

Saarinen *et al.* 20
Sacks, Dr Oliver 120
Sakamoto *et al.* 125
salience 270
Salter, J. 40
Sandelands, L.E. and Buckner, G.C. 283
Scarecrow (exergame) 177
Schiller, Friedrich 5, 156, 157; on play 6
Schwartz Rounds 253–4
Scottish Storytelling Centre 148
Scout Association 244–5, 273
Seedhouse, D. 76
self: coping 228, 231; creative 228, 229–30;
    deprivational effects of illness 242–3;
    essential 228, 232–3; indivisible 228–9;
    physical 228, 233–4; social 228, 231–2;

298 Index

traumatic effects of illness 242
self-actualization 76, 280
self-deprecating humor 168
self-satisfaction, play as 7
Sennett, Richard 156
sense of humor 153
sensory deprivation 25
sensory environment 25, 77
sensory experiences 77–8
sensory satisfaction 76
service learning, community-based 128
services, accessing *see* accessing services
service users 72; hearing impaired 72; involvement in design 214
Setterfield, D. 48
Seven Levels of Consciousness Model (Barrett) 21, 22
sexual health 91–2
sexually-transmitted infections (STIs) 91–2
sexual play 47
Shearing, E. 87
Sheehan (cited University Of Wisconsin Hospitals and Clinics Authority 2015) 216
Shiatsu 205
sickness absence 23
sideways movement 6
Silver (cited Mandeville Legacy 2014) 187
simulation 255–6
'Singing for the Brain' 121
six aspects of health 21, 22
skateboarding 5
Skinner, B.F. 35
skipping rope games 41
sleep 148
smartphone resources 256
smart technology 173
Smith, Donald 148
Smith *et al.* 88–9
social-cognitive learning theory 35
social deprivation 25
social development 34
social health 62–3
social learning theory 267
social media 181–2; age-related usage 174
social model of disability 189
social needs 21
social networking 95
social norms 269–70

social self 228, 231–2
Social Stories 74
social therapy 75, 76, 152–9; craft-based learning 152–3; Glass Studio 154–6, 157; Goethe's 153; play and the celebration of festivals 156–9
socioeconomic status 55
Sørensen *et al.* 161–2
Southern Health Trust 279
Speak Out campaign 64–5
Special Educational Need or Disability (SEND) 33–4
Special Olympics movement 188
spiritual health 63–4, 191
spiritual healthcare 245
spirituality 64, 227, 228, 232, 238; defining 238–9, 240; and healthcare 241–2; illness, healthcare environments and spiritual wellbeing 242–3; Scout Association 244–5
spontaneity 139
sport: Aspire Leisure Centre 193; benefits of 187, 266; and diabetes 87; *see also* disability sport
Sport England 66
sporting activities 93
sport participation 10
sports hall, Aspire Leisure Centre 192
Srinivas, S. 181–2
staff motivation 251
staff wellbeing 251
stand-up comedy 5
Starbuck, W.H. and Webster, E.J. 281
St Clair, M. 5
Steadwood Centre 189
Steen (quoted in Cox) 11
Steiner, Rudolf 39, 76, 77, 152, 156
Sternberg, E. 77
Stern, S. 137
Stevens, Simon 252
stilt-walking 41
stimulation theory of play 24
STIs (sexually-transmitted infections) 91–2
Stitchlinks 85–6, 94
Stoke Mandeville Games 187–8
storyboards 75
storytelling 51–3, 148–9; health literacy 168–9
Storytelling for Empowerment Program 232–3
storytelling model 46

stress: conceiving 47; failure to conceive 48; family life 55–6; workplace 249–50
stress levels 22
stress management: and play 65
stress-related illness 200
Stroke Association 87
strokes 87–8, 120
Study Stack 206–7
substance misuse 90–1
Sugarman, Ian 34–5
suicide rates 24–5
Sultanoff, B. 201
Suomi, S.J. and Harlow, H.F. 24, 25–6
supermarket checkout, dementia assistance 167
Sussex Cancer Centre 75
Sutton-Smith, B. 5; complementary construction of play 6; play theory 7
Sweeney, T.J. and Myers, J. 228
Sweeney, T.J. and Witmer, J.M. 227
swimming, Aspire Leisure Centre 191–2
Symbolism 152

TaiChiCentral 209
'taken up' in play 159
taking notice 13; mental wellbeing 109
Talking Points program 79
Taylor, S.E. 48
Taylor, S.E. and Brown, J.D. 48
teaching: playful 15
tea dances 271
team environments 251
technology 173–4; definition 174–5; digital immigrants 174; digital natives 174; exergames 176–8; gamification of healthcare 178–81; impact on healthcare 174; and play 23; social media 181–2; use in healthcare 175; video games 175–8
temperament 34
testicular cancer 163–4
Thaut, M. 124–5
A Theory of Human Motivation (Maslow) 21
therapeutic coloring books 107
therapeutic knitting 106
therapeutic play intervention 49–50
therapeutic recreation 91
thick theoretical approach 20–1
This Girl Can campaign 66

This is me tool 168
TimeSlips 168–9
tone zones 11
Traditional Chinese Acupuncture 206–7; five phases 206, 207
Traditional Chinese Medicine (TCM) 103; Chinese Herbal Medicine 208–9; conceptualization of illness 204; incorporation into mainstream healthcare systems 204; lack of games or play-based techniques 209; life balance 203; relieving cancer-related fatigue 202; role of play in healing 201; seven emotions of 202; *see also* complementary and alternative medicine (CAM)
trampoline parks 61
transitional space 130
trauma 120
traumatic danger 242
Trent, J. 178
Trevarthen, Professor Colwyn 46
Trudge *et al.* 18
trust, safe environment of 140
Tsiaras, Alexander 144
Twitter 174, 181, 181–2

Unicef 186
United Nations (UN): physical activity 71
United States of America (USA) 258
University of Twente 220
University of West London (UWL) 125
Urist, J. 180–1

van Amstel, F. 220–2
van der Heide, R. 223
Van der Vennet, R. and Serice, S. 107
Van Diest *et al.* 177
van Hecke *et al.* 202
Vaughan Williams, Ralph 129
Vesalius 200
Victorians 144
video games 175–8
virtual communication 73
visible music 40
visual strategies 75
Vygotsky, Lev 36

Wadd *et al.* 89, 90
Walker, Andrew 190

300 Index

walking football 93
walking, health benefits of 270
Walton Centre case study 252–3
Ward, Mary 26
Ward-Wimmer, D. 27
Warland, J. and Smith, M. 258
Watching (opera) 148
water environments 66
Waterworth, J. 217
Watson, J.B. 35
web-based resources 255–6
Weich *et al.* 107
Welfare of Children in Hospital (Ministry of Health) 278
wellbeing 11–13, 26; differences with mental wellness 107; health and 59–67; linking behavioural politics to health and 266–8; and spirituality 242–3; of women starting a family 48–9; *see also* mental wellness
wellness: concept of 227; wheel of 227–8; *see also* indivisible self model of wellness; mental wellness
Western approach to medicine 200
wheel of wellness 227–8
white coat syndrome 73
Whose Shoes boardgame 258–60
Wii fit 176
Wikan, U. 103
Williams, Ian 169

Williams, Z. 107
Wilson-Mulnix, J. and Mulnix, M.J. 101
Winnicott, D.W. 8, 141
Witchen *et al.* 100
words *see* health literacy
working hours: longer 22, 23
Workplace Quality of Life Index (WQLI) 22
workplace stress 249–50
work/play divide 281
work-related illness 250
World Health Organization (WHO): definition of health 70; health inequalities 265; health literacy definition 162–3; mental health 102; physical activity fact sheets 10; support groups 63
Wüest *et al.* 176–7
Wu et al. 256

Yin and Yang 201
yoga 40–1
Yosef, A. 233

Zabelina, D. and Robinson, M.D. 281
ZDoggMD 182
Zeedyk, S. 25
Zeedyk, S. and Robertson, J. 53
Zeilig, H. 124
zuo yue zi 106